T0201074

INTEGRATED CARDIAC SAFETY

INTEGRATED CARDIAC SAFETY

Assessment Methodologies for Noncardiac Drugs in Discovery, Development, and Postmarketing Surveillance

J. Rick Turner, PhD, PGCE, MICR
Chairman, Department of Clinical Research
Campbell University School of Pharmacy
and
Member of the Cardiac Safety Research Consortium

Todd A. Durham, MS
Senior Director of Biostatistics and Data Management
Inspire Pharmaceuticals
and
Adjunct Professor of Clinical Research
Campbell University School of Pharmacy

WILEY

A JOHN WILEY & SONS, INC., PUBLICATION

Library of Congress Cataloging-in-Publication Data is available.

Turner, J. Rick.
    Integrated cardiac safety : assessment methodologies for noncardiac drugs in
discovery, development, and postmarketing surveillance / J. Rick Turner, Todd A. Durham.
        p. cm.
    Includes bibliographical references and index.
    ISBN 978-0-470-22964-4 (cloth)
1. Cardiovascular toxicology. 2. Heart—Effect of drugs on. 3. Drugs—Side
effects—Testing. 4. Drugs—Safety measures. I. Durham, Todd A. II. Title.
    [DNLM: 1. Cardiovascular Diseases—prevention & control. 2. Drug Design.
3. Medication Errors. 4. Product Surveillance, Postmarketing—methods. 5.
Safety Management—methods. WG 120 T948i 2009]
    RC677.T87 2009
    616.1'23061—dc22   2008022807

Printed in the United States of America

10 9 8 7 6 5 4 3 2 1

CONTENTS

PART II CARDIAC FUNCTION AND PATHOLOGY

CHAPTER 3. CARDIAC STRUCTURE AND FUNCTION

CHAPTER 4. CARDIAC PATHOPHYSIOLOGY AND DISEASE

PART III DRUG DISCOVERY AND NONCLINICAL DEVELOPMENT

CHAPTER 5. DRUG DISCOVERY AND DRUG DESIGN

PART VI   BEHAVIORAL DRUG SAFETY

CHAPTER 13.   MEDICATION ERRORS, ADHERENCE, AND CONCORDANCE

PART VII   INTEGRATIVE DISCUSSION

CHAPTER 14.   FUTURE DIRECTIONS IN DRUG SAFETY

FOREWORD

The human heart is a remarkable organ. During an average 80-year lifespan, it beats approximately 3 billion times and produces and utilizes some 30 kg of adenosine triphosphate per day! This rhythmicity on which our cardiovascular health, and indeed our lives, depend is achieved through the remarkably well-coordinated activities of multiple ion channels, both ligand- and voltage-gated, and multiple pharmacological receptors. Given this coordination and the obvious opportunities for interference—physiological, pharmacological, and pathological—it is perhaps equally remarkable that cardiac rhythm disturbances are not more common. However, they are of sufficient frequency and importance, particularly those produced by drugs whose primary actions are designed to be noncardiac, that their frequency and etiology have become of significant concern to both the pharmaceutical industry and drug regulatory agencies worldwide.

As a result of this concern, one specific ion channel has assumed particular distinction in questions of proarrhythmic cardiac safety. The hERG (human ether-a-go-go related gene) channel generates a repolarizing potassium current that maintains cardiac rhythm. It is also, however, a pharmacologically promiscuous entity to which multiple and structurally unrelated drugs—including quinolone antibiotics, antihistamines, antipsychotics, macrolides, and serotonin blockers—bind to produce cardiac rhythm disturbances that are not infrequently fatal, particularly to patients with a genetic predisposition to QT disturbances. As a consequence, hERG may be classified as a "therapeutic antitarget" and the detection of potential drug interactions with this channel is now a routine and early component of the drug discovery process.

However, the complexity and integrated nature of the multiple excitatory and inhibitory inputs that determine cardiac rhythm demands an integrated approach to the assessment of cardiac safety. This issue was certainly brought to the forefront in the CAST and SWORD clinical trials in which Class Ic and Class III antiarrhythmic agents were studied for their efficacy in suppressing sudden cardiac death. These agents turned out to be proarrhythmic. As noted recently by Denis Noble in *The Music of Life: Biology Beyond the Genome* (Oxford University Press, 2006), an excessively reductionist approach to biology too frequently ignores the connectedness of events. Hence, Turner and Durham have titled this book *Integrated Cardiac Safety,* and they provide a very broad description of the assessment of the cardiac safety of noncardiac drugs in the discovery, development, and postmarketing surveillance phases of the overall drug marketing process. The book comprises seven detailed parts. We are first provided with an introduction to cardiac safety assessment and the biology of adverse drug interactions that both introduces the reader to this area and sets the stage for the remainder of the book. Following a part on cardiac function and pathology, we are led logically through parts on the discovery process, the preapproval process (including the QT/QTc studies), and postmarketing assessment methods. The book concludes with chapters on medication errors, still far too common in the United States, and a discussion of future trends in drug safety.

The integrated approach to cardiac safety presented by Turner and Durham should be of interest and value to all concerned with the drug discovery, development, marketing, and surveillance phases of the pharmaceutical endeavor. During the past two to three decades, the pharmaceutical industry has adopted a progressively more integrated approach to the drug discovery process. This book shows the virtue of an integrated approach to the assessment and elimination of cardiac safety issues.

David J. Triggle, PhD
University Professor and SUNY Distinguished Professor
School of Pharmacy and Pharmaceutical Sciences
SUNY at Buffalo

PREFACE

This book discusses assessment methodologies employed in evaluating the cardiac safety of noncardiac drugs, i.e., drugs that are not indicated for cardiac diseases or conditions. Drugs that are prescribed for cardiac diseases or conditions are expected to influence the heart's activity. In contrast, if a noncardiac drug has the propensity to influence the heart's activity, and to do so in a deleterious manner, this is of considerable clinical concern. The potential lethality of later cardiac adverse drug reactions makes assessment of an investigational drug's cardiac safety profile a high priority during premarketing drug development. Equally importantly, once a drug has been approved for marketing, it is essential that its cardiac safety continues to be monitored

Contemporary cardiac safety assessments occur in each of four stages within lifecycle drug development: drug discovery and design; nonclinical research; preapproval clinical development; and postmarketing surveillance. Accordingly, this book adopts a lifecycle perspective to cardiac safety assessment as a fundamental organizational strategy, discussing the methodological approaches that are employed at each stage in sequential order. While these methodologies encompass data analysis, this book's discussions of analytical strategies employed are conceptual in nature rather than computational. A lack of knowledge of (or interest in) computational statistics will not impede your reading of this book.

To date, use of the term cardiac safety in the drug development arena has come to identify one particular aspect of overall cardiac safety, an area that is represented in this book by the term proarrhythmic cardiac safety. A fundamental goal of proarrhythmic cardiac safety is to determine whether an investigational noncardiac drug has the propensity to cause certain kinds of irregular heartbeats, notably ventricular arrhythmias, in patients who may be prescribed the drug if it is eventually approved for marketing. This arrhythmogenesis can result in nonfatal arrhythmias causing syncope (losing consciousness), and it can also prove fatal. Evaluating an investigational drug's proarrhythmic liability is now expected by regulatory agencies.

The methodologies employed in premarketing investigations of proarrhythmic cardiac safety include *in silico* structure-function simulation modeling in the drug design phase, extensive *in vitro* and *in vivo* testing during the nonclinical development program, and extensive electrocardiogram (ECG)

recording and monitoring during the preapproval clinical development program. These activities center on the evaluation of a drug molecule's propensity to precipitate certain alterations in the heart's electrical activity via the employment of cardiac electrophysiology. Electrophysiology is a complex discipline, which is likely one of the main reasons why the field of proarrhythmic cardiac safety became widely regarded as esoteric. This is unfortunate, since a general understanding of all aspects of cardiac safety evaluation is beneficial to clinical researchers, pharmacists, physicians, nurses, students of all of these disciplines, and all allied health professionals. Therefore, this book discusses all of the information needed to obtain a working knowledge of proarrhythmic cardiac safety.

In the preface to the fourth edition of his excellent book entitled *Electrophysiologic Testing*, Fogoros (2006, p. vii) noted that his intentions were "to explain and de-mystify the arcane world of the electrophysiologist to students, residents, cardiology fellows, primary care physicians, cardiologists, nurses, and technicians." In the same manner, one of our intentions in this book is to explain and demystify proarrhythmic cardiac safety. It should be made clear that this book does not attempt to discuss the full spectrum of cardiac electrophysiology: its full realm includes provision of diagnostic capabilities used by physicians in reaching treatment decisions, and we are not clinicians. The evaluation of proarrhythmic cardiac safety requires only a relatively small part of the full discipline of cardiac electrophysiology, i.e., the noninvasive quantification of certain components of the cardiac cycle from the ECG, and consequently this is the only aspect of electrophysiology that is addressed in this text.

In addition to discussing proarrhythmic cardiac safety, this book takes a wider perspective and integrates discussions of two other areas of cardiac safety: these are termed generalized cardiac safety and behavioral cardiac safety. These terms are not used with any particular claim to authoritative nomenclature: it is simply the case that they permit distinction between proarrhythmic, generalized, and behavioral aspects of cardiac safety when such distinction is helpful. The term generalized cardiac safety refers to all cardiac adverse drug reactions with the exception of arrhythmogenic events captured by the term proarrhythmic cardiac safety. Generalized cardiac safety therefore includes fatal heart attacks, major irreversible morbidity (nonfatal myocardial infarctions), debilitating cardiovascular symptoms or events (e.g., transient ischemic attacks, marked fluid retention, and palpitations), and various pathophysiological characteristics that increase the likelihood of cardiac and cardiovascular events (see Borer et al., 2007). While preapproval studies monitor cardiac events, and while investigators remain vigilant for any untoward cardiac responses throughout nonclinical and preapproval clinical development programs, postmarketing surveillance is a key assessment methodology in generalized cardiac safety.

The term behavioral cardiac safety is used to refer to cardiac eventualities where behavioral factors are the primary instigating factor. This category includes medication errors, whereby patients are prescribed, dispensed, and/or administered an unintended drug or drug regimen, and patients' intentional or unintentional lack of adherence to drug regimens. The assessment methodologies employed in the investigation of behavioral cardiac safety are applicable to behavioral drug safety in general, and some aspects of our discussions in Chapter 13 are therefore relatively broad, but specific examples related to cardiac safety are also provided. Behavioral safety is specific to postmarketing situations, since the behavioral factors of interest—errors in prescribing, dispensing, administration (e.g., by health care providers in in-patient settings and nursing homes), and taking one's own medication—occur once a drug is on the market.

The collection of data in behavioral cardiac safety relies predominantly on individuals reporting events that have happened, i.e., errors that they (or others) have made. Historically there has unfortunately been a relatively strong perception of a sense of shame and blame associated with reporting an error. This perception is likely responsible for considerable underreporting of medication errors, and it is the driving force behind the advocacy for the culture of safety, a culture that encourages the reporting of medication errors in a nonpunitive environment so that every effort can be made to reduce the likelihood of future errors.

Each of these three aspects of cardiac safety—proarrhythmic, generalized, and behavioral—has typically been addressed separately by previous publications. This book therefore adopts the unique approach of integrating all of these topics within a single self-contained volume, an approach reflected in the book's title, *Integrated Cardiac Safety*. This integrative approach is also evident in the book's discussions of cardiac safety assessments in all four phases of lifecycle drug development. This breadth of coverage makes the book relevant to a particularly wide audience of health professionals and students. Not everyone needs to be an expert in integrated cardiac safety assessment—and this book alone certainly does not presume to make anyone an expert—but we believe that the topic of cardiac safety is of sufficient importance that everyone interested in drug development and pharmaceutical therapy can benefit from an awareness and knowledge of the fundamentals of this discipline.

To fulfill its goals, the book comprises a self-contained introduction to the nature of cardiac adverse drug reactions and the expansive array of assessment methodologies used in the various fields within integrated cardiac safety. It also contains early chapters that provide background information from diverse underlying disciplines that facilitates the discussions in later chapters. Meaningful discussions of cardiac safety, even at this introductory level, require a certain degree of familiarity with developmental and cell biology, transmission genetics, molecular and medicinal chemistry, bioinformatics and database construction, molecular genetics, genomics, proteomics and pharmacoproteomics, cardiac structure and function, cardiac electrophysiology, and cardiac diseases. To improve the accessibility and flow of the book's material, the overviews of these disciplines are selective and pragmatic, and any of them can be skipped by readers already familiar with one or more of these underlying disciplines without lessening the integrity of the later discussions of cardiac safety. It should also be noted that there is a certain degree of planned repetition in the book: topics are introduced at one point and then integrated with other material at a later point. Additionally, some concepts that were deliberately introduced relatively simply in early chapters are addressed again later in the book in more detail when their importance and relevance to other issues have become clear. While unplanned repetition can be confusing, it is hoped that this planned and progressive strategy will be helpful in assimilating both detail and context.

Because of the book's introductory nature, lists of Further Reading are provided at the end of many chapters for readers who wish to pursue topics of particular interest in more detail. These lists include books and journal articles. Some of the books listed are introductory in nature but focus on just one of the topics discussed in this book. Others are definitive texts that provide authoritative discussions of one or more topics. Some of the journal articles are reviews of published studies, while others present original empirical research: in both cases, we have selected articles from a variety of journals in order to demonstrate the range of journals that cover a given topic.

Throughout the vast majority of the book we have endeavored to present material in an objective manner, an approach that is certainly a reasonable expectation of its readers. However, it is fair to say that some of the topics discussed involve questions that at the time of writing do not have simple and unanimously accepted answers. Accordingly, in several places we have given ourselves license to express our opinions, and we claim neither authoritativeness nor infallibility. You may well disagree with some or even all of these opinions, and we are very comfortable with this possibility. If the opinions expressed here lead you to consider the subject material critically and to arrive at alternative conclusions, and if they encourage classroom discussion among those of you who may be reading the book as a text for a particular course, we will consider this a very worthwhile outcome.

JRT would like to mention an additional influence on his thinking during the writing of this book. Last summer Wiley published *New Drug Development: Design, Methodology, and Analysis* (Turner, 2007). While *New Drug Development* and the present book both address issues in lifecycle drug development, and are therefore related to a certain extent, they were not initially conceived of as a set of two volumes. While fairly brief discussions of safety evaluations were included in *New Drug Development,* that text focused predominantly on methodologies related to the demonstration of efficacy and on conceptual explanations of analytical strategies related to the demonstration of (statistically significant) treatment effects. In one sense, this volume is a continuation of *New Drug Development* in that it addresses drug safety in detail with specific reference to cardiac drug safety, and readers of this book who have also read *New Drug Development* will hopefully see the continuity of thought. However, I am very aware that other readers may not have read the previous book, and it was therefore important to me that this book be self-contained. There is no need to have read *New Drug Development* to be able to follow the present discussions. I am delighted that Todd Durham has joined me on this occasion in the writing of *Integrated Cardiac Safety.* He has brought additional and complementary knowledge and perspectives that have considerably enriched the material presented. This book therefore builds on the professional relationship that Todd and I established during the writing of *Introduction to Statistics in Pharmaceutical Clinical Trials* (Durham and Turner, 2008). Unlike the present book, that text does present computational statistical details for analyses employed throughout a drug's preapproval clinical development program, and does so in a format that we hope is very accessible to anyone wishing to become more familiar with such details.

While the focus of this book is on cardiac safety and some discussions (particularly those related to preapproval evaluation of proarrhythmic cardiac safety) are specific to this domain, much of the discussion also applies to the larger field of drug safety in general. Determining drug safety has many challenges. It is an unfortunate reality that no drug is immune from the possibility of unwanted responses, i.e., adverse drug reactions, in certain individuals. One of the greatest challenges in clinical medicine is that individual patients do not respond uniformly to the same dose of the same drug. A drug's safety is assessed in relation to its efficacy and, when in general use, in relation to its effectiveness (the term used to describe its therapeutic benefit in large populations of patients once it has been given marketing approval). To use a correct but potentially emotional term, a drug must be acceptably safe: its therapeutic benefits must outweigh any risks of harm associated with its administration. That is, it must have a favorable benefit-risk balance and hence be deemed acceptably safe. Such determination necessarily involves assessment and consideration of its safety profile in conjunction with its therapeutic benefit. To receive marketing approval, a regulatory agency must decide that the preponderance of available evidence contained in a marketing application indicates that the investigational drug has demonstrated a favorable benefit-risk balance. To remain on the market, the drug's benefit-risk balance must remain favorable as new information concerning its safety and effectiveness is gathered. Benefit-risk assessments comprise a central and important theme in lifecycle drug development, and they are discussed throughout the book.

Assessment of all aspects of drug safety, including cardiac safety, is a topic of enormous current interest and importance in both preapproval and postmarketing stages of lifecycle drug development. The following are some examples that are discussed in subsequent chapters. During the 1980s and 1990s, a number of drugs were removed from the market following reports of nonlethal and lethal cardiac arrhythmias: these events were the stimulus for the development of regulatory documents governing cardiac safety assessments during the nonclinical and preapproval clinical development programs for new investigational drugs. Memories of the 2004 events surrounding a drug for arthritis are still vivid in drug safety circles (e.g., see Chan and Jones, 2007), and the summer of 2007 was notable for discussions regarding the cardiac safety of a drug used in the treatment of diabetes (e.g., see Home et al., 2007). In September 2007, a paper published in the *Archives of Internal Medicine* reviewed serious adverse drug events reported to the U.S. Food and Drug Administration during the years 1998 to 2005, and its authors concluded that the data presented "show a marked increase in reported deaths and serious injuries associated with drug therapy over the study period" (Moore et al., 2007). Cohen's (2007a) edited volume *Medication Errors* and a report from the Institute of Medicine of the National Academies published in book format in 2007, *Preventing Medication Errors*, addressed the breadth and depth of medication errors (Institute of Medicine, 2007a). Finally here, a segment aired on the television show *60 Minutes* in February 2008 focused on the safety of a drug used during coronary artery bypass grafting (CABG) surgery to reduce bleeding and preserve platelet function (see Mangano et al., 2006, and Schneeweiss et al., 2008, for related discussions).

In late September 2007, the Food and Drug Administration Amendments Act (FDAAA) legislation was approved, and came into being on October 1, 2007. This legislation called for considerably more attention to be paid to postmarketing safety in general, including the more detailed planning and submission of postmarketing surveillance strategies during the approval process. It will be very interesting to see how drug safety assessments, including those for noncardiac drugs, evolve in the coming years as the provisions in this legislation are/may be interpreted, contested, implemented, and funded.

As noted earlier, not everyone needs to be an expert on integrated cardiac safety, and this book does not presume to make anyone an expert. However, we hope that the following discussions will make all readers cognizant of the scope of integrated cardiac safety research, and that it may encourage some readers to enter and/or further pursue this field in their professional careers.

Views expressed in this book are those of the authors and not necessarily those of Campbell University or of Inspire Pharmaceuticals.

Thank you for your interest in this book: we very much hope that you enjoy reading it.

J. Rick Turner and Todd A. Durham
Chapel Hill, North Carolina, June 2008

REFERENCES

Borer, J.S., Pouleur, H., Abadie, E., et al., 2007, Cardiovascular safety of drugs not intended for cardiovascular use: Need for a new conceptual basis for assessment and approval, *European Heart Journal*, 28:1904–1909.

Chan, K.A. and Jones, S.C., 2007, NSAIDS—COX-2 Inhibitors—Risks and benefits. In Mann, R. and Andrews, E. (Eds.), *Pharmacovigilance*, 2nd edition, Chichester, UK: John Wiley & Sons, 583–602.

Cohen, M.R. (Ed.), 2007, *Medication errors*, 2nd edition, Washington, D.C: American Pharmacists Association.

Durham, T.A. and Turner, J.R., 2008, *Introduction to statistics in pharmaceutical clinical trials*, London: Pharmaceutical Press.

Fogoros, R.N., 2006, *Electrophysiologic testing*, 4th edition, Malden, MA: Blackwell Publishing.

Home, P.D., Pocock, S.J., Beck-Nielsen, H., et al. for the RECORD Study Group, 2007, Rosiglitazone evaluated for cardiovascular outcomes: An interim analysis, *New England Journal of Medicine*, 357:28–38.

Institute of Medicine, 2007, *Preventing medication errors*, Washington, DC: National Academies Press

Mangano, D.T., Tudor, I.C., and Dietzel, C., 2006, The risk associated with aprotinin in cardiac surgery, *New England Journal of Medicine*, 354:353–365.

Moore, T.J., Cohen, M.R., and Furberg, C.D., 2007, Serious adverse drug events reported to the Food and Drug Administration, 1998–2005, *Archives of Internal Medicine*, 167:1752–1759.

Schneeweiss, S., Seeger, J.D., Landon, J., et al., 2008, Aprotinin during coronary-artery bypass drafting and risk of death, *New England Journal of Medicine*, 358: 771–783.

ACKNOWLEDGMENTS

The format of this book evolved during extensive communications with three outstanding editors at Wiley. The original book proposal was received by Steve Quigley. He provided extremely useful review comments and then graciously steered the proposal to Thom Moore, who equally graciously steered it to Jonathan Rose: both Steve and Thom felt that the book would find its best Wiley home in Jonathan's area of responsibility. Jonathan has been a constant source of advice and encouragement throughout the project. I also thank Christine Punzo, the book's production editor.

Several colleagues have provided assistance in the preparation of individual chapters (responsibility for any inaccuracies remains ours alone) and in allowing us to use information from their presentations at various conferences: Drs. Michael Adams, Marilyn Agin, Chris Blanchette, Gary Bowers, Tim Callaghan, Bob Cisneros, Borge Darpo, George Diamond, John Finkle, Christina Hewitt, Richard Kovacs, Jeff Litwin, Pierre Maison-Blanche, Joel Morganroth, Jonathan Sackner-Bernstein, Larry Satin, Pete Siegl, Wendy Stough, Hugo Vargas, Paulina Voloshko, and Bill Wheeler. The book was prepared in camera-ready format by Ms. Barrie Ward, President of The Perfect Page (see http://www.theperfectpage.net).

When writing any book that synthesizes a wide range of topics, authors owe a debt of gratitude to all of the researchers who conducted and reported the original research that is cited in the book. In this case, we owe an additional debt of gratitude to the authors who have written and edited the many books and review articles we cite. Relatedly, because JRT has read the work of a large number of authors over a long period of time, I am aware of the possibility that I might, quite unintentionally, have failed to cite individuals whose work I read some time ago and which demonstrably influenced my thinking. If anyone recognizes such an omission, I sincerely apologize, and I will be extremely happy to rectify this in any future editions.

Deep appreciation for their love and support is expressed to our wives, Karen Turner and Heidi Durham, to whom the book is dedicated. Loving companionship and playful encouragement during the midnight writing hours were provided by our respective four-legged family members Misty and Mishadow, and Rachel and Daisy.

ABBREVIATIONS

A	adenine	CHMP	Committee for Medicinal Products for Human Use
ADOPT	A Diabetes Outcome Progression Trial	CI	confidence interval
AE	adverse event	CIOMS	Council for International Organizations of Medical Sciences
AERS	Adverse Event Reporting System		
AIDS	acquired immunodeficiency syndrome	CLASS	Celecoxib Arthritis Safety Study
ANCOVA	analysis of covariance	C_{max}	maximum concentration/ systemic exposure
APPROVe	Adenomatous Polyp Prevention On Vioxx (trial)		
As_2O_3	arsenic trioxide	CMS	Concerned Member State
AUC	area under the curve across all time	CO	cardiac output
		COX	cyclooxygenase
		COX-2	cyclooxygenase-2
		CPMP	Committee of Proprietary Medicinal Products
BLA	Biologicals License Application		
		CSRC	Cardiac Safety Research Consortium
bpm	beats per minute		
		CTA	Clinical Trial Application
C	cytosine	CV	cardiovascular
Ca^{2+}	calcium ion	CVM	Center for Veterinary Medicine
CABG	coronary artery bypass grafting		
		CYP	cytochrome P450
CBER	Center for Biologicals Evaluation and Research		
		d	dalton
CBI	Center for Business Intelligence	DBP	diastolic blood pressure
		DNA	deoxyribonucleic acid
CDER	Center for Drug Evaluation and Research	DREAM	Diabetes Reduction with Ramipril and Rosiglitazone Medication (trial)
CDRH	Center for Devices and Radiological Health		
CEO	chief executive officer	DSMB	data safety monitoring board
CFSAN	Center for Food Safety and Applied Nutrition		

EAD	early afterdepolarization	I_{Kr}	potassium current that flows through the hERG ion channel
eag	ether-a-go-go gene		
ECG	electrocardiogram		
EHRs	electronic health records	IND	Investigational New Drug Application
EMEA	European Medicines Agency		
		IOM	Institute of Medicine
ERMS	European Risk Management Strategy	IPD	individual patient/ participant data
EU	European Union	IRB	Investigational Review Board
FDA	Food and Drug Administration	IRT	Interdisciplinary Review Team
FDAAA	Food and Drug Administration Amendments Act	ISoP	International Society of Pharmacovigilance
		ISS	Integrated Summary of Safety
FDAMA	Food and Drug Administration Modernization Act	ITT	intent-to-treat (population in data analysis)
FTE	full-time equivalent	IUT	Intersection-union Test
FTIH	first-time-in-human (study)	JNC	Joint National Committee on Prevention, Detection, Evaluation, and Treatment of High Blood Pressure
FTIM	first-time-in-man (study): alternate name for above		
G	guanine		
GAO	General Accountability Office	K^+	potassium ion
		KcsA	*Streptomyces lividans* potassium ion channel
H_A	alternative hypothesis		
HDLc	high-density lipoprotein cholesterol	LDLc	low-density lipoprotein cholesterol
hERG	human ether-a-go-go related gene	LL	lower limit
		lpm	liters per minute
Hg	mercury	LQTS	long QT syndrome
HGP	Human Genome Project		
H_0	null hypothesis	MAA	Marketing Authorisation Application
ICH	International Conference on Harmonisation	MAP	mean arterial (blood) pressure
IHCIS	Integrated Healthcare Information Services	mAb	monoclonal antibody
		m-cells	midmyocardial cells
IHGS	International Human Genome Sequencing (Consortium)	MedDRA	medical dictionary for regulatory affairs
		MI	myocardial infarction

ml	milliliter	QRS	QRS complex on the ECG
MPDSC	Medical Products Development Strategy Committee	QSAR	quantitative structure-activity relationship
mRNA	messenger RNA	QT (interval)	time from the onset of the QRS complex to the offset of the T-wave on the ECG
MthK	*Methanobacterium thermoautotrophicum* potassium ion channel		
mV	millivolt	QTc	QT interval corrected for heart rate
		QTcB	QTc calculated using Bazett's formula
Na⁺	sodium ion		
NCA	National Competent Authorities	QTcF	QTc calculated using Fridericia's formula
NCE	new chemical entity (alternatively, NME, new molecular entity)	QTcI	QT calculated using individual data
NDA	New Drug Application	RiskMAP	risk minimization action plan
NDC	National Drug Code		
NEJM	New England Journal of Medicine	rDNA	recombinant DNA
		RECORD	Rosiglitazone Evaluated for Cardiac Outcomes and Regulation of Glycaemia in Diabetes (trial)
NIH	National Institutes of Health		
NSAID	nonsteroidal anti-inflammatory drug	REMS	risk evaluation and mitigation strategies
ODS/OSE	Office of Drug Safety/ Office of Surveillance and Epidemiology	RMS	Reference Member State
		RNA	ribonucleic acid
		RR	relative risk resting (heart) rate (in the calculation of QTc)
OR	odds ratio		
OTC	over the counter		
		RR (interval)	the time from the R-wave of one heartbeat to that of the next on the ECG
PCA	passive cutaneous anaphylaxis		
PDUFA	Prescription Drug User Fee Act	S	transmembrane segment in an ion channel (e.g., S1, S2)
PEM	prescription-event monitoring		
PhRMA	Pharmaceutical Researchers and Manufacturers of America	SAE	serious adverse event
		SAR	structure-activity relationship
PK/PD	pharmacokinetic/ pharmacodynamic	SBP	systolic blood pressure
		SCD	sudden cardiac death

SEER	Surveillance, Epidemiology, and End-results	TPE	T_{peak} to T_{end}
		TPR	total peripheral resistance
		TQT	thorough QT/QTc (study)
SNP	single nucleotide polymorphism	TRIaD	triangulation, reverse use dependence, and instability
SQTS	short QT syndrome		
		UK	United Kingdom
T	thymine	UL	upper limit
TdP	torsades de pointes		
TDR	transmural dispersion of repolarization	VIGOR	Vioxx Gastrointestinal Outcomes Research (trial)
T_{max}	time of maximum concentration/systemic exposure	WHO	World Health Organization

1

THE IMPORTANCE OF CARDIAC SAFETY ASSESSMENTS

1.1　INTRODUCTION

The importance of assessing the cardiac safety of noncardiac drugs, i.e., those that are not intended to treat cardiac conditions, has become very clear in recent years. A drug's propensity to influence the operation of the heart's electrical system in a certain deleterious manner is one of the most common causes of discontinuing a new drug's development program, failure to obtain marketing approval from a regulatory agency for a new drug, and removal of the drug from the market after approval (see Morganroth and Gussak, 2005). Some drugs lead to delayed cardiac repolarization, an occurrence that is explained in detail in due course and that plays a putative role in precipitating potentially lethal cardiac arrhythmias. Another occurrence of concern, and one that has prompted high-profile postmarketing regulatory actions in recent years, is discussion of potential links between a drug and other cardiac events such as fatal and nonfatal heart attacks. Assessments of cardiac safety have therefore become extremely important in contemporary drug development and pharmaceutical therapy.

　　This chapter provides an overarching introduction to the book's content. The process of new drug development is reviewed, along with the process of postmarketing surveillance. The term drug development is frequently used to describe the research and development that is done before an application requesting marketing permission is filed with a regulatory agency. Postmarketing surveillance refers to the monitoring of the drug's safety and therapeutic effectiveness once it has received marketing approval from a regulatory agency and is being prescribed by physicians and used by their patients. An additional term is also useful in the context of this book: the term lifecycle drug development embraces both premarketing and postmarketing activities. A drug's development in the sense of improving its safety and/or effectiveness profiles does not stop at the point of marketing approval. Data collected during the drug's use in large patient populations can lead to meaningful improvements in the drug. The term lifecycle drug development therefore emphasizes that it is vital to remain vigilant about the drug's effects from the very beginning of the drug discovery phase throughout the entire time that the drug is on the market and hence available for prescription to patients: this term captures the spirit of this book very well.

Integrated Cardiac Safety: Assessment Methodologies for Noncardiac Drugs in Discovery, Development, and Postmarketing Surveillance. By J. Rick Turner and Todd A. Durham
Copyright © 2009 John Wiley & Sons, Inc.

So too does the term integrated cardiac safety. A central tenet of this book is that it is beneficial to discuss the assessment methodologies used to collect information on cardiac safety at four stages of lifecycle drug development—drug discovery and design, nonclinical development, preapproval clinical development, and postmarketing surveillance—in one book, and to integrate this information to the greatest degree possible. The assessment methodologies used at these stages are quite different from each other, and an introduction to each methodology is therefore appropriate before discussing the information each provides. The term integrated cardiac safety also reflects another of the book's intentions, i.e., to bring together three areas within the overall spectrum of cardiac safety that are typically discussed separately. In this book these areas are termed proarrhythmic, generalized, and behavioral cardiac safety. Each of these areas is introduced in this chapter.

1.2   LIFECYCLE DRUG DEVELOPMENT

As Turner (2007) noted, the process of bringing a new drug to marketing approval is a lengthy, expensive, and complex endeavor. While precise quantification of "lengthy" and "expensive" is difficult, it is sufficient to note that respective values of 10–15 years and US$1.3 billion are realistic and informative approximations in 2008. As noted in Section 1.1, a drug's life history can be meaningfully categorized into four stages. Safety assessments during these four stages can be meaningfully integrated since the safety of a drug is addressed at all four stages in its lifecycle. While these stages of investigation generally occur in the order in which they are listed, it is important to note that additional research falling within the remit of previous phases can be generated by the occurrence of safety concerns in a later phase. This scenario is particularly relevant when safety concerns are identified in postmarketing surveillance.

1.2.1   Drug Discovery and Design

Drug discovery and design can be thought of as the work done from the time of the identification of a therapeutic need to the time the lead drug candidate, the drug molecule deemed most likely to safely effect the desired therapeutic benefit, has been identified and optimized. *In silico* modeling has become an important aspect of this research. A drug candidate may be a small molecule or a biological macromolecule such as a protein or nucleic acid. Drug discovery activities vary between small molecules and macromolecules, but once a drug candidate has been identified and moves into the drug development phase, the regulatory governance of nonclinical and clinical trials and the marketing approval process are very similar in both cases. Discussions in this text focus on the discovery of small-molecule drugs.

The term drug design is used throughout this book since contemporary research in small-molecule drug discovery incorporates *in silico* methodologies that employ predictive structure-function modeling in attempts to engineer a drug molecule that will successfully (therapeutically) interact with its target biological structure within the body while not interacting with nontarget biological structures.

1.2.2   Nonclinical Development

Once optimized, the drug candidate moves forward to a nonclinical development program, at which time the term investigational drug is commonly used. The term nonclinical development includes the nonhuman animal research that is currently necessary before permission will be given by regulatory agencies to test a new drug in humans, and also the additional nonhuman research that is done in parallel with preapproval clinical trials. Nonclinical research involves both *in vitro* and *in vivo* testing, and gathers critical information concerning drug dose, frequency, and route of administration as it relates to beneficial pharmaceutical therapy. Investigation of toxicity is also very important in nonclinical development. Some of the more lengthy, more complex, and more expensive nonhuman animal testing is typically not started until initial human testing reveals that the drug has a good safety profile in humans, and therefore has a reasonable chance of being approved for marketing if it also proves to be safe and effective in later clinical trials.

While human pharmacological therapy is the ultimate goal, understanding a drug's nonclinical biological activity is critical to subsequent rationally designed, ethical human trials. The term efficacy is used in preapproval clinical trials to refer to the desired therapeutic (biological) effect of the candidate drug, as discussed in the next section.

1.2.3   Preapproval Clinical Development

The pharmaceutical clinical trials conducted in a preapproval clinical development program examine the safety and efficacy of the drug in human participants. The term participant is used in this book to refer to anyone taking part in a clinical trial, while the term patient is reserved for individuals receiving pharmacological therapy from their personal physicians. Some participants may take part in a clinical trial at the recommendation of their physicians. These individuals are patients in the sense that they were under individual medical care from their physician at the time they commenced their participation in the trial, and they may well return to the same physician for further medical care upon their completion of participation in the trial. However, while they take part in a clinical trial, the term participant is appropriate.

The term efficacy refers to how well a drug achieves its intended therapeutic action during clinical trials. An investigational antihypertensive drug that does indeed lower blood pressure demonstrates efficacy, and the greater the drop in blood pressure, the greater the efficacy of the drug. It should be noted here that the term effectiveness also refers to how well a drug works, but it can be meaningfully distinguished from the term efficacy. Efficacy is evaluated during tightly controlled clinical trials that include a total of perhaps 3,000 to 5,000 participants. While this total may seem a large number, a marketed drug may be prescribed to hundreds of thousands of patients. These patients will comprise a much more diverse set of individuals than the set of people who took part in the clinical trials, and they will likely take the drug in a less controlled (more realistic) manner. The term effectiveness relates to how well the drug works in the patient population taking the drug.

This book does not address the assessment of efficacy in detail since it focuses on drug safety. However, as introduced in Section 1.6, meaningful assessment of drug safety is operationalized in terms of assessing a drug's benefit-risk balance, and a drug's efficacy/effectiveness must therefore be considered alongside its safety when making the benefit-risk assessments that are of fundamental importance in lifecycle drug development. Discussions of efficacy assessments can be found in many books, including Durham and Turner (2008), Kay (2007), Piantadosi (2005), Senn (2007), and Turner (2007).

A drug's safety profile captures side effects that are caused by the drug: the terms adverse events and adverse drug reactions are typically used in preclinical trials and postmarketing surveillance, respectively. Since no drug can be guaranteed immune from side effects, a drug's safety profile is assessed in every phase of its development. The term toxicity profile is sometimes used in this context since, as just noted, every drug is likely have some unwanted side effects. Initial safety evaluations are conducted in healthy adult participants in first time in human (FTIH) studies. If all goes well in these trials, the investigative drug is administered to relatively small numbers of participants with the medical disease or condition of interest. If all goes well in these trials, subsequent trials are conducted in which the investigative drug is administered to a much larger number of participants with the disease or condition of interest. These larger trials are undertaken towards the end of a preapproval drug development program with the goal of providing an answer to a specific research question concerning the efficacy of the drug. The safety and efficacy data collected in these trials facilitate a regulatory agency's deliberations concerning the possible approval of the drug for marketing.

Preapproval clinical trials are often categorized into various phases, with any given trial being identified as belonging to one of them. These categories include Phase I, Phase II, and Phase III trials. A traditional description of preapproval phases is as follows:

> ➤ Phase I trials. Pharmacologically oriented studies that typically look for the best dose to employ. Comparison to other treatments is not typically built into the study design.
> ➤ Phase II trials. Trials that look for evidence of activity, efficacy, and safety at a fixed dose. Comparison to other treatments is not typically built into the study design.
> ➤ Phase III trials. Trials in which comparison with another treatment (e.g., placebo, an active control) is a fundamental component of the design. These

trials are undertaken if Phase I and Phase II studies have provided preliminary evidence that the new treatment is safe and effective.

A more informative alternative system has been suggested by the International Conference on Harmonisation (ICH) of Technical Requirements for Registration of Pharmaceuticals for Human Use. The ICH is an amalgamation of expertise from various regulatory agencies and pharmaceutical-related organizations across the world. It publishes guidance documents on many aspects of clinical research. The ICH Guidance E8 provides an approach to classifying clinical studies according to their objective, as shown in Table 1.1. This book presents subsequent discussions of clinical trials using this descriptive terminology.

Table 1.1 The ICH Classification of Clinical Trials

Objective of Study	Study Examples
Human Pharmacology Assess tolerance. Describe or define pharmacokinetics (PK) and pharmacodynamics (PD). Explore drug metabolism and drug interactions. Estimate [biological] activity.	Dose-tolerance studies. Single and multiple dose PK and/or PD studies. Drug interaction studies.
Therapeutic Exploratory Explore use for the targeted indication. Estimate dosage for subsequent studies. Provide basis for confirmatory study design, endpoints, methodologies.	Earliest trials of relatively short duration in well-defined narrow patient populations using surrogate of pharmacological endpoints or clinical measures. Dose-response exploration studies.
Therapeutic Confirmatory Demonstrate/confirm efficacy. Establish safety profile. Provide an adequate basis for assessing benefit/risk relationship to support licensing [marketing approval]. Establish dose-response relationship.	Adequate and well-controlled studies to establish efficacy. Randomized parallel dose-response studies. Clinical safety studies. Studies of mortality/morbidity outcomes. Large simple trials. Comparative studies.
Therapeutic Use Refine understanding of benefit/risk relationship in general or special populations and/or environments. Identify less common adverse reactions. Refine dosing recommendation.	Comparative effectiveness studies. Studies of mortality/morbidity outcomes. Studies of additional endpoints. Large simple trials. Pharmacoeconomic studies.

Source: ICH E8: *General Considerations for Clinical Trials*

1.2.4   Postmarketing Surveillance

After a drug is approved for marketing, additional data concerning its safety and effectiveness are collected. As noted in the previous section, it is likely that the number of patients taking a marketed drug will be much larger than the total number of participants who took part in preapproval therapeutic confirmatory trials. This occurrence has a major implication for drug safety assessment: rare and potentially very serious side effects that were not seen during preapproval trials (it is probabilistically very unlikely that they would have been) may be seen at this point. These adverse drug reactions need to be identified and investigated.

Postmarketing surveillance monitors reports of adverse drug reactions and thus compiles extended safety databases (terms such as pharmacovigilance and pharmacoepidemiology studies are used in this context in other books, as discussed in Section 10.2). Postmarketing surveillance therefore plays a critical and integral role in lifecycle drug development: its goal is to ensure that all members of a target disease population receive the greatest possible protection from adverse drug reactions.

1.3   THE INTERNATIONAL COMMITTEE ON HARMONISATION

Regulatory agencies in many countries across the world oversee the development, marketing, and postmarketing use of drugs (and other medical interventions, including surgery and medical devices, not discussed in this book). The current regulatory environment is largely a result of the work of the ICH, an amalgamation of expertise from various agencies and organizations across the world.

The ICH arose since the regulations for submitting documentation requesting marketing approval of a drug were historically quite different between countries. Data requirements around the world were dissimilar, meaning that studies often had to be repeated to satisfy national regulatory requirements if marketing permission was desired in multiple countries. This lack of uniformity meant that nonclinical and clinical studies had to be repeated, resulting in additional and unnecessary use of animal, human, and material resources. It also meant that bringing a drug to market in various countries took longer than necessary, delaying its availability to patients.

Harmonization of regulatory requirements was pioneered by the European Community (now the European Union, EU) in the 1980s as it moved towards the development of a single market for pharmaceuticals. The success achieved in Europe demonstrated that harmonization was feasible. The harmonization process was then extended to include Japan and the United States. The ICH was formed from a government body and an industry association from each of these regions. These bodies and associations are:

> ➤ The European Commission, and the European Federation of Pharmaceutical Industries and Associations;

➢ The Japanese Ministry of Health, Labour and Welfare and the Japan Pharmaceutical Manufacturers Association;
➢ The United States Food and Drug Administration (specifically, the Center for Drug Evaluation and Research and the Center for Biologics Evaluation and Research) and the Pharmaceutical Research and Manufacturers of America.

1.3.1 Goals of the International Committee on Harmonisation

The ICH has several goals, including:

➢ To maintain a forum for a constructive dialog between regulatory authorities and the pharmaceutical industry on differences in technical requirements for marketing approval in the EU, the United States, and Japan in order to ensure a more timely introduction of new drugs and hence their availability to patients.
➢ To facilitate the adoption of new or improved technical research and development approaches that update or replace current practices. These new or improved practices should permit a more economical use of animal, human, and material resources without compromising safety.
➢ To monitor and update harmonized technical requirements leading to a greater mutual acceptance of research and development data.
➢ To encourage the implementation and integration of common standards of documentation and submission of regulatory applications by disseminating harmonized guidelines.
➢ To contribute to the protection of public health from an international perspective.

1.3.2 Guidances Issued by the International Committee on Harmonisation

The ICH has produced many guidance documents for sponsors to use in various aspects of drug development research and documentation, including drug quality, safety, and efficacy. These guidances are arranged in four categories:

➢ Quality (designated by the letter Q)
➢ Nonclinical Safety (S)
➢ Clinical Efficacy and Clinical Safety (E)
➢ Joint Safety/Efficacy (Multidisciplinary, M)

Guidances that discuss evaluations of safety issues in both nonclinical and clinical research include those listed in Table 1.2. (The safety guidances that fall in the "E" category are sometimes listed separately from the safety guidances that fall in the "S" category. See the ICH web site, http://www.ich.org, for more detailed information on all their guidances.)

Table 1.2 ICH Guidelines Addressing Safety Issues

Guidance (Yr. Finalized)	Title
S1A (1996)	The Need for Long-term Rodent Carcinogenicity Studies of Pharmaceuticals
S1B (1998)	Testing for Carcinogenicity of Pharmaceuticals
S1C (1995)	Dose Selection for Carcinogenicity Studies of Pharmaceuticals
S1C(R) (1997)	Guidance on Dose Selection for Carcinogenicity Studies of Pharmaceuticals: Addendum on a Limit Dose and Related Notes
S2A (1996)	Specific Aspects of Regulatory Genotoxicity Tests for Pharmaceuticals
S2B (1997)	Genotoxicity: A Standard Battery for Genotoxicity Testing of Pharmaceuticals
S3A (1995)	Toxicokinetics: The Assessment of Systemic Exposure in Toxicity Studies
S3B (1995)	Pharmacokinetics: Guidance for Repeated Dose Tissue Distribution Studies
S4A (1999)	Duration of Chronic Toxicity Testing in Animals (Rodent and Nonrodent Toxicity Testing)
S5A (1994)	Detection of Toxicity to Reproduction for Medicinal Products
S5B (1996)	Detection of Toxicity to Reproduction for Medicinal Products: Addendum on Toxicity to Male Fertility
S6 (1997)	Preclinical Safety Evaluation of Biotechnology-derived Pharmaceuticals
S7A (2001)	Safety Pharmacology Studies for Human Pharmaceuticals
S7B (2005)	The Non-clinical Evaluation of the Potential for Delayed Ventricular Repolarization (QT Interval Prolongation) by Human Pharmaceuticals
S8 (2006)	Immunotoxicity Studies for Human Pharmaceuticals
M3 (1997)	Nonclinical Safety Studies for the Conduct of Human Clinical Trials for Pharmaceuticals
E1A (1995)	The Extent of Population Exposure to Assess Clinical Safety: For Drugs Intended for Long-term Treatment of Non-life-threatening Conditions
E2A (1995)	Clinical Safety Data Management: Definitions and Standards for Expedited Reporting
E2C (1997)	Clinical Safety Data Management: Periodic Safety Update Reports for Marketed Drugs
E2C Addendum (1997)	Addendum to ICH E2C Clinical Safety Data Management: Periodic Safety Update Reports for Marketed Drugs
E2D (Draft 2003)	Postapproval Safety Data Management: Definitions and Standards for Expedited Reporting
E2E (2005)	Pharmacovigilance Planning
E14 (2005)	Clinical Evaluation of QT/QTc Interval Prolongation and Proarrhythmic Potential for Non-Antiarrhythmic Drugs

1.4 REGULATORY AGENCIES

There are many regulatory agencies around the world that are responsible for the governance of new drug development in their respective countries. Accordingly, following the practice employed in Turner (2007), the general phrase regulatory agency is used wherever possible in this book. On certain occasions, however, specific agencies are discussed. Since both authors of this book live and work in the United States, and since each of us has had involvement in the Food and Drug Administration (FDA) and FDA-related activities, it is fair to say that more text is probably allocated to the FDA than to other regulatory agencies. Nevertheless, the postmarketing-related work of the European Medicines Agency (EMEA: this agency was previously called the European Medicines Evaluation Agency, and this organization's widely known acronym was retained when its name was modified) is discussed in some detail: the EMEA has recently been ahead of the FDA in some very salient areas of regulation. We hope that readers in other countries will recognize that our FDA-specific discussions almost always address issues of international regulatory concern. Additionally, the Further Reading section at the end of this chapter contains references that provide discussion of regulatory activity in the EU, several individual countries within the EU, and Japan.

1.4.1 The Food and Drug Administration

The regulatory agency responsible for the governance of new drug development in the United States is the FDA. The FDA is housed within the Public Health Service, part of the Department of Health and Human Services. Redefined in the 1997 FDA Modernization Act, the FDA's relatively broad mission includes providing reasonable assurances that foods and cosmetics (both of which are regulated products) are safe, and that drugs and devices (also regulated products) are safe and effective. Several program centers facilitate the FDA's operations, including:

➢ The Center for Drug Evaluation and Research (CDER)
➢ The Center for Biologics Evaluation and Research (CBER)
➢ The Center for Veterinary Medicine (CVM)
➢ The Center for Devices and Radiological Health (CDRH)
➢ The Center for Food Safety and Applied Nutrition (CFSAN)

The FDA becomes involved in new drug development when nonclinical research conducted by a sponsor starts to indicate that the investigative drug has potential benefits in humans (Ascione, 2001). Regulatory oversight does not apply to drug discovery and design, and some of the earlier aspects of nonclinical development are not conducted under regulatory oversight either. However, many later aspects of nonclinical development and all aspects of clinical development are conducted under regulatory governance. This governance also includes manufacturing processes.

There are many regulatory requirements for new drug development and approval. Before a sponsor submits a request for a drug to be registered for human use, a tremendous amount of highly specified laboratory testing, nonclinical work, and clinical trials need to be performed. In all cases, the procedures and results must be documented appropriately. From a regulatory perspective, if the research is not documented, for all intents and purposes it has not been done.

This applies to nonclinical development as well as clinical development. Nonclinical work is reported to the FDA in an Investigational New Drug Application (IND). This document is reviewed to see if clinical work should be allowed to start. Once the clinical development program is completed, all of the developmental work will be reported to the FDA in a New Drug Application (NDA) or a Biologicals License Application (BLA). If the review of these enormous documents goes well, the drug will be approved for marketing.

The new drug development and approval process includes several principal steps (Regulatory Affairs Professionals Society, 2005; see also 2007):

> ➢ Nonclinical testing.
> ➢ Submission of an IND.
> ➢ FDA review of the IND.
> ➢ Preparation and submission of an NDA or a BLA following clinical research.
> ➢ FDA review and approval of the NDA or BLA.

While the ICH publishes an extensive list of guidances, individual regulatory agencies also publish guidance documents. For example, the FDA publishes Guidances for Industry that can be located via the FDA's web site (http://www.fda.gov). Web sites for guidances published by the EMEA are provided in the next section.

1.4.2   The European Medicines Agency

The EMEA is headquartered in London. This agency coordinates the evaluation and supervision of medicinal products throughout the EU, thereby bringing together the scientific resources of the EU member states (27 at the time of writing in 2007).

The regulatory documentation submission process is not identical in different countries, and this is exemplified by differences between FDA and EMEA processes. In the European system a Clinical Trial Application (CTA) is submitted by the sponsor at the point when an IND would be submitted to the FDA. Since a CTA is protocol specific, one CTA must be filed for each clinical study protocol, which means that the number of individual CTAs increases during a clinical development program. Additionally, CTAs are based on summary information only.

When a sponsor's clinical development is completed the sponsor submits a Marketing Authorisation Application (MAA), the vehicle used for both small molecule drugs and biologics. Two submission routes are available (in general) from which the sponsor may choose:

➤ The centralised procedure.
➤ The decentralised procedure.

The centralised procedure, which has been in place since 1995, leads to a single EU Scientific Opinion, which is then translated into a pan-EU decision by the European Commission. While this procedure is mandatory in some cases (e.g., for biotech drugs, and drugs intended for oncology, human immunodeficiency virus (HIV), diabetes, and neurodegenerative disease indications), it is also gaining popularity for all new chemical entities.

The decentralised procedure has been in place since 2006. The review of the MAA is conducted by a single agency, called the Reference Member State (RMS). However, other EU countries in which the sponsor wishes to market the drug receive a copy of the MAA and are involved in confirming the assessment made by the RMS. These additional agencies are called Concerned Member States (CMSs). The decentralised procedure has its roots in the earlier mutual recognition procedure that was put in place in 1995. The mutual recognition procedure operated in a similar way except that the CMSs did not receive the whole MAA until after the RMS had approved the product. In both the decentralised and the mutual recognition procedure, EMEA and the Committee for Medicinal Products for Human Use (CHMP) do not get involved unless the RMSs and CMSs cannot reach a consensus decision.

In the case of many new chemical entities ([NCEs], those for which the centralised procedure is not mandatory), choosing between the centralised and decentralised procedure involves many factors, and the decision is a strategic milestone involving medical practice, manufacturing plans, the nature of the product, market forces, and the size, resources, and strengths of the sponsor in the EU (see Harman, 2004, for more details).

Similarly to the FDA, CHMP and its Expert Working Parties provide scientific and regulatory guidelines that apply across the EU to complement ICH guidances. (Regulatory agencies in other countries and regions may develop guidelines as needed.) Thus, while considerable progress towards harmonization has been made, it is still important for those seeking global regulatory approvals to consider regional and national regulatory guidance. (For further information see   http://www.emea.europa.eu/htms/human/humanguidelines/efficacy.htm   and http://www.emea.europa.eu/htms/general/contacts/CHMP/CHMP_WPs.html.)

1.5   THE ROLE OF BENEFIT-RISK ASSESSMENT

The engine that drives new drug development is typically an unmet medical need, which is ultimately an unmet biological need (some new drugs are developed to address a medical need that is not being optimally addressed by existing drugs). That is, a drug is needed for the treatment or prevention of patients' biological states that are of clinical concern. Efficacy considerations in clinical trials and effectiveness considerations in postmarketing surveillance are therefore important. However, as highlighted by this book's content, so too are safety considerations. The ultimate goal of new drug development, then, is to produce a biologically active drug that is reasonably safe, well tolerated, and useful in the treatment or prevention of the disease or condition of concern. The word reasonably in the previous sentence may initially seem strange, but all drugs are likely to have side effects. The important goal, therefore, is to ensure a reasonable benefit-risk ratio, or benefit-risk balance.

1.5.1   THE EMPLOYMENT OF RATIOS IN LIFECYCLE DRUG DEVELOPMENT

The formation and calculation of mathematical ratios is a useful way to compare two quantities in many circumstances, including several in clinical research and drug development. Imagine that a sports team has won 15 games and lost 5 games in a season. How can the team's performance be captured in a relational manner? One way is to say that it won 10 more games than it lost. Another way is to calculate the ratio of games won to games lost. This is done simply and meaningfully by dividing the number of games won by the number of games lost. In this example, the number of games won is considered the numerator in this division, and the games lost is considered the denominator. Therefore, we have:

$$\frac{15 \text{ games}}{5 \text{ games}} = 3.00 \qquad (1.1)$$

That is, the team won three times as many games as it lost.

Note here that the calculation could have been done the other way round, as shown in Equation 1.2. That is, we could have chosen the number of games lost as the numerator and the number of games won as the denominator:

$$\frac{5 \text{ games}}{15 \text{ games}} = 0.33 \qquad (1.2)$$

The interpretation here would be that the team lost one-third as many games as it won. This statement, while also mathematically true, does not seem to flow as easily as the statement associated with Equation 1.1, i.e., the statement that the team won three times as many games as it lost. This example is provided here simply to illustrate that the choice of numerator and denominator is important for meaningful dissemination of information, a subject that is discussed in considerably more detail in Chapter 8.

1.6   BENEFIT-RISK ESTIMATES

As noted in Section 1.2.3, while not addressed in this book, the assessment of efficacy is needed in the process of benefit-risk estimation. The term benefit-risk estimate addresses precisely the same concept as the term benefit-risk ratio, but does so in a more meaningful manner in the present context. While the mathematical calculation that compares benefit to risk is correctly thought of as a ratio since we wish to compare benefit (the numerator) with harm (the denominator), the term ratio can imply a degree of precision that is not actually possible in benefit-risk assessment.

The calculation that is performed here can be more meaningfully expressed as

$$\text{Benefit-risk estimate} = \frac{\text{Estimate (probability and degree) of benefit}}{\text{Estimate (probability and degree) of harm}} \qquad (1.3)$$

This expression of the calculation that is conducted makes explicit that the two values that are placed into the equation and hence used in the ensuing calculation (the numerator and the denominator) are estimates, not precisely known quantities. Therefore, the result of this calculation is also an estimate. It is certainly true that, for any two values placed into this formula, a precise mathematical answer will be given, but since this answer is the result of a computation involving two estimates the answer is an estimate too.[1]

The term benefit-risk balance is also used in this book. A favorable benefit-risk balance is one in which the estimate of benefit is sufficiently greater than the estimate of harm, and an unfavorable benefit-risk balance is one in which the estimate of benefit is not sufficiently greater than the estimate of harm. To be considered reasonably safe, a drug needs to have a favorable, or acceptable, benefit-risk balance, whatever acceptable is deemed to be by a regulatory agency or a physician (see the following two sections).

It should also be noted here that a drug's benefit-risk balance can vary across time. Several occurrences can prompt a reevaluation of the benefit-risk balance. Identification of additional risk at a later time point (perhaps from postmarketing surveillance) reduces the benefit-risk estimate (the denominator in Equation 1.3 becomes greater). This is probably the occurrence that comes more readily to mind when considering this topic. However, the benefit-risk estimate can also be reduced, i.e., the benefit-risk balance made less favorable or acceptable, if the benefit decreases (the numerator in Equation 1.3 becomes smaller). This occurrence prompts the question: in what circumstances would the estimate of benefit be considered to have become reduced? One possibility is that postmarketing surveillance reveals that the effectiveness of the drug in the large population of patients taking it is less than was expected on the basis of the efficacy seen in the preapproval clinical trials that led to the drug's marketing approval.

Another scenario in which a drug's benefit-risk estimate can be reduced is the subsequent availability of a second drug with an equal benefit estimate and a lower

---

[1]This logic is analogous to that for using the term sample-size estimation rather than sample-size calculation when determining how many participants to employ in a clinical trial (see Turner, 2007, pp. 127–135).

risk estimate. This means that the original drug no longer offers a unique therapeutic benefit. Therefore, while the estimate of risk for the original drug remains the same, the estimate of its relative benefit is decreased by the availability of the second drug that possesses an equal benefit estimate and a lower risk estimate. In this scenario, as in the previous one, the original drug's benefit-risk estimate is decreased by a numerator that is smaller. However, the reason for the decrease in the benefit estimate is different.

Benefit-risk determinations, i.e., benefit-risk estimations in our nomenclature, are central and critical components of both regulatory and clinical decisions. Regulatory decisions have an impact on a potentially extremely large patient population, i.e., they have public health implications, and clinical decisions have an impact on individual patients on a case-by-case basis. Both kinds of decisions are extremely important. The scenarios in the previous paragraph attest to the need to consider several factors in benefit-risk estimations. In real life, this process is far less clear-cut than indicated in these scenarios, and far less clear-cut than frequently intimated in (often sensationalist and inaccurate) media coverage of pharmaceutical topics.

1.6.1   Benefit-risk Estimations by Regulatory Agencies

Once an NDA is submitted to a regulatory agency at the end of a clinical development program, the regulatory agency is faced with a decision: does it approve the drug for marketing? As will be discussed in considerably more detail in Section 8.10, the information that the regulatory agency must use to make this decision, while gathered from a seemingly large number of subjects, cannot be definitive.

As noted in Section 1.2.3, the information before regulatory agencies at this point has been obtained from a relatively small number of subjects, on the order of 3,000–5,000. While this may initially seem a sizable number, it is dwarfed by the number of patients who may take the drug if it is approved for marketing. The regulatory agency therefore is placed in the position of having to decide, on the basis of how a relatively small number of participants responded to the drug in clinical trials, whether the drug is likely to be sufficiently more beneficial than harmful to the hundreds of thousands (or more) of patients who may take it. This decision is based on a benefit-risk estimate. The clinical trials provide an estimate of the likely benefit to these patients and also an estimate of the likely harm. These data are the information that forms the basis of the regulatory agency's benefit-risk estimate, and thus the basis of their decision to give or not to give marketing approval.

Regulatory agencies also have the responsibility of deciding if a marketed drug should be removed from the market on the basis of safety concerns (this topic is discussed in Chapters 10–12). Just like the decision to approve a drug for marketing, the decision to remove a drug from the market is not a decision that can be reached with absolute certainty. It is a relative decision based on the likely harm to patients, the likely benefit to patients, and the ramifications of removing the drug from the market. Once it is removed, patients for whom the drug was effective and who suffered no ill effects do not have access to it. Depending on the availability or not of suitable alternative therapies, these patients may be harmed by no longer having access to beneficial treatment.

1.6.2   Benefit-risk Estimations by Physicians

Once a drug has been approved for marketing, it can be prescribed by physicians to their patients. When deciding upon a treatment regimen for an individual patient, a physician has to perform a benefit-risk estimation. Several pieces of information are used in the estimation process, including:

> All the available research data on a drug.
> The physician's knowledge of the patient's condition and medical history.
> The physician's clinical experience and clinical judgment in this situation.
> The patient's thoughts and feelings.

Having weighed the probability and degree of benefit to the patient against the probability and degree of harm, the physician has to decide, in conjunction with the patient, whether to prescribe the drug or not. That is, clinical decisions need to balance the relative weights of safety and efficacy considerations. If a higher dose of a given drug is considerably more effective than a lower dose and it only leads to a minimal increase in very mild side effects, a clinician may decide that, on balance, it is worth recommending the higher dose to the patient. Conversely, if a higher dose of a given drug is only minimally more effective than a lower dose and it leads to a considerable increase in moderate or severe side effects, a clinician may recommend the lower dose to the patient.

Clinical decisions involve an extra degree of complexity since, as noted, they are linked to the probability of the outcome occurring as well as the nature of a particular outcome. Consider the example of a physician and patient deciding together whether a new drug would be a useful therapy for the patient. Imagine that clinical research during the drug's development indicates that a particular side effect is likely to occur in 5% of patients who take the drug. If this drug would be particularly useful in the management of the patient's condition and the side effect is relatively benign (e.g., occasional moderate headaches), the clinician and the patient may decide that the risk of the side effect is worth taking. The side effect is relatively unlikely, and its occurrence would be manageable.

Consider now a similar scenario in which a different side effect also has a 5% probability of occurring, but that side effect is extremely debilitating. The patient and the clinician may make a different decision this time. On balance, the potential benefit of the drug may not outweigh the risk of experiencing the relatively unlikely but very undesirable side effect. The issue of balancing the probability of benefit with the probability of harm is a central element of clinical practice, and the probability of benefit always needs to outweigh the probability of harm. Determining just how much the probability of benefit needs to outweigh the probability of harm in a given situation is the province of the physician's clinical judgment and the physician-patient relationship.

1.6.3   Similarities and Differences in Regulatory and Clinical Benefit-risk Estimation

While the basic process of using a benefit-risk estimate to make a decision is the same for a regulatory agency and for a physician, there is an important distinction. The regulatory agency is making a decision that it considers to be in the best interests of the whole population with the disease or condition that the drug is intended to treat, i.e., as noted earlier, it has public health as its focus. The physician is making a decision he or she considers to be in the best interests of a specific individual patient. While physicians have many patients, and are also interested in the larger picture of public health, they must practice their clinical interventions one patient at a time.

1.7   FORMALIZED DRUG SAFETY IS A RELATIVELY YOUNG DISCIPLINE

Orchestrated drug safety monitoring is still a relatively young discipline that can be traced to activities that followed the thalidomide tragedy in the 1960s. The drug thalidomide was first marketed in Germany for the treatment of insomnia and vomiting in early pregnancy in 1956. In 1961, there was a sizable increase in the incidence of congenital birth defects noted in that country. The defects typically noted were an absence or reduction of the long bones of the limbs in conjunction with normal or rudimentary hands and feet. Very unfortunately, however, the association of these defects with the use of thalidomide was not recognized for several years after the drug was marketed, and thousands of babies worldwide suffered from this congenital condition. This tragedy prompted widespread acceptance that greater control of medicines was necessary to prevent recurrences in the future (West, 1991).

   Over the next several years, many countries adopted new approaches to assessing drug safety. First, legislation was introduced requiring that a drug's safety be assessed before the drug was marketed: some companies conducted clinical trials on their new drugs, but this was not a legal requirement. Second, systems for collecting information concerning the occurrence of adverse drug reactions from both medical professionals and the pharmaceutical industry were established. West (1991, p. 89) described this activity as "the foundation stone of safety surveillance and the start of regulatory authorities playing a significant role in ensuring drug safety."

   The last 40 years have seen a lot of progress in safety surveillance, and this progress is detailed in subsequent chapters. Many parts of this book adopt a chronological approach, providing a historical framework to show how this progress came about and allowing us to see how and why we are where we are today. Most important, this perspective also allows us to look forward. It is fair to say that we still have room for many improvements in drug safety, and this historical approach is hopefully beneficial in facilitating discussions of where we would like to be in the future, and how best to get there in an effective and timely manner.

1.8 INTEGRATED CARDIAC SAFETY

This book brings together three domains of cardiac safety—proarrhythmic, generalized, and behavioral—that together form integrated cardiac safety. Such integration is not typical in texts addressing cardiac safety, and, perhaps of particular note, behavioral cardiac safety is not typically addressed in texts addressing proarrhythmic and/or generalized cardiac safety. It is a quite different aspect of integrated cardiac safety, and, like proarrhythmic cardiac safety, it is certainly broad enough and important enough to warrant its own dedicated texts. However, we have written this book in the belief that everyone concerned with and involved in the provision to patients of drugs that can improve their health (and their quality of life) can benefit from an awareness of all three facets of integrated cardiac safety.

1.8.1 Proarrhythmic Cardiac Safety

The history of formalized proarrhythmic cardiac safety is even shorter than that of overall orchestrated drug safety as discussed in the previous section. While individual articles in scientific journals have been published for several decades and have been increasingly published for the last 15 years or so, books bringing together various aspects of proarrhythmic cardiac safety are a recent phenomenon. Seven such books are listed here, and all of them are highly recommended (they are cited in full, and in the usual alphabetical order, in the References). The first four are:

2002:   Yap and Camm, *Drug-induced long QT syndrome.*

2003:   Gussak and Antzelevitch (Eds.), *Cardiac repolarization: Bridging basic and clinical science.*

2004:   Camm, Malik, and Yap, *Acquired long QT syndrome.*

2005:   Morganroth and Gussak (Eds.), *Cardiac safety of noncardiac drugs: Practical guidelines for clinical research and drug development.*

It is also instructive to quote a few lines from each. It should be noted that these quotes contain terms with which you may not be familiar at this time. This is Okay: you will be very familiar with them once you have read this book. Morganroth and Gussak (2005, pp. vii and viii) noted that their book was "designed to present current preclinical, clinical, and regulatory principles to assess the cardiac safety of new drugs based primarily on their effects on the ECG" and to be "a primary reference for drug developers as well as academicians consulting in this arena." The individual chapters in their edited book, like those in the Gussak and Antzelevitch (2003) volume, provided detailed discussions of many aspects of this field, and one of our book's goals is to provide you with the background knowledge necessary to benefit fully from reading more advanced works in this research field.

In their Introduction, Yap and Camm (2002, p. 1) observed that:

> Drug effects are the most common cause of acquired long QT syndrome (LQTS)...In recent years, it has become apparent that a spectrum of noncardiac drugs, such as nonsedating antihistamines, macrolide antibiotics, antipsychotics, and others can cause QT prolongation and aggravate torsades de pointes. Of concern is that the proarrhythmic risk of many of these drugs was not detected during the developmental phase and was recognized only after the drug had been marketed for many years.

In their Preface, Gussak and Antzelevitch (2003, p. ix) noted the following:

> The past decade has seen an explosion of knowledge and radical changes in our understanding of ventricular repolarization as an integral part of the cardiac electrophysiologic matrix; a topic which, until now, has not been covered in depth. *Cardiac repolarization: Bridging basic and clinical science* presents comprehensively the latest developments in the field of cardiac electrophysiology with a focus on the clinical and experimental aspects of ventricular repolarization, newly discovered clinical repolarization syndromes, electrocardiographic phenomena, and their correlation with the most recent advances in basic science.

Camm, Malik, and Yap (2004, p. vi) noted similarly that:

> This book is written with the intention of providing a detailed review on acquired long QT syndrome, from drug-induced QT prolongation to cardiac and noncardiac causes of QT prolongation. Detailed attention is paid to the mechanism of drug-induced QT prolongation and the clinical methodology of measuring myocardial repolarization which is crucial in the assessment of the proarrhythmic risk of a particular drug.

Likewise, Morganroth and Gussak (2005, p. vii) commented that:

> *Cardiac safety of noncardiac drugs: Practical guidelines for*
> *clinical research and drug development* is designed to present the
> current preclinical, clinical, and regulatory principles to assess the
> cardiac safety of new drugs based primarily on their effects on the
> ECG. Practical guidance to define cardiac safety at all stages of
> clinical research and drug development are featured and discussed
> by internationally recognized experts with academic, industrial,
> and regulatory experience.

It is also informative here to note three other books. Two of these resulted from Novartis Foundation symposia, and the third is a volume in the Wiley-VCH book series entitled "Methods and Principles in Medicinal Chemistry."

> 2003:   Chadwick and Goode (Eds.), *Development of the cardiac*
>   *conduction system.* (Novartis Foundation Symposium 250)
>
> 2005:   Chadwick and Goode (Eds.), *The hERG cardiac potassium*
>   *channel: Structure, function and long QT syndrome.* (Novartis
>   Foundation Symposium 266)
>
> 2006:   Triggle, Gopalakrishnan, Rampe, and Zheng (Eds.), *Voltage-gated*
>   *ion channels as drug targets.*

In the early 1990s, Morganroth (1993) observed that "At present, our knowledge base about the relation of the QT interval and torsades de pointes is grossly incomplete." Twelve years later, discussing a chapter by Morganroth and Gussak (2005), Shah (2005a, p. 259) referred to Morganroth's observation and commented as follows:

> Unfortunately, despite extensive research for more than a
> decade since, this still remains the same today. It is therefore not
> surprising that more than any other drug-induced adverse reaction,
> it has been responsible in recent times for the withdrawal of many
> drugs from the market.

1.8.2   Generalized Cardiac Safety

As noted in the Preface, the term generalized cardiac safety is used in this book to refer to all cardiac adverse drug reactions with the exception of arrhythmogenic events captured by the term proarrhythmic cardiac safety. Events falling within our category called generalized cardiac safety include fatal heart attacks, major irreversible morbidity (e.g., nonfatal myocardial infarctions), debilitating cardiovascular symptoms or events (e.g., transient ischemic attacks, marked fluid retention, and palpitations), and various pathophysiological characteristics that increase the likelihood of cardiac and cardiovascular events (see Borer et al., 2007).

While cardiac and cardiovascular parameters are certainly monitored during preapproval drug development programs, formal generalized cardiac safety assessment typically starts once a drug is marketed (using essentially the same postmarketing surveillance methodologies used in proarrhythmic postmarketing surveillance). Chapter 12 addresses generalized cardiac safety by way of three case studies involving high-profile instances in the last few years where the cardiac safety of specific drugs was questioned. One of these case studies addresses drugs generally known as coxibs, anti-inflammatory agents, and another addresses drugs known as thiazolidinediones, agents used in the treatment of diabetes.

1.8.3   Behavioral Cardiac Safety

The third aspect of cardiac safety discussed in this book is termed behavioral cardiac safety. This term is used to refer to cardiac adverse events where behavioral factors are the primary instigating factor. This category includes medication errors whereby patients are prescribed, dispensed, and/or administered an unintended drug or drug regimen and patients' intentional or unintentional lack of adherence to legitimately prescribed drug regimens. Chapter 13 therefore discusses the roles of physicians, pharmacists, and nurses in pharmacotherapy: as Dowell (2004, p. 50) noted, "the term clinician can meaningfully be applied to professionals in each of these healthcare domains since each may be in the position of discussing the use of or authorising the supply of medicines." The category of behavioral cardiac safety also includes the behavior of the patient in terms of how he or she actually takes medication that has been accurately prescribed and dispensed. The term adherence is one term that is used to address this issue, and patients vary considerably in their adherence to an appropriately prescribed drug regimen.

The assessment methodologies employed in the investigation of behavioral cardiac safety are applicable to behavioral drug safety in general, and so behavioral drug safety is discussed in general, but with specific examples related to cardiac safety. Behavioral safety is largely specific to postmarketing situations, since many of the behavioral factors of interest—errors in prescribing, dispensing, administration (e.g., by health care providers in in-patient settings and nursing homes), and taking one's own medication—occur once a drug is on the market. One area of behavioral safety that is not specific to postmarketing involves the preparation of clinical trial drug products, the pharmaceutical delivery vehicles via which the investigational drug and a comparator treatment (e.g., a placebo) are administered to participants in preapproval clinical trials.

As discussed in more detail in due course, one of the major problems in clinical medicine is that not everyone reacts in the same manner to the same approved and marketed drug. In the vast majority of cases, a very large percentage of patients will safely experience a beneficial therapeutic effect, a small percentage may safely experience no therapeutic benefit, and a (very) small percentage may experience an adverse drug reaction. This unfortunate occurrence can happen despite full due diligence on the part of the pharmaceutical company that developed the drug, the regulatory agency that approved the drug for marketing, and the physicians who prescribed the drug to patients who experienced the adverse drug reactions. As noted in the Institute of Medicine's report on the future of drug safety (2007b, p. 27), "The approval decision does not represent a singular moment of clarity about the risks and benefits associated with a drug—preapproval clinical trials do not obviate continuing formal evaluations after approval" (Part III of this book focuses on precisely such continuing formal evaluations). The main reasons that certain patients experience adverse drug reactions to drugs that were prescribed in full accordance with evidence available from all currently employed diagnostic tools, and with the highest degree of clinical judgment on the part of the prescribing physician, are individual genetic differences that influence the way a drug is metabolized and the degree to which a drug interacts with nontarget biological structures. These topics are discussed in due course: For now, the main point is that everyone involved in providing drugs to patients who experience proarrhythmic or generalized cardiac adverse drug reactions performed to the very best of their ability.

Unfortunately, this is not the case in behavioral cardiac adverse drug reactions. As noted previously, the field of behavioral cardiac safety includes studying the occurrence of medication errors, errors whereby patients are prescribed, dispensed, and/or administered an unintended drug or drug regimen that leads to a cardiac adverse drug reaction. Medication errors occur much more frequently than one might think: tens of thousands of people in the United States die each year from medication errors. Having made these statements, statements that can certainly appear harsh and judgmental—the word errors has a habit of sounding judgmental, an issue that is discussed in some depth in Chapter 13—it is extremely important to note that judgments are the last thing needed in this context. The physicians who prescribe, pharmacists who dispense, and nurses who administer drugs to patients are human beings, and human errors happen. Indeed, we should expect human errors to occur. The fundamental issue here is the design and implementation of safety systems that eliminate (or minimize to the greatest degree possible) the occurrence of errors by building in enough checks so that errors occurring early in the process are caught and rectified before the patient takes the drug at the end of the process. Health care is a high-risk field: patients can and do die from medication errors. However, it is not the only high-risk field (think about landing a military aircraft on the deck of an aircraft carrier on a pitch black night in very heavy seas). Safety systems have evolved to a much greater degree in other high-risk situations, and the need for the continuing evolution of health care safety systems is discussed in Chapter 13.

Chapter 13 also examines the role of the patient in medicine taking. This takes discussions into the realms of adherence—how closely the patient's pattern of taking prescribed medication matches the prescribed regimen—and concordance, which focuses on the interaction between physician and patient at a holistic level. Patients' psychosocial and behavioral characteristics can significantly influence which medicines they are willing to take and how they take them once prescribed, and the greater the degree of open discussion between the physician and the patient the better.

Some books that address these issues are listed here in chronological order (again, full details are provided in the References).

2000:   Institute of Medicine, *To err is human: Building a safer health system.*

2003:   World Health Organization, *Adherence to long-term therapies: Evidence for action.*

2004:   Bond (Ed.), *Concordance.*

2004:   Institute of Medicine, *Patient safety: Achieving a new standard for care.*

2005:   Bosworth, Oddone, and Weinberger (Eds.), *Patient treatment adherence: Concepts, interventions, and measurement.*

2006:   O'Donohue and Levensky (Eds.), *Promoting treatment adherence: A practical handbook for health care providers.*

2007:   Park and Liu (Eds.), *Medical adherence and aging: Social and cognitive perspectives.*

2007:   Cohen (Ed.), *Medication errors,* 2nd edition.

2007:   Institute of Medicine, *Preventing medication errors.*

1.9   TEACHING AND LEARNING OBJECTIVES OF THIS BOOK

Differentiation between teaching and learning is an interesting philosophical challenge, and one that is beyond the scope of this book. In practical terms, we would like to convey certain information to our readers: we will try to teach you about, and we hope that you will learn about, research activities in the field of integrated cardiac safety. Whether one therefore regards the following points as teaching or learning objectives, we hope that reading this book will facilitate your appreciation of the following points that provide an effective agenda for subsequent discussions:

> Obtaining the full benefits from integrated cardiac safety assessment requires an integrated approach that makes use of optimum quality information to make optimum quality benefit-risk assessments throughout a drug's lifecycle. This assessment starts during drug design, occurs in nonclinical and clinical research, and extends throughout the drug's time on the market.

> *In silico* structure-function prediction research conducted during contemporary drug design aims to engineer safety into new molecular entities by engineering cardiotoxicity out of them.

> The ICH Guidance S7B, *The Non-clinical Evaluation of the Potential for Delayed Ventricular Repolarization (QT Interval Prolongation) by Human Pharmaceuticals*, directs nonclinical cardiac safety research addressing a candidate drug's proarrhythmic liability.

> The ICH Guidance E14, *Clinical Evaluation of QT/QTc Interval Prolongation and Proarrhythmic Potential for Non-antiarrhythmic Drugs*, directs clinical trials addressing an investigational drug's proarrhythmic liability.

> Postmarketing surveillance methodologies play a crucial role in monitoring for the occurrence of proarrhythmic and generalized cardiac adverse drug reactions.

> In addition to adverse drug reactions that can result from appropriately taken medication, medication errors (errors of prescription, dispensing, and administration) lead to a large number of adverse drug reactions. Developing and implementing safety systems throughout pharmaceutical (and all areas of) health care must be a high priority.

As noted on several occasions, the discussions in this book are at the introductory level. Accordingly, lists of Further Reading are provided at the ends of chapters for those of you who would like to take your study of integrated cardiac safety (or any component thereof) to the next level. The sources in the following section, the further reading for this chapter, are presented in the typical alphabetical order. In some of the subsequent chapters that focus on specific areas within integrated cardiac safety, the sources are presented in chronological order to provide a mini-history of developments in the respective areas.

1.10   FURTHER READING

Arnold, B.D.C., 2004, Regulatory aspects of pharmacovigilance. In Talbot, J. and Waller, P. (Eds.), *Stephens' detection of new adverse drug reactions*, 5th edition, Chichester, UK: John Wiley & Sons, 375–451.
[This chapter contains discussion of the Council for International Organizations of Medical Sciences, the ICH, and regulatory activities in the EU, France, Germany, the United Kingdom, Japan, and the United States.]

Harman, R.J., 2004, *Development and control of medicines and medical devices,* London: Pharmaceutical Press.
[This book discusses the roles of UK and pan-European regulatory authorities.]

Lee, C-J., Lee, L.H., Wu, C.L., Lee, B.R., and Chen, M.L, 2006, *Clinical trials of drugs and biopharmaceuticals*, Boca Raton, FL: CRC/Taylor & Francis.

Mann, R. and Andrews, E. (Eds.), 2007, *Pharmacovigilance,* 2nd edition, Chichester, UK: John Wiley & Sons.
[This volume provides instructive information on regulatory activities in the EU, the United Kingdom, France, Germany, the Netherlands, New Zealand, Japan, and the United States.]

Rang, H.P. (Ed.), 2006, *Drug discovery and development: Technology in transition*, Philadelphia: Churchill Livingstone/Elsevier.

Regulatory Affairs Professionals Society, 2007, *Fundamentals of U.S. Regulatory Affairs,* 5th edition, Rockville, MD: Regulatory Affairs Professionals Society.

Rogge, M.C. and Taft, D.R. (Eds.), 2005, *Preclinical drug development*, Boca Raton, FL: CRC/Taylor & Francis.

Smith, C.G. and O'Donnell, J.T. (Eds.), *The process of new drug discovery and development,* 2nd edition, New York: Informa Healthcare.

Talbot, J. and Waller, P. (Eds.), *Stephens' detection of new adverse drug reactions,* 5th edition, Chichester, UK: John Wiley & Sons.

Turner, J.R., 2007, *New drug development: Design, methodology, and analysis*, Hoboken, NJ: John Wiley & Sons.

2

THE BIOLOGICAL BASIS OF ADVERSE DRUG REACTIONS

2.1   INTRODUCTION

Drug safety is concerned with assessing unwanted drug responses that are of clinical relevance. As Turner (2007) noted, clinical relevance is intimately related to biological relevance, which places biological considerations at the heart of this book. Useful drugs treat or prevent biological states of clinical concern, but they must also be reasonably safe (recall the discussion in Section 1.5). Therapeutic efficacy is the result of the interaction between a drug and its target biological structure, and the consequent beneficial cascade of biological information that changes a patient's biology for the better. Unfortunately, drugs can also lead to undesirable biological consequences. Adverse drug reactions result from an interaction between a drug and a nontarget biological structure and the consequent cascade of biological information. Therefore, before discussing the nature of these undesirable consequences and the methodologies for their prediction and assessment, it is appropriate to become familiar with the biological structures and systems activated by a drug.

This chapter starts at the level of atoms and molecules and then moves to biological structures and systems: an understanding of molecular biology is extremely helpful for subsequent discussions concerning unwanted cardiac responses to noncardiac drugs. It should be noted here that biological considerations are presented from a pragmatic perspective and in a stylized format. In keeping with the goal of writing a self-contained book on integrated cardiac safety, this introduction is written for readers who will benefit most from it. Readers who are already well versed in these subjects may prefer to move on to Chapter 3.

2.2   INDIVIDUAL VARIATION IN RESPONSES TO DRUGS

One of the greatest problems in pharmaceutical medicine is that all patients do not respond in the same manner to the same drug. This phenomenon is called individual variation. When a given drug is administered to different patients for whom it is appropriate, as determined by the best diagnostic techniques currently available, many of these patients will safely experience a therapeutic benefit. However, there

Integrated Cardiac Safety: Assessment Methodologies for Noncardiac Drugs in Discovery, Development, and Postmarketing Surveillance. By J. Rick Turner and Todd A. Durham
Copyright © 2009 John Wiley & Sons, Inc.

are other possible outcomes that may be experienced by relatively small numbers of patients:

> Individual patients may not show a beneficial therapeutic response. Increasing the dose may lead to a beneficial response in some cases.
> Individual patients may show an undesirably excessive therapeutic response (e.g., becoming hypotensive instead of normotensive following the administration of an antihypertensive drug). A lower dose of the same drug may work well in some cases. In this scenario the unwanted response is the result of excessive activation of the target biological structure. That is, the mechanism of action of the unwanted response is understood.
> A number of patients may show relatively serious adverse drug reactions that result from the drug's interaction with nontarget biological structures. Some of these mechanisms of action are known, and others remain unknown at the present time.

The key question here is: why do individual patients react differently to the same drug? An understanding of the causes of this individual variation requires knowledge of the biological underpinnings of drug responses. This knowledge and understanding are being continuously enhanced by tremendous advances in molecular biology. Molecular biological aspects of drug responses are discussed later in this chapter following an overview of some basic biology. The order in which topics are presented here is not typical of traditional biology or biochemistry courses, but is tailored specifically to enhance appreciation of biological discussions in subsequent chapters.

2.3 DEOXYRIBONUCLEIC ACID

The acronym DNA is now so well known that it often appears in books, media coverage, and television shows with no accompanying definition: when is the last time you saw or heard the words deoxyribonucleic acid? Every time we watch a contemporary detective show on television we are almost waiting to hear about the DNA evidence that indicates or refutes a suspect's guilt. However, despite the ubiquity of this acronym, it is probably reasonable to say that DNA's nature and function are less well known. Since genetics plays an influential role in both beneficial and unwanted responses to drug therapy it is appropriate to review DNA at this point.

Deoxyribose nucleic acid is a very large molecule and is legitimately called a macromolecule. Each word in its name is descriptive of its nature. Ribose is one form of sugar, along with glucose, fructose, sucrose, and others. The prefix "deoxy-" (the "D" in DNA) specifies a ribose that has lost one of its oxygen atoms at a specific site in the molecule. Nucleic acids (the "N" and the "A") are a group of complex compounds derived from carbohydrates, purines, and pyrimidines (discussed shortly), and phosphoric acid. Nucleic acids are found in all living cells. They are also found in viruses, which are not actually alive until they hijack another cell's genetic material and make it work for them (Nobel laureate Sir Peter Medawar has called viruses "a piece of nucleic acid surrounded by bad news" [cited by Bryson, 2004, p. 385]).

2.3.1   Bases

Each DNA macromolecule contains many copies of four bases, known as adenine ("A"), guanine ("G"), thymine ("T"), and cytosine ("C"). Each of these is a molecule in its own right, comprised of carbon, hydrogen, oxygen, and nitrogen atoms. These four bases can be meaningfully split into two categories:

> ➤ Adenine and guanine, both of which are purines.
> ➤ Thymine and cytosine, both pyrimidines.

Pyrimidines are chemical structures that are composed of one ring of carbon atoms, and purines are chemical structures composed of two rings.

2.3.2   Nucleotides

Both pyrimidines and purines are capable of joining together (bonding) with a deoxyribose molecule that also contains a phosphate group. The combination of each of the four bases—adenine, guanine, thymine, and cytosine—with a deoxyribose molecule leads to the formation of four different nucleotides. Using the purine and pyrimidine categorization system again, there are two purine nucleotides, adenine and guanine, and two pyrimidine nucleotides, thymine and cytosine.

As ring chemical structures, these four molecules are relatively flat, a characteristic that makes the DNA macromolecule very strong since these nucleotides can stack up in a compact fashion. This planar geometry of individual nucleotides is in marked contrast to the eventual and very complex three-dimensional shape of DNA. The three-dimensionality of macromolecules is extremely pertinent to the following discussions.

2.3.3   Polynucleotide Strands

A polynucleotide strand is made up of hundreds of thousands of individual nucleotides linked together. The nucleotides in a polynucleotide strand are combined in a specific manner. The forces that hold atoms and hence molecules together are called bonds, and bonds occur between specific atoms in specific ways. Nucleotides in a strand are held together by bonds between the sugar component of one nucleotide and the phosphate component of the other nucleotide. Since each nucleotide has both a sugar component and a phosphate component it can bond to one nucleotide "above" it and another nucleotide "below" it, allowing a polynucleotide chain to be formed.

It is important to emphasize that molecules are three-dimensional in nature. Representing three-dimensional structures on two-dimensional pages of a book is a challenge, and chemists, biologists, and illustrators have devised many ingenious methods of doing so (computer programmers have also devised such methods for *in silico* representations of biochemical activity presented on a two-dimensional computer screen that present a convincing appearance of three-dimensionality). Despite this extremely useful two-dimensional representation of molecules in textbooks, however, we must remember that we are dealing with three-dimensional molecules, a tremendously important determinant of molecular interactions.

The phosphates and sugars form a column that is called the backbone of the strand. Imagine one strand running across the top of a book page, as represented in Figure 2.1.

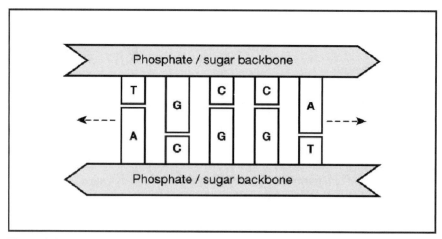

Figure 2.1. Representation of a section of DNA.

The base of each nucleotide—adenine, guanine, thymine, or cytosine—can then be thought of as extending towards the center of the page. Imagine now a second strand that runs along the bottom of the page. Again, the phosphates and sugars form the backbone of the strand. Imagine that the bases of the nucleotides in this second strand also extend towards the center of the page. That is, for each strand, the phosphates and sugars form a column on the "outside" and the nucleotide bases project towards the "inside." The magic of DNA's double helix arrangement is facilitated by this molecular organization.

2.3.4   The Double Helix

Each DNA macromolecule is comprised of two strands of nucleotides that are attached together. This molecular structure and the ensuing molecular geometry of DNA lead to its characteristic double helix nature. Once formed, single strands of DNA like to be matched with, and attached to, another strand. The process of matching and attaching is nonrandom and governed by certain rules. Imagine that the bases of the strand running along the top of Figure 2.1 are reaching out with open arms to the bases of the strand along the bottom of the figure. Each base wants to be matched with and attached to another base. However, there two hard-and-fast rules:

> ➤ An adenine base can only be matched with and attached to a thymine base.
> ➤ A guanine base can only be matched with and attached to a cytosine base.

The term complementary bases reflects this arrangement: each of the four nucleotide bases has a complementary base to which it becomes attached. An extremely important consequence of this is that, once the sequence of nucleotides in one strand is known, the sequence of nucleotides in the other strand is also known.

This adenine-thymine and guanine-cytosine pairing strategy also means that, in each pairing, one purine nucleotide (adenine or guanine) is paired with one pyrimidine nucleotide (thymine or cytosine, respectively). The relevance of this arrangement is again related to three-dimensional geometry. As noted in Section 2.3.1, pyrimidine bases comprise a single ring, while purine bases comprise two rings. Hence, pyrimidine bases are smaller than purine bases. Imagine the (impossible) scenario in which a pyrimidine base on the left-hand backbone was able to attach to a pyrimidine base on the right-hand backbone, and a purine base on left-hand backbone was able to attach to a purine base on the right-hand backbone. Imagine also that pyrimidine bases each measure one unit of length, while purine bases each measure two units of length. Once any two pyrimidine bases were attached to each other, the total distance between the two backbones would be the combined length of the two pyrimidine bases, i.e., two units of length. On the other hand, once any two purines were attached to each other, the total distance between the two backbones would be the combined length of the two purine bases, i.e., four units of length. This would mean that the distance between the backbones would vary, depending on the nature of each base-base pairing, with the consequence that the overall DNA macromolecule would have an extremely irregular three-dimensional structure.

In contrast, the actual arrangement within the DNA macromolecule ensures geometrical regularity. Each base pairing occurs between one purine base and one pyrimidine base, which means each pairing results in a total length of three units of length and, therefore, that the total distance between the two backbones is always three units of length. This regularity has two very important consequences. First, it facilitates spatial compression. The DNA macromolecules are able to coil very tightly within a cell, which means that a molecule that would be very long if arranged in a simple linear fashion can be compacted into a very short length. Second, errors in replication are less likely.

2.3.5   Replication

While this book does not deal with the genetic process of replication directly, it is worth noting here that replication is the process by which DNA is able to produce an exact copy of itself. First, the two polynucleotide chains that comprise a DNA molecule split apart from each other. Each then becomes reattached to a new partner, and the partner is an exact copy of its original partner. This occurrence is governed by the rules we have just discussed: adenine only binds with thymine, and guanine only binds with cytosine. Therefore, two precise copies of the original DNA macromolecule are formed. These two copies can then replicate and result in four copies of the original. The exponential nature of replication means that one DNA macromolecule can produce an extremely large number of copies of itself, enough for an entire organism.

Chromosomes are strands of DNA that contain genes. In humans (and other higher organisms) a full set of chromosomes is contained in the nucleus of each cell. Humans have a total of 46 chromosomes, comprised of 2 sex chromosomes and 44 autosomal chromosomes. Sex chromosomes, as their name indicates, determine the individual's sex: two X chromosomes yield a female, and one X and one Y chromosome yield a male. The term autosomal simply differentiates the other chromosomes from the sex chromosomes. The total complement of chromosomes is arranged into pairs, 1 pair of sex chromosomes and 22 pairs of autosomal chromosomes. The individual chromosomes in each pair are considered homologous (identical in shape and size), and they can be referred to as homologs. Each pair of homologous chromosomes carries the same genes. At each location along each chromosome (think in terms of the same address on each chromosome: see Dawkins, 1999) there will be one of a number of possible variations of the same gene. These alternate versions are called alleles.

2.3.6   Autosomal Dominant or Autosomal Recessive Inheritance

Imagine that a specific gene has two alleles, represented by the uppercase letter G and the lowercase letter g. At a certain address on each of two homologous chromosomes there will be one of these alleles. There are four possible combinations:

➤ G and G
➤ G and g

> ➤ g and G
> ➤ g and g

The combination of the two alleles determines what phenotype results from this pairing of alleles. If the allele G is dominant (and the allele g is therefore recessive), the phenotype encoded for by the G allele will occur for each of the first three combinations. Only in the fourth combination, where the recessive allele is present on both chromosomes, will the phenotype encoded for by the g allele occur. This occurrence is of particular relevance in this book in terms of the autosomal dominant or autosomal recessive inheritance of certain cardiac disorders discussed in Chapter 4.

2.4   TRANSMISSION GENETICS AND MOLECULAR GENETICS

Genetics, itself a relatively young science, is concerned with how traits are passed from one generation to the next. Since the advent of genomics, a more recent science that is discussed in more detail shortly, the term transmission genetics has come to represent what had previously been called simply genetics. The mathematics of transmission genetics were first described by Mendel in 1866 (see Edelson, 1999). The study of genes themselves is called molecular genetics. The focus of molecular genetics includes the physical and chemical structure of DNA. The information contained within our DNA codes for all of our individual characteristics. This includes eye color, blood type, susceptibility to disease, and, of particular relevance in this book, likely responses to drugs. When molecular genetic study moves from studying individual genes to studying the entire complement of the genome, the term genomics becomes appropriate (e.g., see Dale and von Schantz, 2002). The Human Genome Project is discussed shortly, but first it is meaningful to consider the transmission genetic work of T.H. Morgan and his colleagues conducted with another organism.

2.5   THE PIONEERING WORK OF MORGAN USING *DROSOPHILA MELANOGASTER*

Genetic experiments using *Drosophila melanogaster,* the fruit fly, were first conducted in 1901 at Harvard University, but were taken to the next level at Columbia University by Morgan starting in 1907 (see Watson, 2004, pp. 12–13).

Fruit flies have marked advantages for use in transmission genetic research. They are abundant in nature, and they are easily fed and accommodated. Moreover, they are prodigious reproducers. They have a generation time of 10 days, and females produce around 300 eggs each (of which half are female). In the space of a single month (three generation times), one fruit fly couple can lead to 150 (half of 300) times 150 times 150 flies, i.e., over 3 million flies (Watson, 2004).

Since there was no current knowledge of established genetic differences in 1907, it was hard to for Morgan to know where to start. As Watson (2004, p. 13) commented, "you cannot do genetics until you have isolated some distinct characteristics to track through the generations." A search for mutant genes was therefore started. Mutant genes, i.e., variations from the normally occurring genes, lead to distinct characteristics. This search led to the discovery of some flies with white eyes (the normal color being red). Morgan then started what has become a long tradition in *Drosophila* research, namely, giving descriptive names to mutant genes. This gene was called white. Names subsequently given to other genes have also been colorful, but in a different sense of the word. (Readers who have heightened political correctness sensibilities, consider yourselves forewarned.) The web site http://tinman.vetmed.helsinki.fi/eng/drosophila.html lists some of these names. One of these genes, known as the ether a-go-go gene (eag), has around 20 alleles. A human gene that is related to this gene is of particular relevance in this book and it is discussed in the next chapter.

In addition to identifying the genetic influence responsible for certain characteristic traits in flies possessing these genes, Morgan's work laid the groundwork for one of the central components of the Human Genome Project and all of the genome projects undertaken for different organisms. In the course of studying genes located on the same chromosome, Morgan and his students found that chromosomes actually break apart and re-form during the production of sperm and egg cells. This process of breaking and re-forming shuffles gene copies between members of a chromosome pair. In contemporary language, this breaking and re-forming is called recombination. It occurs naturally in the reproductive process, but the technique can now be used to create new segments of DNA by the technologies of recombinant DNA engineering.

The study of recombinant events facilitates the mapping of the positions of particular genes along a given chromosome. Recombination involves breaking (and re-forming) chromosomes. Because genes are arranged like beads along a chromosome string, a break is statistically much more likely to occur between two genes that are far apart (with more potential breakpoints intervening) on the chromosome than between two genes that are close together. If, therefore, we see a lot of reshuffling for any two genes on a single chromosome, we can conclude that they are far apart. In contrast, the rarer the reshuffling, the closer together the genes likely are. This basic and immensely powerful principle underlies all of genetic mapping. It was of fundamental importance in the Human Genome Project, and it is a central technique in research on genetic diseases.

2.6   GENES AND THE HUMAN GENOME PROJECT

The original proposal for the Human Genome Project was made in 1990 by the Office of Health and Environmental Research, U.S. Department of Energy. This department had long been interested in the effects of nuclear radiation on human genetics, and they proposed a joint venture with the National Institutes of Health (NIH). The original timeline was 15 years, but the goal was actually accomplished in less time and under budget, partly because of competition from private companies, including Celera Genomics (Palladino, 2006).

In June 2000, scientists from the Human Genome Project and from Celera Genomics announced in a press conference held with President Clinton that a "working draft" of the human genome was assembled. In February 2001, leading scientists from the Human Genome Project and Celera Genomics announced that initial papers describing their work would be published in the journals *Nature* and *Science*, respectively (IHGS Consortium, 2001; Venter et al., 2001). In April 2003, the International Human Genome Sequencing Consortium announced that its work was completed and that, with the exception of a few very small gaps, all base pairs in the human genome were identified and placed in sequence (see IHGS Consortium, 2004).

2.6.1 The Human Genome: So Much DNA, So Few Genes

Only a decade or so ago, it was widely thought that the human genome may contain upward of 100,000 genes. However, following the completion of the Human Genome Project, current authoritative estimates are in the 20,000–25,000 range, a remarkably lower estimate than the aforementioned 100,000 genes.

Human DNA contains approximately 3 billion base pairs, but the 20,000–25,000 genes comprise only a small percentage (on the order of 2% to 5%) of these base pairs. As Taylor and Bristow (2006, pp. 74–75) noted:

> The "genes" themselves are only a modest part of the whole genome. It is clear that some of the "non-translated" DNA is required for genes to function normally, but the function of large portions of our DNA remains enigmatic. Equally remarkable, perhaps, is that humans do not use all of their genes at any one time, so far less than 25,000 genes are utilized on a day-to-day basis.

Necessary genes are transcribed by being translated into messenger ribonucleic acid (mRNA) intermediates, these are subsequently translated into functional proteins.

2.6.2 Finding Genes Is Not Easy

Finding our genes is not straightforward task. Overall, less than 5% of the human genome codes for proteins: the rest is noncoding and comprises long stretches of base pairs that are often repeated. As Watson (2004, p. 197) noted, "protein-coding regions are but strings of As, Ts, Gs, and Cs embedded among all the other As, Ts, Gs, and Cs of the genome—they do not stand out in any obvious way." To make things even more difficult when locating genes, the base pairs that comprise a gene are not arranged in an uninterrupted linear sequence. In 1977, Dr. Richard J. Roberts discovered protein-coding (exon) and noncoding (intron) regions within a gene, research for which he was awarded the 1993 Nobel Prize in Medicine (see Roberts, 1993). An elegant editing process called RNA splicing removes these noncoding chunks of genetic material and connects the relevant segments together to create mRNA. The mRNA then ensures that amino acids are successfully strung together in the correct order to make proteins. Proteins are therefore made from the genetic instructions coded in the DNA molecule.

A typical human gene has eight introns that lie between the exon coding sections. The human gene dystrophin is spread across approximately 2.4 million base pairs and has 79 introns that separate the coding sections. Moreover, of the 2.4 million base pairs in this gene, less than 1% encodes the actual protein (Watson, 2004). Given these difficulties in identifying individual human genes, knowledge of the genomes of other species has proved a considerable help. Table 2.1 presents genomic data for humans and other organisms of interest in the context of this book.

TABLE 2.1. Approximate Genomic Data for Humans and Other Organisms of Interest

Organism and Date Genomic Data Obtained	Size of Genome (base pairs)	Number of Genes	Percentage of Genes Shared with Humans
Humans (2004)	3 billion	20,000–25,000	(100%)
Dog (2003)	6 billion	18,000	75%
Fruit fly (2000)	165 million	14,000	50%
Mouse (2002)	2.5 billion	30,000	80%
Rat (2004)	2.75 billion	22,000	80%

Source: Adapted from Palladino (2006).

The number of genes for each of the other organisms in the table is strikingly similar to the number of genes for humans. Studying the genomes of these other organisms (particularly the mouse) is advancing our understanding of the human genome. Individual genes of interest in this book are preserved to a great degree across different species. For example, the functional parts of the human and mouse genomes are "remarkably similar" (Watson, 2004, p. 199). In contrast, the nonfunctional regions are much less similar. This means that "looking for similarity in sequence between the human and mouse data is therefore an effective way of identifying functional areas, like genes" (Watson, 2004, p. 199).

2.6.3   Individual Differences in the Human Genome

Since every individual on the planet is unique (the special case of multiple identical births, e.g., twins and triplets, is discussed shortly in Section 2.8), how are we to conceptualize the meaning of the human genome? The documented human genome can be conceptualized as a reference human genome. A remarkable observation is that the vast majority of each individual's genome is identical, and so, from that perspective, the documented human genome represents each of us very well. However, as noted, we are all unique, and so the documented genome does not (cannot) capture the individual differences that make each of us who we are. Given that the vast majority of each individual's genome is identical, our differences in height, sense of humor, and any other trait you care to think of are driven by a small portion of our shared genome.

2.6.4   Single Nucleotide Polymorphisms

The term single nucleotide polymorphism (SNP, pronounced "snip") contains two defining criteria. First, it refers to a single nucleotide (an individual base pair) that can differ between individuals. Second, the word polymorphism indicates that a particular single nucleotide change of interest is shared by at least 1% of the population.

2.7   PROTEOMICS AND TRANSCRIPTOMICS

Since the completion of the Human Genome Project (HGP), the disciplines of proteomics and transcriptomics have emerged. Watson (2004, p. 217) noted the following:

> In the wake of the HGP, two new postgenomic fields have duly emerged, both of them burdened with unimaginative names incorporating the "-omic" of their ancestor: proteomics and transcriptomics. Proteomics is the study of the proteins encoded by genes. Transcriptomics is devoted to determining where and when genes are expressed—that is, which genes are transcriptionally active in a given cell.

Gene expression is discussed in the following section.

Soloviev et al. (2004, p. 218) also addressed the nature of the developing field of proteomics:

> Characterization of the complement of expressed proteins from a single genome is a central focus of the evolving field of proteomics. Monitoring the expression and properties of a large number of proteins provides important information about the physiological state of a cell and an organism. A cell can express a large number of different proteins and the expression profiles (the

number of proteins expressed and the expression levels) varies in different cell types, explaining why different cells perform different functions.

Bernot (2004, p. 133) noted that "In the same way that genomics represents the study of genomes, the transcriptome consists of establishing the expression of messenger RNAs on the grand scale."

Proteomics and transcriptomics, quite literally, bring the instructions encoded by individual genes within the genome from blueprint (or from recipe: see Dawkins, 1999) to life. Using older terms, ones that have represented certain academic disciplines for quite a while, Watson (2004) noted that genetics focuses on heredity, the information contained in a fertilized egg that is passed down to an individual from the previous generation, while developmental biology focuses on the use of that information. He also noted that "interactions between proteins and DNA, and between proteins and other proteins, lie at the heart of how cells detect and respond to signals, express genes, replicate, repair, and recombine their DNA, and so on—as well as how those processes are regulated" (Watson, 2004). Given the central importance of proteins in the biology of pharmacotherapy of adverse drug reactions, proteins are discussed in some detail in this chapter.

2.8   GENE EXPRESSION

As noted earlier, genes code for proteins. That is, they contain the information that enables a sequence of amino acid residues to be joined together to form a protein. When a gene's protein is actually manufactured, the gene is said to be expressed. As noted in Section 2.6.1, gene expression involves genes being transcribed by being translated into mRNA intermediates, and these intermediates are then translated into functional proteins. However, as also noted in that section, not all human genes are expressed at any one time, meaning that far fewer than the 20,000–25,000 human genes are utilized on a day-to-day basis. Moreover, some of the genes that play critical roles during embryonic development remain largely unused in adult life. Others are not used during early development and are only expressed later in development or even in adulthood (Taylor and Bristow, 2006).

With very few exceptions, the body's cells that contain a nucleus (nucleated cells) share an identical genome, i.e., identical genetic information for the construction of proteins. This means that any and every cell in the body contains the information needed to become any kind of cell. This observation leads to a very reasonable question: during cell differentiation, why do some cells become muscle cells, others part of our nervous system, and so on? That is, how does exactly the same blueprint within different cells cause those cells to display enormous variety in their structure and function?

One of the ways that tissues and cells differentiate is by expressing different sets of genes. One estimate is that human cells use approximately 50% of the genes within them (see Jongeneel at al., 2003, and the discussion by Taylor and Bristow, 2006). Some genes are expressed in many cells, while others have very specific roles within a specific organ. Genes that tend to be expressed in all cells and perform general functions are known as housekeeping genes. Protein products from these housekeeping genes are essential for the functioning of the cell. Jongeneel's research group estimated that one-third of our genes may fall in this category. In contrast, about one-quarter of our genes code for proteins with highly specific functions. These genes are less widely expressed, and their proteins are therefore less widely used. They may be expressed within a specific organ, or even expressed within only a subset of cells within an organ.

In vertebrates, sophisticated gene switches play a role in gene expression. Regulatory proteins flank genes and bind to DNA to turn the adjacent gene on or off. These regulatory proteins and their role in determining whether a particular gene is turned on (expressed) or not at a given point in time facilitate the complexity of vertebrate life (Watson, 2004).

Another aspect of gene expression that facilitates the complexity of life in higher organisms is the fact that a given gene can yield many different proteins, not just the single protein that is classically associated with that gene. Two processes are involved here:

➤ Alternative splicing.
➤ Posttranslational modification.

As discussed in Section 2.6.2, the term splicing refers to the joining together of different exons along a section of DNA that comprise a gene, the introns separating these coding sections being removed. Usually exactly the same set of exons is joined together to form the mRNA that produces a specific protein. Alternative splicing occurs when slightly different sets of exons are spliced together, resulting in different proteins.

The term posttranslational modification refers to biochemical changes that may be made to the proteins after they have been produced (Watson, 2004). Posttranslational modification is discussed in Section 2.16.

The number of proteins in our proteome is therefore considerably larger than the number of genes in our genome (this is true of many other higher organisms). This phenomenon is the result of "the simple although not widely appreciated fact that multiple, distinct proteins can result from one gene" (Holmes et al., 2005). The journey from genome to proteome is not a straightforward one. Holmes et al. (2005) represented this journey in a multistep process, starting with a gene of interest in the genome:

➤ DNA replication results in many gene forms;
➤ RNA transcription leads to pre-mRNA;
➤ RNA maturation results in mature mRNA;
➤ Protein translation results in an immature protein;

> ➤ Protein maturation results in a mature protein in the proteome: posttranslational modifications are possible here.

The tremendous diversity of proteins in the proteome is facilitated by multiple possible means of protein expression. At each stage in the multistep process just described, alternative mechanisms produce variants of the standard product. The combination of possible variations in the multistep process results in an enormous potential diversity in the resulting proteome (Holmes et al., 2005). These processes mean that the 20,000–25,000 human genes can produce many more proteins (estimates range upward of 1 million).

Environmental factors, such as food and alcohol, can also have sizable impacts on gene expression. While the genomes of identical multiple births are the same, the genes expressed by members of multiple identical births are not likely identical for various reasons, including environmental ones. That is, the complement of proteins within members of multiple identical births will not be identical. Augen (2004) noted that this occurrence makes each person's totality of metabolic pathways unique. This makes them unique in all sorts of ways. Of particular relevance to our discussions, it means that they may well respond differently to a given drug.

2.8.1   Cardiac Gene Expression

While gene expression in general is of considerable importance in many fields of investigation, gene expression in several biological entities—such as ion channels, other drug target and off-target biological structures, and metabolic enzymes—is of particular relevance in this book. Gene expression in the heart is of particular interest. Within the human heart, it has been estimated that around 40% of genes within cells are expressed (see Taylor and Bristow, 2006). The term proteome is widely (and correctly) used to refer to an organism's total putative collection of proteins. However, it can also be meaningfully applied to cells, organelles, and organs. As Jamshidi et al. (2007, p. 270) observed:

> The proteome of a biological system (an organelle, a cell, or an organism) is characterized by its protein content, posttranslational modification states, localization, and abundance. Therefore, proteomic data are dependent on the environmental and internal conditions of the system.

The expression of genes may be modulated by cardiac events such as a myocardial infarction (Taylor and Bristow, 2006). If such changes in expression occur, the proteins present in cardiac cells will be different, and therefore it is reasonable to assume that the cells may no longer perform in the same manner. This may be one mechanism whereby different cardiac and cardiovascular diseases are comorbid: one event may change molecular genetic functioning, thereby leading to, or at least predisposing a second event (see also Asano et al., 2002; Lowes et al., 2002; Yasumura et al., 2003).

2.9   PROTEINS

The word protein derives from the Greek word *proteios*, meaning "of first importance." This is a suitable lineage for this work, given the enormous importance of proteins. Holmes et al. (2005, p. 446) addressed their importance in this manner:

> Although much attention has been paid to the sequencing aspects of genome projects, the eventual end goal of these projects actually is to determine how the genome builds life through proteins. DNA has been the focus of attention because the tools for studying it are more advanced and because it is at the heart of the cell, carrying all the information—the blueprint—for life. However, a blueprint without a builder is not very useful, and the proteins are the primary builders within the cell.

While genes code for proteins, genes and proteins do not actually communicate directly in this process: the intermediary called RNA plays a critical role here. It is noteworthy that this nucleic acid has not reached the public consciousness to the same degree as the nucleic acid DNA, and that the acronym RNA has therefore not attained the widespread recognition afforded to the acronym DNA. (If this book were to play any small role in raising awareness of the vitally important role this macromolecule plays in life, and making the acronym RNA more well known, JRT would be very pleased.) Ribonucleic acid is a DNA equivalent, since it can store and replicate genetic information. Importantly, it is also a protein equivalent, since it can catalyze critical chemical reactions. Section 2.6.2 discussed the creation of proteins. There are 20 naturally occurring amino acids, listed in Table 2.2. Since proteins are made from amino acids, the function of each protein is encrypted in its amino acid sequence.

TABLE 2.2. Naturally Occurring Amino Acids

Alanine	Glycine	Proline
Arginine	Histidine	Serine
Asparagine	Isoleucine	Threonine
Aspartic acid	Leucine	Tryptophan
Cysteine	Lysine	Tyrosine
Glutamic acid	Methionine	Valine
Glutamine	Phenylalanine	

2.9.1   Protein Structure

As Wishart (2005, p. 224) commented, proteins are perhaps the most complex chemical entities in nature: "No other class of molecule exhibits the variety and irregularity in shape, size, texture, and mobility that can be found in proteins." Proteins are described using a model comprising primary, secondary, and tertiary structures. The primary structure represents the sequence of a protein, the string of amino acids that comprise it. The individual amino acids in this chain are termed residues, and these residues are joined together (covalently connected together) by peptide bonds to form chains. This string of amino acids is initially shapeless and not biologically active. The nature of the chemical bonds and the chemical nature of various amino acid side chains mean that proteins do not exist simply as an extended string of amino acids. As Wishart (2005, p. 224) expressed it, "proteins have a natural proclivity to form more complex structures."

Secondary structures are formed by short stretches of residues. These substructures make up sequentially proximal components of proteins, and they have shapes. A complex combination of attractive and repulsive forces between close and more distant parts of the structure affects the resultant shape of secondary structures, and predicting the secondary structure from knowledge of the linear amino acid sequence alone remains a tremendous challenge. The tertiary structure addresses the overall three-dimensional structure of the protein, the spatial packing of secondary structures (Ofran and Rost, 2005). Both secondary and tertiary structures can be categorized into several different classes (see Wishart, 2005).

Certain proteins of particular interest in this book are discussed shortly. At this point, it is worth noting two general properties of proteins:

> ➤ Any change to any part of the structure of a protein will have an impact on its biological activity (Thomas, 2003). Proteins can comprise many amino acids. Changes in an amino acid that is a long way from the protein's active site (the specific region of the protein that is responsible for its particular function) can exert a major influence on that function.
> ➤ Once a protein is formed, it does not exist as a linear chain of its constituent amino acids. It folds into very complex geometries.
> ➤ Taking the previous point a (large) step forward, Kennelly and Rodwell (2006a, p. 36) noted that proteins are "conformationally dynamic molecules that can fold and unfold in a time frame of milliseconds, and can undergo unfolding and refolding hundreds or thousands of times in their lifetime."

2.10   CELLS

The Raleigh, North Carolina *News & Observer* (October 7, 2007) carried a story entitled "What Is Life?" One of the subheadings was "Breakthroughs in the creation of synthetic organisms stimulate the debate over the definition of life."

Philosophical deliberation on the definition of life is considerably outside the scope of this book, but some of the article's contents are quite *apropos* here. Synthesizing a cell requires knowledge of a biological (naturally occurring) cell's nature. This nature is captured in the article's discussion of the "three major hurdles to creating synthetic life," which represent three central qualities of a biological cell:

> A container, or membrane, that functions as a defining boundary and that keeps out certain molecules while retaining others, including those that allow the cell to multiply.
> A genetic system that controls the functions of the cell.
> A metabolism that extracts materials from the environment as food and then changes food into energy.

The following discussions touch on most of these topics inasmuch as they relate to the topic of cardiac safety. Discussions of metabolism at this point in the book relate more to the degradation of certain molecules, i.e., drug molecules, than to the transformation of other molecules into energy. However, discussions of the nature of diabetes in Section 12.3.1 touch on the metabolism of energy storage and use in relation to the effects of a lack of insulin on normal physiological functioning in this regard.

Devlin (2006) discussed the origins of cellular life. Initially, the elements carbon, hydrogen, oxygen, nitrogen, sulfur, and phosphorus formed simple chemical compounds. These compounds included water (represented as H_2O, indicating a molecule incorporating two hydrogen atoms and one oxygen atom) and organic molecules, molecules that include the element carbon. Larger molecules were then formed, including, in time, a complex molecular structure capable of self-replication.

Further developments led to increasing biological sophistication. As Devlin (2006, p. 2) commented:

> With continued formation of ever more complicated molecules, the environment around some of these self-replicating molecules became enclosed by a membrane. This development gave these primordial structures the ability to control their own environment to some extent. A form of life had evolved, and a unit of three-dimensional space—a cell—had been established.

This quote contains two sentiments of particular relevance to later discussions. First, cell membranes, and more specifically certain structures located within cell membranes, are of considerable importance in cardiac safety. Second, as noted earlier, biological activity occurs in three-dimensional space.

No matter how complex an organism is, the cell is the basic unit of life. In higher organisms, activity within the cell can be very sophisticated. All discussions in this book are directed towards the investigation of cardiac adverse drug reactions in patients taking prescription medications, and so the organism of primary interest is the human being. However, several other organisms (e.g., fruit flies, dogs, and rodents) are also discussed since much useful information (and, in some cases, information required by regulatory agencies) can be obtained from studying them. All of these organisms have eukaryotic cells, cells that have an outer membrane and additional membranes within the cell that surround the cell's nucleus and other intracellular organelles. These intracellular membranes create distinct cellular compartments, in which various different and highly organized processes occur. A major function of the outer membrane is to create a relatively stable intracellular environment. The additional internal membranes take this process a step further, creating and protecting various intracellular environments in which different chemical reactions that require different environmental conditions can occur simultaneously (Devlin, 2006).

2.10.1   The Importance of Intracellular Water

Water is a major constituent within cells and is the one common component within the individual microenvironments created by intracellular membranes. As Devlin (2006, p. 4) noted, "Substances required for the cell's existence are dissolved or suspended in water. Life on earth exists because of the unique physiochemical properties of water." Water makes up about 60% of the lean body mass of the human body (Murray and Granner, 2006). Extracellular fluid constitutes around one-third of total body water, and intracellular fluid constitutes about two-thirds. Intracellular fluid provides the environment for the cell to:

- ➢ Make, store, and utilize energy.
- ➢ Repair itself.
- ➢ Replicate.
- ➢ Perform special functions.

2.10.2   The Importance of Ions

When molecules dissolve in water, their constituents exist as ions, positively and negatively charged particles related to the atoms that formed the molecule. For example, common table salt is made up of molecules of sodium chloride. Each molecule is comprised of one sodium ion (Na^+) and one chlorine ion (Cl^-). When salt is dissolved in water, the two ions separate. Molecules made up of ions are called electrolytes since their electric charges make it possible for them to conduct electric currents. Two ions of particular interest in this book are positive ions formed from two elements in the same chemical family:

- ➢ K^+: potassium ions
- ➢ Na^+: sodium ions

In addition to containing ions, cells contain a variety of other molecular entities, including proteins. Table 2.3 provides a comparison of the mean concentrations of potassium ions, sodium ions, and proteins in intracellular and extracellular fluid (see Murray and Granner, 2006, p. 423).

TABLE 2.3. Mean Concentrations in Mammalian Intracellular and Extracellular Fluid

Substance	Intracellular Fluid	Extracellular Fluid
K^+	140 mmol/dL	4 mmol/dL
Na^+	10 mmol/L	140 mmol/dL
Protein	16 g/dL	2 g/dL

2.11 CELL MEMBRANES

Cells are surrounded by membranes, and the same is true of distinct intracellular compartments. Outer membranes called plasma membranes enclose the whole cell, and inner membranes within the cell enclose various intracellular organelles. The plasma membrane represents the boundary between the cell and the extracellular milieu. The outer surface of plasma membranes is in contact with a variable external environment, and the inner surface is in contact with a relatively constant environment provided by the cell's cytoplasm. This relatively constant environment allows the cell to conduct its cellular business.

The two sides of plasma membranes have different chemical compositions and functions. As noted, the outer surface of the membrane encounters a variable environment, while its inner surface is in contact with a relatively constant environment. This constancy results from the fact that membranes prevent many substances from entering the cell while permitting select ions and organic molecules to pass through the membrane as necessary.

Cellular membranes within the cell separate various components of the cell. As noted, the intracellular environment is relatively constant. The membranes surrounding the distinct compartments within the cell take this consistency one step further by ensuring that the environments within these compartments stay consistent, even though the environment within one component may differ from that within another. To achieve this environmental consistency, cellular membranes operate similarly to plasma membranes. They prevent rapid movements of many molecules, including water, from one compartment to another, while also having specialized capabilities that allow molecules to be transported as appropriate to modulate the concentration of substances within their compartments.

2.12 PROTEINS IN CELL MEMBRANES

Cell membranes are made up of lipids and proteins. Every membrane possesses a different set of proteins, meaning that there is no standard membrane structure.

Plasma membranes may comprise up to 100 proteins, while inner membranes may have considerably less (Murray and Granner, 2006). Proteins are the major functional molecules of membranes, and examples include:

> Ion channels.
> Receptors for endogenous molecules (molecules originating inside the body), including internal chemical messengers.
> Receptors for exogenous molecules (molecules originating outside the body), including drugs.
> Enzymes.

Such protein function is involved in the generation of biological signals that affect processes of interest in this book. These include:

> Translocation of ions and small molecules across membranes.
> Signal reception via receptors for both small molecules (such as small-molecule drugs) and large molecules (such as proteins that facilitate intercell communication and biologics).

While plasma membranes, as noted, prevent many molecules from passing through the membrane, they contain specific transport mechanisms, or pores, through which certain ions and organic molecules pass from one side of the membrane to the other. These transport mechanisms are comprised of transmembrane proteins that are embedded in the cell's membrane, passing through the membrane and therefore being in contact with molecules on the intracellular side and the extracellular side of the membrane. Communication between a cell and other cells in its surroundings is based almost exclusively on these mechanisms, and communication, i.e., transmembrane signaling, can occur in both directions.

Transmembrane proteins are embedded in the membrane in a specific manner: they have a defined orientation, and this orientation is defined by the protein's primary structure. Some of these proteins function as ion channels that facilitate translocation of ions from one side of the membrane to the other (ion translocation occurs in both directions). Other membrane proteins function as biological structures that bind with endogenous molecules such as hormones and neurotransmitters (see Sections 3.5.1 and 3.6.1). This binding results in a signal being passed into the cell. Other receptors bind with drugs and similarly generate biological signals that pass into the cell. While many of these signals lead to biological cascades of information that culminate in therapeutic benefits, we are currently concerned with biological processes that lead to adverse drug reactions.

In addition to these ion channels and ligand-binding receptors that are located in certain membrane domains, membranes contain domains for proteins involved in catalytic activity. Our interest lies with the catalytic activity of one particular category of enzymes, metabolic enzymes. Once an orally administered drug has been absorbed into the bloodstream and is on its way to a target biological structure, and from our current perspective also on its way to nontarget biological structures, the drug has to face an onslaught by metabolic enzymes that attempt to break it down. The drug is an intruder, a xenobiotic, and the body's defense mechanisms are not aware that it has been administered with the intent of producing a beneficial therapeutic response.

Membranes are located in many organelles and are involved in many processes, and genetic mutations affecting their constituent proteins can lead to a wide array of diseases and disorders and can influence a drug's effects.

2.13   ION CHANNELS

As Schultz (2006, p. 358) observed, "Structured molecular complexes of multiple protein subunits are common in biology." Ion channels are one example of a structured molecular complex. They occur in the membranes of many cells, and most cells have a variety of ion channels, including the Na^+ and K^+ channels that are of particular relevance in this book. Ion channels facilitate electrical signals in neurons and in other excitable cells including cardiac muscle cells, i.e., myocardial cells. Ion channels located in plasma membranes have a multiple-subunit structure that facilitates their function. These include transmembrane glycoprotein subunits, including α-subunits and β-subunits. There can be multiple similar subunits, and there can be combinations of different subunits. The transmembrane domains of many transmembrane proteins are called α-helix subunits. Multiple α-helix subunits can be organized to form a tubular structure, a channel or pore, which can serve as a passageway for movement of ions or molecules through the membrane (Devlin, 2006). Since ions carry an electric charge (either positive or negative), movement of ions through these channels changes the electrical gradient between the cell's intracellular and immediate extracellular environments, propagating a biological signal.

Properties of ion channels include (Murray and Granner, 2006, p. 422):

  ➤ As just noted, they are composed of transmembrane protein subunits. The functional components of the channels of particular interest in this book are largely α-helices, but other subunits provide structural stability for the channels, and may modulate their activity (see Section 4.3.4).
  ➤ They are usually highly conserved across species.
  ➤ Most are highly selective for one ion.
  ➤ Mutations in genes encoding them can cause specific diseases.
  ➤ Their activities are affected by certain drugs.

This list of properties provides an effective agenda for many of our subsequent discussions.

2.13.1   Operational Features of Ion Channels

It is of interest to know something about the features of ion channels that lead to
their properties as noted in the previous section. These features include (Murray and
Granner, 2006, p. 422):

> ➢ Their overall structure: how are they made, and which proteins comprise
>   them.
> ➢ Their gating properties: how the channels are "opened" and "closed."

Since ions channels are typically highly conserved across species, studying
channels in other species provides insights into the workings of human ion channels.
The considerable progress made in elucidating the structure and function of ions
channels in species such as *Aeorpyrum pernix* has proved useful. Techniques such
as site-directed mutagenesis (changing the form of a gene at a particular location)
and x-ray crystallography have been used to garner this information.

Two ion channels of interest in this book's discussions are the Na^+ and K^+
channels. Sodium ion channels are of particular importance in cardiac depolarization
(cardiac cells "firing" or contracting) and potassium ion channels are of particular
importance in cardiac repolarization (cardiac cells getting ready to fire again). These
channels are members of a large superfamily of ion channels. They are ion-specific
in that they favor the translocation of specific ions through the channels, and they
are voltage-gated, a term explained in the next section.

Informative research has been conducted on the *Aeorpyrum pernix* sodium
ion channel. This channel is made up of four domains, each with six transmembrane
segments. The four domains are homologous (similar) domains, and each
domain contains six transmembrane segments numbered S1 through S6. This
results in a total of 24 transmembrane segments, connected by both intracellular
and extracellular loops. Ion channels are composed of specific transmembrane
glycoprotein subunits. These transmembrane segments facilitate the translocation of
some ions from the intracellular side of the membrane to the extracellular side of the
membrane, and vice versa for other ions. The glycoprotein segments are arranged in
a more-or-less circular manner in the membrane, with a funnel-like channel, or ion-
conducting aqueous pore, formed through the middle of the α-subunits. A schematic
representation of a sodium ion channel is presented in Figure 2.2.

Movement of ions through this pore is dependent on each ion's concentration
gradient from one side of the membrane to the other. Ions move from the higher
concentration to the lower concentration. Consequently (and in contrast to some
other translocation processes, such as ion pumps that are also located in membranes),
this process does not require metabolic energy.

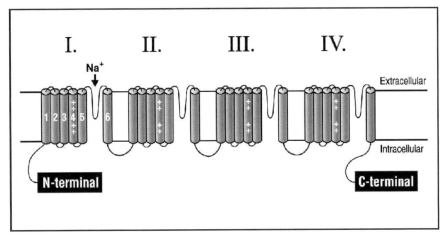

Figure 2.2. The monomeric sodium channel.

2.13.2   The Gating Properties of Ion Channels

Ion channels can be voltage-gated or ligand-gated. The Na^+ and K^+ channels are voltage-gated. Voltage-gated ion channels are controlled by transmembrane electrical potential. They have a sensor domain (sensor) in the protein that detects membrane potential and transfers the energy to the channel domain to control its gate. For example, depolarization of the plasma membrane leads to the opening of Na^+ channels.

In *Aeorpyrum pernix,* transmembrane segment S4 and part of transmembrane segment S3 operate as the voltage sensor. There are four of these in each channel, linked to the gate, and the channel is therefore voltage-gated. The gate part of the channel is constructed from four S6 helices, one from each of the four subunits. Movement of part of the channel in response to changing voltage effectively closes the channel or reopens it. Reopening allows a current of ions to cross the membrane.

2.14   RECEPTORS

As noted in Section 2.12, cell membranes contain receptors for endogenous and exogenous molecules. The tremendous diversity in proteins, and their specificity of shape and electrical charge, may be the reason for the evolution of their role as receptors.

2.14.1   Receptors for Endogenous Molecules

Cardiac adrenergic receptors receive (bind) stimuli from naturally produced neurotransmitters and hormones. These chemical messengers are used by the nervous and the endocrine systems, respectively. These receptors and their interactions with neurotransmitters and hormones are discussed in the following chapter.

2.14.2   Receptors for Exogenous Molecules

Many drugs exert their influence by associating with receptors located in the plasma membrane of a cell, and these receptors have become a central focus of investigation in understanding the molecular basis of drug action, both therapeutic and in causing adverse drug reactions. Receptors are responsible for the selectivity of a drug's action. The molecular size and shape of a drug molecule determine whether, and with what affinity, it will bind to a particular receptor: there is an enormous amount of chemically different receptors. Slight alterations in the chemical structure of a drug can dramatically increase or decrease its affinities for different classes of receptors, with resulting alterations in therapeutic and toxic effects.

It is important to note that there is no biological difference between target and nontarget receptors: the delineation is purely one of intent. Target receptors are those with which we intend a drug to interact and thus to lead to a therapeutic effect. Nontarget receptors are defined as those with which a given drug's interaction was not intended. This may cause an adverse drug reaction.

2.15   ENZYMES

Individual differences in drug metabolism can be influenced by molecular genetic and gene expression differences in drug-metabolizing systems. Enzymes are biological polymers and comprise the largest class of proteins. They act as catalysts for almost all of the chemical reactions that occur in living organisms and therefore make life as we know it possible (Kennelly and Rodwell, 2006b). Catalysts are not consumed or permanently altered as a consequence of their participation in a reaction.

Almost all steps in biological reactions are catalyzed by enzymes. Enzymes reduce the activation energy required for each of the stages in these reactions by a considerable amount: they catalyze the conversion of one or more compounds (substrates) into one or more different compounds (products) and enhance the rates of the corresponding noncatalyzed reactions by factors of 10^6 or more. Reducing the activation energy required for the reaction makes it much easier for the substrate to become the product, thereby enormously increasing the rate at which the product is created from the substrate. Most reactions that occur within a cell would not occur spontaneously under the physical conditions (pH, temperature, and ionic milieu) of the cell since the activation energy required would be too high, and so enzymes are extremely important (see Weiner, 2006).

Catalysis takes place at the enzyme's active site, a specific location on the enzyme macromolecule. As noted several times already, biological molecules are three-dimensional structures, and enzymes are no exception. The active site is a small component of the enzyme. Most of the amino acid residues that comprise the macromolecule do not come into contact with the substrate, serving instead as a backbone that allows the active site to be configured appropriately in three-dimensional space so that it can align with the functional (active) groups of the substrate that it catalyzes. As Weiner (2006, p. 375) noted, "the distances and angles between the catalytic residues of the enzyme and the substrate must be exact to permit catalysis to occur." This is why enzymes are extremely selective catalysts, selecting for a single substrate (or very small group of them) and the type of reaction catalyzed. The three-dimensional nature of enzymes, and hence of their active sites, facilitates catalysis by shielding the substrates from solvents, i.e., stabilizing them, while they are catalyzed into their respective products (Kennelly and Rodwell, 2006b, pp. 50–51).

Two notable qualities of enzymes, then, are:

➤ They are substrate specific: as just noted, they catalyze only one (or very few) substrates, and they do so in a specific manner.
➤ They are extremely efficient: i.e., they have high catalytic efficiency.

These properties reflect the existence of environments that are "exquisitely tailored to a single reaction" (Kennelly and Rodwell, 2006b, pp. 50–51). This environment is created by the enzyme, and is typically a molecular cleft or pocket, i.e., a relatively extensive three-dimensional space that shields the substrate from solvents and facilitates catalysis. This is termed the active site of the enzyme. A part of the substrate molecule that will not be chemically altered during the ensuing reaction binds to part of the enzyme's active site. This binding holds the substrate molecule in a specific three-dimensional orientation, one that perfectly aligns those portions of the substrate molecule that will be chemically altered during the ensuing reaction with the functional groups of the enzyme responsible for carrying out the reaction. The degree of alignment required explains why a given enzyme only catalyzes one (or very few) substrates: it can only catalyze molecules that have certain precise molecular geometries (Kennelly and Rodwell, 2006b).

2.15.1 Metabolic Enzymes

Metabolic enzyme activity in the liver is one of the body's main neutralization strategies for drugs, substances that the body recognizes as xenobiotics. Drug molecules, i.e., the substrates of interest here, are catalyzed into products called metabolites. Mulder (2006) noted that drug metabolism can be divided into three phases:

➤ Phase 1 metabolism. The chemical structure of the compound is modified by oxidation, reduction, or hydrolysis. This process forms an acceptor group.

➤ Phase 2 metabolism. A chemical group is attached to the acceptor group. This typically generates metabolites that are more water-soluble and are therefore more readily excreted.

➤ Phase 3 metabolism. Transporters carry the drug or metabolites out of the cell in which Phase 1 and Phase 2 metabolism has occurred.

In Phase I metabolism the major oxidative drug-metabolizing pathway is catalyzed by cytochrome P450 (CYP) enzymes (Mulder, 2006). Genetic differences between individuals in drug metabolism can be largely explained by genetic influences on drug-metabolizing enzymes. Genetic mutations (variations in DNA sequence) can lead to changes in the enzyme's biological activity. If the enzyme becomes less effective or ineffective, the concentration of the drug in the bloodstream will remain higher and could lead to toxic effects (beneficial effects that become too beneficial). Less effective or ineffective enzymatic activity can result in two ways: mutations that result in a needed enzyme not being made or mutations that result in incorrect manufacture of the enzyme. In addition, gene multiplication may lead to increased expression of a particular enzyme in certain individuals. This leads to the "very extensive metaboliser" phenotype (Mulder, 2006, p. 43).

2.16   POSTTRANSLATIONAL MODIFICATION

As noted in Section 2.9, there are only 20 amino acids encoded genetically. Proteins (polypeptide chains) are assembled from these amino acids. However, once they have been incorporated into proteins, these constituent amino acids can be modified in a process called posttranslational modification. This process leads to the formation of many different amino acid derivatives in proteins. These modifications may be permanent or easily reversible (Glitz, 2006).

As we have seen, membrane proteins can function as ion channels, receptors (for endogenous chemical messengers and for drugs), and enzymes. Proteins in all of these classifications can undergo posttranslational modifications. These modifications include:

➤ Glycosylation
➤ Hydroxylation
➤ Acetylation
➤ Phosphorylation
➤ Methylation
➤ Iodination
➤ Sulfonylation

Glycosylation is the most frequent posttranslational modification. The process of glycosylation involves the enzymatic attachment of sugars to the amino acid, and around 50% of proteins have sugars attached (Murray, 2006). Membrane proteins are often glycosylated, and mutations affecting the process of glycosylation can alter their function.

2.17   GENETIC MUTATIONS AS CAUSES OF CHANGES IN THREE-DIMENSIONAL MOLECULAR GEOMETRY

From this book's perspective, genetic mutations can be conceptualized as causing changes in the geometry of the protein they code for. Mutations can change the protein directly, and mutations can result in differences in posttranslational modifications: both can alter the protein's function. While only a small number of amino acids in a protein may be modified, the modification can often have a major role in the function of the protein. Since members of all protein classifications are often glycosylated, mutations affecting the process of posttranslational glycosylation may alter their structure and therefore their function.

A small change in a protein's structure can have a very considerable effect on its function. A mutation in a single amino acid within a protein comprised of many amino acids can alter the structure of the protein when it folds and assumes its three-dimensional shape. Of particular importance is the geometry of the active site of the protein molecule, the site that is involved in actually carrying out the protein's function. This site can be very small in relation to the whole protein molecule, but mutations anywhere in the molecule (e.g., in an amino acid that is a long way from the active site) can influence the function of the active site. To carry out its function, the active site must display precisely the right three-dimensional geometry: the "right" geometry is the geometric arrangement that will permit the three-dimensional interaction with whatever it is that the protein interacts with to carry out its function.

Consider first the case of a therapeutic drug and its target receptor. Drug molecules are also three-dimensional entities. A drug molecule can be thought of as an active site that is supported on an organic backbone. That is, most of the atoms in the drug molecule provide three-dimensional structural support for the relatively small number of atoms that comprise the molecule's three-dimensional active site. For the active site of the drug to interact correctly with the active site of the protein that functions as its target receptor, the two three-dimensional active sites must make a precise match (think of this as a very sophisticated atomic version of two spacecraft successfully docking in orbit around the earth). Any mutation in the protein that functions as this receptor may alter the receptor's structure and alter the geometry of its active site. Two possible consequences of the resulting less than perfect geometrical match are that the drug passes on a less powerful biological signal (it is less effective), and that the drug is not able to pass on a signal at all (it is completely ineffective).

Now consider the case of a drug and a nontarget receptor. Under normal circumstances, i.e., when that receptor's protein is formed as usual, the drug's active site and the receptor's active site may not match at all, and therefore the drug does not interact with the receptor and no biological signal is generated. However, genetic mutation may lead to substitution of a different amino acid somewhere within the protein. This structural change may lead to a functional change such that the receptor's active site now does indeed match the drug's active site. Therefore, the drug interacts with the nontarget receptor, an unintended biological signal is generated, and an adverse drug reaction may occur.

Next, consider the case of an ion channel, a channel that allows the passage of ions that are involved in biological signaling necessary for a healthy function to take place. A given drug's active site may not interact at all with the normal protein that comprises the ion channel, and therefore it has no effect on the channel's function. However, mutations in the protein may lead to a different result. The structural changes that result from an amino acid substitution (a different amino acid from the normal one) in the protein comprising the ion channel may create an active site that does indeed interact with an active site on the drug. One result of this three-dimensional docking interaction is that the channel may not function as usual, meaning that the ion flow through the channel is not as usual. This means that the biological signal produced by the usual flow of ions is changed. This change in the biological signal can lead to adverse drug reactions. Drugs can affect the function of ion channels. However, a given drug may have a harmful effect via its interaction with a given ion channel, if the ion channel has been formed by a protein with a certain mutation. That is, certain ion channels are genetically predisposed to be susceptible to interactions with drugs, leading to adverse drug reactions.

Finally, consider the case of metabolic enzymes, and an enzyme that breaks down a particular drug molecule and renders it inactive. A genetic mutation in the protein that comprises the enzyme can lead to alterations that cause the enzyme to be less effective or ineffective. It should also be noted that a different genetic influence, the extent of expression of a gene that codes for an enzymatic protein, can play a role here. Less than usual expression of the normal enzyme can lead to less enzymatic activity, and hence to a greater drug response. A greater than usual expression of a metabolic enzyme can lead to a drug being degraded to a greater extent than usual and a lesser drug response.

Change in three-dimensional geometry as a result of genetic mutation is one of the explanations for the individual differences in how people react to drugs. Consider the case of adverse drug reactions. The vast majority of patients who are prescribed a drug may have normal versions of the nontarget receptor in question. This version of the nontarget receptor does not interact with the drug, and no resultant adverse effects are seen. However, a small percentage of them may have a mutant form of this receptor, a form that permits interaction with the drug molecule's active site, leading to an adverse drug reaction.

2.18   MECHANISMS OF ACTION

It is possible that a given drug may be very safe and very effective, and that we do not know how it exerts its beneficial therapeutic effect. If there is sufficient evidence of its safety and efficacy, it is possible that this drug might be approved for marketing and prescribed very successfully. However, there are many good reasons why it is advantageous to know a drug's mechanism of action. That is, it is advantageous to know with which biological structures the drug interacts to elicit its beneficial therapeutic effect, and, from our current perspective, with which biological structures the drug interacts to elicit adverse drug reactions.

These observations lead us to the concept of biological plausibility. When designing a new drug molecule, it is very helpful (and arguably necessary) to understand the biological changes that lead from a state of health to a state of disease. Once these pathways are elucidated, it becomes possible to approach the search for a beneficial drug molecule from a rational basis: the drug molecule needs to intervene somehow to prevent the biological changes that lead to the disease, to reverse them, or at least to ameliorate them. Understanding an investigational drug's biological mechanisms of action helps researchers to decide if the drug molecule may be useful in treating the disease or condition, and therefore to devote the necessary resources to the development of the drug molecule.

It is also advantageous to know how an adverse drug reaction is elicited if we wish to take steps to prevent it from happening. An understanding of the biology presented in this chapter will allow you to follow subsequent discussions that describe the mechanism of action that leads certain drugs to elicit one cardiac adverse drug reaction of particular interest in genetically susceptible individuals. This adverse drug reaction is the elicitation of a potentially lethal form of cardiac arrhythmia called torsades de pointes, discussed in Section 4.2.3. Knowledge of this mechanism of action facilitates extensive research during drug development to identify investigational drugs that may lead to this adverse drug reaction, and to stop further development or to attempt to modify the chemical structure of the drug molecule such that it will still lead to its desired therapeutic benefit but not lead to this adverse drug reaction

We will also consider other cases where a drug may or may not elicit certain cardiac adverse drug reactions, but if it does, we are not certain of the mechanism of action by which it does so. This relative lack of knowledge of the mechanism of action makes it more difficult to address the issue of a drug's possible involvement in directly leading to an adverse drug reaction. A lack of biological plausibility in any proposed mechanism of action is not helpful.

2.19   THE PROMISE OF PRECISION PHARMACEUTICAL MEDICINE

Genetic variation between individuals regarding these proteins of interest is not represented by normal clinical signs or biochemical tests. From this book's perspective, it manifests itself only when the patient is prescribed a drug and suffers an adverse drug reaction. The identification of individuals who are genetically predisposed (genetically susceptible) to adverse drug reactions to a particular drug would provide extremely useful (and potentially lifesaving) information to the individuals' physicians, and alternative therapeutic modalities could be used to help these patients. This process is not currently a routine part of clinical practice, but this situation may change in the future when advances in proteomic knowledge and technology result in gene-chip systems that facilitate the practice of precision medicine by identifying in advance how a patient will respond to a particular drug.

2.20   SUMMARY

This chapter has provided an overview of biological considerations relevant to subsequent discussions. This section provides a summary of the key points.

- ➤ Three biological structures of particular interest in the study of cardiac adverse drug reactions are ion channels, drug receptors, and enzymes.
- ➤ These structures are comprised of proteins that are embedded in cell membranes.
- ➤ Ion channels permit the flow of electrically charged particles called ions from one side of the membrane to the other. As will be discussed further in the next chapter, translocation of ions leads to electric currents flowing into and out of a cell.
- ➤ Drug-induced alterations in ion channel function can lead to adverse drug reactions.
- ➤ Endogenous chemical messengers interact with receptors on cell membranes to transmit their message to the cell.
- ➤ Drugs interact with drug receptors on cell membranes and lead to biological signals. Drug interactions with target receptors lead to beneficial (therapeutic) effects. Drug interactions with nontarget receptors receptor lead to unintended effects that may be adverse drug reactions.
- ➤ Metabolic enzymes break down drugs into metabolites. On occasions, these metabolic products are active compounds, but our focus is on cases where they are not active. The enzymes therefore lessen the effect of the drug.
- ➤ Genetic mutations causing changes in amino acids that comprise proteins and differences in gene expression can lead to alterations in the net function of enzymes. Enzymatic function can become greater than usual or less than usual. This can cause a drug to be less effective or to remain in the body longer and therefore exert its effect longer (i.e., is it more effective, potentially adversely so).

3

CARDIAC STRUCTURE AND FUNCTION

3.1 INTRODUCTION

This chapter provides an overview of healthy cardiac structure and function, setting the scene for the following chapter's overview of cardiac pathophysiology and diseases of particular interest in this book. These reviews provide the context in which to examine cardiac adverse drug reactions in later chapters. While our primary focus is the heart, the intimate relationship between the heart and the vasculature means that it is also beneficial to discuss some aspects of the cardiovascular system.

As Turner (1994) noted, the heart is a supreme example of biomechanical engineering, and, under normal circumstances, it operates with elegant economy. As acute metabolic demand varies with increases and decreases in skeletal muscular activity, so too does cardiac activity. The skeletal musculature therefore receives commensurate supplies of blood, and hence of oxygen, to facilitate its physical activity. This intimate and biologically sensible relationship is facilitated by the autonomic nervous system and its chemical messengers, neurotransmitters.

Key topics discussed in this chapter include the chambers of the heart and their pattern of contraction during cardiac cycles; the cardiac conduction system and the electrical stimuli that govern cardiac activity; cellular depolarization and repolarization; and the recording of cardiac electrical activity at the body surface by the electrocardiogram (ECG).

3.2 THE HEART

The human heart is a strong muscular pump, a bit bigger than a fist, located in the middle of the chest. It is actually a dual pump, made up of a right-hand side and a left-hand side. Each side has an upper chamber called an atrium and a lower chamber called a ventricle.

The right atrium collects deoxygenated blood returning from the body and sends it via the right ventricle to the lungs. Carbon dioxide collected from the body's cells is removed and a new supply of oxygen added to this blood, which returns to the left atrium. This oxygen-rich blood passes into the left ventricle. The blood ejected from the left ventricle flows into the aorta, one of the "great vessels." This artery then distributes blood throughout the body via a network of other

Integrated Cardiac Safety: Assessment Methodologies for Noncardiac Drugs in Discovery, Development, and Postmarketing Surveillance. By J. Rick Turner and Todd A. Durham
Copyright © 2009 John Wiley & Sons, Inc.

arteries. Blood flows from arteries into smaller arterioles and then into even smaller body tissue capillaries, where the exchange of oxygen and carbon dioxide occurs. Deoxygenated blood leaving the capillaries flows first into venules, then into the larger veins, and back to the right-hand side of the heart.

Arteries are located relatively deep inside the body and they have relatively thick walls. There is considerable blood pressure inside arteries, as discussed in Section 3.4.2. Since complex organs have an extensive microcirculation to facilitate their activities, blood needs to be ejected from the left ventricle into the systemic (whole body) circulation with a certain degree of pressure to ensure that blood can subsequently be propelled through these organs' microcirculation upon arrival there. Veins are located relatively close to the surface of the body, have relatively thin walls, and have much lower blood pressure inside them than arteries. When blood is drawn for clinical tests or for donation to a blood bank, the blood is collected from a vein, typically at the inside of the elbow. Veins are much easier to access than arteries, and the lower pressure means that a small amount of blood can be drawn safely. In contrast, accidental laceration of an artery can cause relatively profuse bleeding and, in some cases, lead to death in a short time.

3.2.1   The Myocardium

The heart muscle is called the myocardium. This muscle surrounds both sides of the heart and influences the flow of blood through all four heart chambers by its regular pattern of squeezing and then relaxing. This pattern of squeezing and then relaxing is called the heartbeat.

Lower organisms have tubular hearts that function as a one-way pump, operating by peristaltic contractions. In contrast, fully developed human hearts have chambers and one-way valves. Chamber hearts are more powerful than tubular hearts. As indicated in the previous section, humans and other higher organisms have increased resistance to blood flow in the microcirculation of organs such as the liver and kidney, which means that blood must be ejected into the systemic circulations with enough force to address this need. In chamber hearts, the atria facilitate efficient filling of the ventricles, and the ventricles become the "power pumps" (Moorman and Christoffels, 2003, p. 29). An additional requirement of a chamber heart is the need for one-way valves at both the inflow and the outflow of a chamber. When a chamber relaxes, it has to be prevented from refilling from the downstream compartment, and when it contracts, backflow into the preceding compartment has to be prevented (Moorman and Christoffels, 2003). The valves in the heart that control the passage of blood from the atria to the ventricles and prevent regurgitation are as follows:

➤ The tricuspid valve is between the right atrium and the right ventricle.
➤ The pulmonary valve is between the right ventricle and the pulmonary artery.

> ➤ The mitral valve is between the left atrium and the left ventricle.
> ➤ The aortic valve is between the left ventricle and the aorta.

Atrial contractions are not particularly forceful since blood simply has to be moved into the nearby ventricles (when standing, gravity assists in this process). In contrast, the ventricles need to contract relatively forcefully. The left ventricle contracts more forcefully than the right ventricle: It has to eject blood against the higher pressure contained in the systemic circulation, whereas the right ventricle ejects blood against the lower pressure in the pulmonary circulation that takes blood from the heart to the lungs and back.

3.2.2 Coronary Circulation

The heart has its own set of blood vessels that supply it with blood and oxygen. A reasonable question here is: why would the heart, which is full of blood, need its own blood supply? The answer is that only those cells on the surfaces of the insides of the left atrium and left ventricle (the two chambers that contain blood full of oxygen) could potentially get oxygen from the blood inside the chambers. Therefore, a specialized network of vessels called the coronary circulation supplies the whole heart.

The first arteries to branch off the aorta are the coronary arteries. The word corona means "crown": The right coronary artery and the left coronary artery surround the heart like a crown. The right coronary artery supplies blood to the right side and usually the bottom of the heart. The left coronary artery divides into two branches, the anterior descending branch and the circumflex branch. The anterior descending branch supplies blood to the left side of the heart, and both the anterior descending branch and the circumflex branch supply blood to the rear of the heart. By curling around the heart and dividing into smaller and smaller branches, the coronary arteries are able to supply every muscle fiber in the myocardium with blood and, hence, oxygen.

3.2.3 Heartbeat and Heart Rate

Heart rate is the number of heartbeats, or cardiac cycles, in a given period of time, typically one minute. Each heartbeat has two phases, one of contraction and one of relaxation. The phase of contraction is called systole (pronounced "sis-toll-ee") and the phase of relaxation is called diastole (pronounced "di-ass-toll-ee"). When a male adult is sitting down quietly, the resting heart rate is typically around 70 beats per minute (bpm). For a female adult, this value is typically a little higher. This relationship is a largely function of the typical weight of males and females. Females tend to be less heavy. (A related observation is that as weight or body size decreases in different species, heart rate typically increases.)

The heart rate goes up during physical work and exercise. Heart rates of over 200 bpm can occur in young people during strenuous exercise. Higher heart rates than usual are also seen when a person has a fever. During fever, when a person's body temperature rises, heart rates of 140–160 bpm are common even when the person is lying still. The heart rate can also go up during stress. In contrast, the heart rate slows down when we get cold. When a person is suffering from hypothermia, the heart rate can be dangerously low. In this case, the body does not receive enough blood to keep all the cells healthy.

3.4   CARDIOVASCULAR PARAMETERS OF INTEREST

Four cardiovascular parameters of interest are:

- ➢ Stroke volume.
- ➢ Cardiac output.
- ➢ Blood pressure.
- ➢ Total peripheral resistance of the systemic vasculature.

3.4.1   Stroke Volume and Cardiac Output

Each time the heart beats, it pumps a certain amount of blood out into the arteries. The blood pumped per heartbeat is called the stroke volume. Stroke volume is typically measured in milliliters (ml) per beat, and a typical stroke volume is on the order of 60–100 ml. The total amount of blood pumped per unit of time is called the cardiac output. Like heart rate, cardiac output is usually represented in intervals of one minute, and is measured in liters per minute (lpm). A typical cardiac output for an adult resting quietly is about 5 to 6 lpm. This can increase severalfold as needed during physical activity and also during emotional stress.

3.4.2   Arterial Blood Pressure

There is continuous pressure in the arteries of the circulatory system to drive blood through the arteries. This pressure is known formally as arterial blood pressure, but in practice this term is typically shortened to blood pressure, a convention followed in this book. (As noted earlier, venous pressure is much lower than arterial blood pressure and has fewer ramifications for disease development than does atypical arterial blood pressure). The level of blood pressure fluctuates during each cardiac cycle. Pressure is highest during systole (contraction), when blood is ejected from the left ventricle into the aorta, and lowest during diastole (relaxation). Systolic blood pressure (SBP) represents the maximum pressure in the arterial system, which occurs as the ventricles contract and eject blood, and diastolic blood pressure (DBP) represents the lowest pressure in the arterial system between heartbeats.

The unit of blood pressure measurement, millimeters of mercury, originates from the earliest ways of measuring blood pressure. A catheter was placed into the brachial artery in the arm, and the blood was channeled to the bottom of a tube of mercury (Hg is the chemical symbol for mercury). The blood pressure at any point in time caused the column of mercury to rise to a certain height. This height was measured in millimeters, hence the unit mmHg. Given the fluctuation in pressure during each cardiac cycle, the height of the mercury column varied during the cycle. A modified, noninvasive version of this procedure is used when health professionals employ a stethoscope, a blood pressure cuff, and a sphygmomanometer.

To measure blood pressure using this equipment, the cuff is placed around the upper arm and inflated to a fairly high pressure (perhaps 180 mmHg) and the stethoscope is placed over the inside of the elbow. The goal is to inflate the cuff sufficiently so that the brachial artery, the main artery in this region, is temporarily collapsed. This means that no blood can flow through the artery because the pressure in the cuff is greater than the pressure propelling blood through the arterial system. If this is achieved, the health professional taking the readings will not be able to hear anything through the stethoscope because there is no blood flow. The cuff pressure is then gradually reduced, thereby reducing the external pressure applied to the brachial artery. Eventually, a pressure is reached when blood starts to spurt through the artery during each heartbeat. The sounds that are made by the gushing blood (called Korotkoff sounds after the method's founder) can be heard using the stethoscope. This pressure is defined as SBP. As the cuff continues to be deflated, the blood flows more and more easily until the flow becomes smooth. Once blood flows smoothly, Korotkoff sounds are no longer heard. The pressure at which flow becomes smooth and Korotkoff sounds disappear is defined as the DBP.

Commonly cited healthy blood pressure values for adults are a SBP value of 120 mmHg and a DBP of 80 mmHg. Such blood pressure measurements would typically be written as "120/80 mmHg" and stated as "120 over 80." Young women tend to have somewhat lower blood pressures than young men, and blood pressures typically rise with age in both men and women in industrialized countries.

3.4.3   Pulse Pressure and Mean Arterial Pressure

Two other noteworthy blood pressure parameters are pulse pressure and mean arterial pressure. Pulse pressure is the arithmetic difference between SBP and DBP, calculated as SBP minus DBP. The previously cited values of 120 over 80 would therefore yield a pulse pressure of 40 mmHg.

Mean arterial pressure (MAP) is a way of expressing a representative pressure across the entire cardiac cycle, and is calculated as DBP plus one-third of the pulse pressure:

$$MAP = DBP + 1/3(SBP - DBP) \tag{3.1}$$

It should be noted that, while the word mean is the first word in the term MAP, this value is not the arithmetic mean of SBP and DBP (which would be 100 mmHg for values of 120 over 80). This mean is a weighted mean that gives more influence to DBP than to SBP, a reflection of the fact that approximately two-thirds of the duration of the cardiac cycle is spent in diastole (relaxation) and one-third in systole (contraction). The values of 120 over 80 therefore lead to a MAP of 93.33 mmHg.

3.4.4   Total Peripheral Resistance of the Systemic Vasculature

Total peripheral resistance of the systemic vasculature (TPR) is of considerable importance because, along with cardiac output (CO), it is one of the two primary determinants of blood pressure. The simultaneous measurement of MAP and CO allows the derivation of TPR from the following formula:

$$TRP = MAP/CO \tag{3.2}$$

Rearranging this formula to place MAP as the parameter being calculated leads to the following formula:

$$MAP = CO \times TPR \tag{3.3}$$

This formula reflects the fact that arterial blood pressure can be thought of as representing a manifestation of the interaction between the heart and the vasculature (Obrist, 1981). If either CO or TPR increases while the other remains constant, an increase in MAP will result. A given change in blood pressure, therefore, can be the result of a change in CO, a change in TPR, or a combination of a change in both.

3.5   THE AUTONOMIC NERVOUS SYSTEM

The nervous system can be meaningfully divided into the central nervous system and the peripheral nervous system. The autonomic nervous system, of primary interest here, is part of the peripheral nervous system. It can be thought of as being in charge of basic survival functions that are under involuntary control, including cardiac function. Heart rate is primarily controlled by nuclei in the hindbrain, located in the brainstem (it is possible to learn to exert influence on heart rate using breathing regulation strategies and biofeedback, but our hearts typically function under involuntary control). The brainstem evolved some 500 million years ago, and is concerned with biological stability and survival. In a lifetime of 75 years, a person's heart beats on the order of 3 billion times without conscious instruction.

The autonomic nervous system comprises the sympathetic nervous system and the parasympathetic nervous system. These branches of the autonomic system can be regarded as being concerned with mobilization of the body and calming of the body, respectively. The heart (like many other organs) is innervated by both the sympathetic system and the parasympathetic system, and its activity at any point in time is the net result of two opposing influences, one to beat faster and one to beat slower.

3.5.1   Neurotransmitters

The autonomic system uses chemical messengers called neurotransmitters to transmit its instructions to the heart. The sympathetic system uses norepinephrine (noradrenaline), while the parasympathetic system uses acetylcholine. Both sympathetic and parasympathetic nerves release their neurotransmitters very close to their target organs, including the heart. Each time neurotransmitters are released, they transmit their respective messages to the target organ for a very brief time. Stimulation of the target organ can therefore be very brief, or it can be more prolonged if the nerves release neurotransmitters for a period of time.

3.6   THE ENDOCRINE SYSTEM

While our discussions focus primarily on nervous system innervation of the heart, the influence of the endocrine system should also be noted. The endocrine system consists of glands throughout the body that secrete chemical messengers called hormones into the bloodstream. The hormone epinephrine (adrenaline) is secreted into the bloodstream by the adrenal glands, located above the kidneys. When epinephrine reaches the heart it conveys the same instruction, i.e., beat faster, as the sympathetic neurotransmitter norepinephrine.

Two brain regions that are more recent in their evolution, the thalamus and the hypothalamus, are well connected to the endocrine system (they are also connected to the nervous system). These structures are involved in emotion. While their influence on cardiac activity is more driven by perceptions and emotions than by the pure need to maintain biological stability, it can nevertheless be a considerable influence. Many of us have experienced an increased heart rate during periods of psychological stress.

3.6.1   Hormones

Hormones are chemically very similar to neurotransmitters, and some chemicals act as hormones for the endocrine system and as neurotransmitters for the nervous system. However, hormones pass on their messages in a different way than neurotransmitters. When released from an endocrine gland, hormones travel around the body in the bloodstream and can therefore affect several different organs in turn. Additionally, once released into the bloodstream, they exert their effects for several hours. Thus, while nervous excitation via neurotransmitters can be very brief or more prolonged, hormonal excitation of organs is typically more long-lasting.

3.7   OVERVIEW OF THE CARDIAC CONDUCTION SYSTEM

The cardiac conduction system facilitates the flow of electrical stimuli across tissues in the heart. It can be studied by employing the medical specialty of cardiac electrophysiology. Cardiac electrophysiology is a complex discipline that facilitates clinical diagnosis of cardiac abnormalities and pathophysiology. It can also be used in a much simpler manner to obtain information that is of particular relevance to our discussions.

This overview is geared toward the latter use of cardiac electrophysiology. The description in the following sections is not intended to provide an account of diagnostic cardiac electrophysiology (we are not clinicians). Accordingly, we do not present an array of ECG figures or attempt to describe clinical diagnostic strategies. However, since ECG recordings are used in drug development research to investigate potential alterations in one particular aspect of the ECG, the QT interval (Figure 3.1) shows a stylized ECG and indicates this aspect.

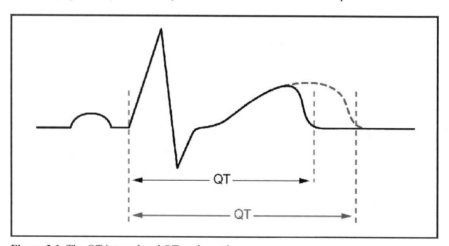

Figure 3.1. The QT interval and QT prolongation.

The QT interval is defined by the onset of the QRS complex and the offset of the T-wave. It should be emphasized that these landmarks have deliberately been made very clear on the stylized ECG presented in Figure 3.1. In real life, these landmarks can be difficult to identify, and strategies that make use of sophisticated computer algorithms have been developed for this purpose (see Chapter 7). This chapter's overview of the cardiac conduction system, and of the use of cardiac electrophysiology to investigate potential QT interval prolongation, is intended to provide a basic level of understanding that will facilitate later discussions of certain cardiac adverse drug reactions.

As Rentschler et al. (2003, p. 195) noted, the tissues in the cardiac conduction system "comprise the 'smart components' of the vertebrate heart, responsible for setting and coordinating the rhythmic pumping of cardiac muscle through the generation and propagation of electrical impulses." Proper conduction of these electrical impulses through the conduction tissues results in coordinated activation and contraction of the heart. The atria contract first to fill the ventricles with blood, followed by contraction of the ventricles to pump blood into the systemic circulation and the pulmonary circulation

The nature of myocardial muscle is of interest. The body contains several types of muscle tissues:

> Skeletal muscle, which is striated. This musculature operates under voluntary control.
> Smooth muscle, such as that found in the intestines. This musculature operates under involuntary control and is intrinsically rhythmic.
> Myocardial muscle, which is striated. This musculature operates under involuntary control, but it lacks its own intrinsic rhythmicity.

The term striated refers to the striated appearance of the muscle during light microscopic studies. This appearance results from the high degree of organization of muscle cells (most muscle fiber cells are aligned in a structured manner).

Myocardium muscle is therefore intermediate in its histological structure between intrinsically rhythmic and involuntary smooth muscle and the voluntary skeletal muscle. The initiation and coordination of the normally rhythmical cardiac contraction depend on a specialized component of the myocardium, the cardiac conduction system. This system facilitates the flow of the heart's electrical impulses. The timing and pattern of these impulses determine the heart's rhythm, orchestrating the sequence of myocardial muscle contraction during each heartbeat. This muscle contraction sequence is important for optimizing stroke volume and hence cardiac output, and "Derangements in this rhythm often impair the heart's ability to pump enough blood to meet the body's demands" (Fogoros, 2006, p. 3).

3.7.1   The Sinoatrial Node and the Atrioventricular Node

The mechanism of automaticity refers to the process by which the normal heart rate is generated. The sinoatrial node, located near the top of the right atrium, is regarded as the heart's natural pacemaker. It generates the cardiac impulse, a depolarizing impulse or current, which is rapidly propagated throughout the atrial myocardial muscle, causing atrial contraction, i.e., this impulse spreads throughout the atrial muscle cells, causing them to contract. The impulse also reaches the atrioventricular node, which is responsible for slowing down the impulse, thereby delaying its arrival at the ventricular myocardial muscle cells. This impulse delay allows the atrial chambers the necessary time to pump blood in the atria into the ventricles (i.e., to fill the ventricles with blood) before the impulse continues on to the ventricles and causes them to contract: Ventricular contractions that occur before they have been filled with the blood in the atria result in inefficiency in pumping blood into the systemic and pulmonary circulations.

After the appropriate delay, the cardiac impulse needs to be propagated rapidly throughout the ventricular myocardium. A specialized linkage system between the atrial and ventricular muscles conveys the impulse. This axis is the only link between atrial and ventricular muscular masses. The electrical impulse is conducted via this axis, which spreads through the ventricular myocardium in a system comprising the Purkinje fibers. Ventricular contractions results from this impulse (Anderson and Ho, 2003).

The heart rate pace set by the sinoatrial node must be able to vary during the day to keep up with changing metabolic demands. When more oxygen is needed, the heart is required to beat faster to increase the cardiac output and hence the oxygen supply to working muscles. This regulation of heart rate is facilitated by sympathetic and parasympathetic nerve fibers that innervate the sinoatrial and atrioventricular nodes (the rest of the heart's electrical system is predominantly innervated by the sympathetic nervous system). An increased sympathetic tone (increased sympathetic excitation) influences the heart to beat more quickly, while an increased parasympathetic tone influences the heart to beat more slowly. As noted in Section 3.5, the actual heart rate at a given point in time results from the balance of these opposing influences.

3.8   THE CARDIAC TRANSMEMBRANE POTENTIAL

Cardiac cells are surrounded by a membrane, and the cell's intracellular environment has a negative electrical charge compared with the cell's immediate extracellular environment. The voltage difference across the cell membrane is termed the transmembrane potential. Between contractions, the resting transmembrane potential level for cardiac cells is on the order of −80 millivolts (mV) to −90 mV. The greater negativity inside the cell results from an accumulation of negatively charged ions inside the cell.

When a cardiac cell is electrically stimulated, ion channels in the cell's membrane open and close rapidly (some more rapidly than others). This activity facilitates the translocation of various ions into and out of the cell. This translocation of ions results in a fluctuating transmembrane potential. At each point in time, the change in transmembrane potential from the resting level is the net result of the electrical charges carried by all of the incoming and outgoing ions. The resulting voltage fluctuations can be graphed against time to yield the cell's action potential.

3.9   PHASES OF THE ACTION POTENTIAL

Figure 3.2 shows a stylized action potential for a Purkinje fiber cell.

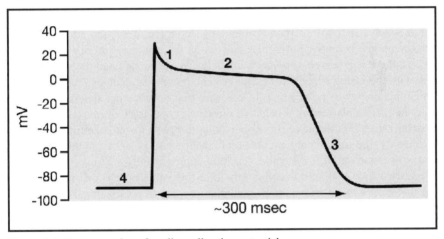

Figure 3.2. Representation of cardiac cell action potential.

The typical action potential for each type of cardiac cell is somewhat different, but the action potentials for two cardiac cell types of particular interest here, atrial muscle and ventricular muscle, are not dissimilar to that of a Purkinje fiber cell, as shown in Figure 3.2.

Five phases of the action potential are shown in Figure 3.2, i.e., phase 0 through phase 4. At different time points during the cardiac cycle, ions are being translocated through several structures in the cell's membrane, including sodium, potassium, and calcium ion channels and biological structures called ion pumps. This activity leads to many ionic currents, and phases 0 through 4 result from the net flow of various ions into and out of the cell during different time points in this cycle. The discussions in this book are deliberately simplified: we do not discuss calcium channel currents or ion pumps, and we focus on one particular repolarizing potassium ionic current, I_{Kr}. The use of the letter I in this field derives from the use of this letter in physics to represent a current: electrophysiology can be regarded as one form of applied physics. The I_{Kr} current is the rapid ("r") component of the repolarizing I_K current. [There is also a slow ("s") component, I_{Ks}, which is listed in Table 4.1, but our discussions focus on I_{Kr}.] This I_{Kr} current can have a major influence on the overall electrical activity of the heart, and therefore on cardiac function and performance. It can also be impacted by noncardiac drugs, as will be seen in due course.

Since the full complexity of ionic currents during the action potential is not essential for present discussions, it is conceptualized here in terms of three general phases (see Fogoros, 2006): These phases are:

➢ Depolarization.
➢ Repolarization.
➢ The resting phase.

Before commencing the discussion of these phases, however, it is helpful to become conversant with certain terminology. As noted in Section 3.8, the resting transmembrane potential for cardiac cells is on the order of −80 mV to −90 mV. That is, there is a degree of polarization between the outside and the inside of the cell, with the inside being more negative. The process of depolarization is one in which this degree of polarization is lessened. Since the resting state is a negative state, i.e., it is polarized in a negative direction, depolarization makes the degree of polarization less negative. In other words, it moves towards zero polarization. In actuality, the transmembrane potential reaches zero polarization and then goes past zero polarization for a while, reaching approximately +30 mV. The process of repolarization that starts very shortly after this value of +30 mV is attained is one that moves the transmembrane potential's degree of polarization back towards where it started. That is, the transmembrane potential moves back towards −80 mV to −90 mV.

Both of these alterations in transmembrane potential, depolarization and repolarization, are achieved by translocation of K^+, Na^+, and calcium ions (Ca^{2+}) into and out of the cell (as previously noted, calcium ions, while also very important in the overall scheme of cardiac electrophysiology, are not discussed here for simplicity's sake: our main focus in proarrhythmic cardiac safety concerns a potassium ion channel). Note that the ions being translocated are positively charged ions. To make the inside of the cell more positively charged (i.e., less negatively charged), there has to be a net movement of positively charged ions into the cell. Conversely, to make the inside of the cell more negatively charged, there has to be a net movement of positively charged ions out of the cell. Therefore, inward movement of positively charged ions results in a depolarizing influence, while outward movement of positively charged ions results in a repolarizing influence.

3.9.1 Depolarization

Sections 2.13.1 and 2.13.2 introduced the structure and function of the cardiac sodium ion channel. Depolarization occurs when rapidly acting sodium ion channels in the myocardial cell membrane are stimulated to open. At this time, Na^+ ions rush into the cell, leading to a rapid change in the transmembrane potential in a positive direction. That is, the transmembrane potential moves towards zero polarization (and, as noted in the previous section, actually goes past zero to become positively polarized for a brief period of time). As Fogoros (2006, p. 6) noted, "When we speak of the heart's electrical impulse, we are speaking of this depolarization."

The voltage spike resulting from a given cell's depolarization tends to cause adjacent cardiac cells to depolarize by causing their sodium channels to open. Once a cardiac cell is stimulated to depolarize, an electrical impulse is propagated across the heart, cell by cell, by a wave of depolarization. The speed of a cell's depolarization is reflected by the slope of phase 0 of the action potential, as shown in Figure 3.2: the steeper the slope (i.e., the closer it is to vertical), the faster the rate of depolarization. The speed at which the electrical impulse is propagated is dependent upon the speed of depolarization of the initiating cell. The greater the rate of depolarization of the initiating cell, the sooner the next cell will depolarize, and so on. The rate of depolarization therefore determines the speed at which the electrical impulse is propagated across the heart. The speed of impulse propagation across cardiac tissue is called the conduction velocity.

3.9.2 Repolarization

A cardiac cell that has recently been depolarized (i.e., the cell has recently contracted) cannot be depolarized again until it has been repolarized. Given that cardiac cells must continue to contract for us to stay alive, it is important that they be able to depolarize again very soon. Therefore, the cells must become repolarized very quickly. To achieve repolarization, the net direction of ionic flux must be reversed such that there is a net flow of positively charged ions out of the cell, bringing the cell back to its negatively charged resting transmembrane potential. The time taken by the process of repolarization is called the refractory period. Its length corresponds roughly to phases 1 through 3 of the action potential, i.e., the width of phases 1 through phase 3 in the time domain.

As noted in the previous section, depolarization is the result of rapid inward movement of Na^+ ions. That is, it results from Na^+ ionic currents flowing through sodium ion channels. In contrast, repolarization is mainly influenced by K^+ ionic currents resulting from the outward movement of K^+ ions through potassium ion channels. Multiple forms of potassium channels mediate repolarization of cardiac action potential by conducting various K^+ ionic currents. One of these currents, I_{Kr}, is the current of particular relevance to our discussions in proarrhythmic cardiac safety.

3.9.3   The Resting Phase

For the majority of cardiac cells, phase 4, the resting phase between action potentials, is a quiet time in that there is no net movement of ions across the cell membrane. For some cells, however, this is not the case. These cells have small movements of ions back and forth across the cell membrane during phase 4, with the net result that there is a gradual increase in transmembrane potential. When the transmembrane potential is high enough in these cells (i.e., when it reaches the threshold voltage), the appropriate channels are activated and the cells depolarize. Just like the regular depolarization of the majority of cardiac cells, this depolarization can stimulate nearby cells to depolarize in turn, which means that the spontaneously generated electrical impulse is propagated across the heart. Cells capable of producing spontaneous depolarization initiate phase 4 of the action potential, and this phase 4 activity leading to spontaneous depolarization is called automaticity.

3.10   ONE REPOLARIZING CURRENT OF SPECIFIC INTEREST IN PROARRHYTHMIC CARDIAC SAFETY

As noted at the end of Section 3.9.2, the I_{Kr} repolarizing current is of particular interest in cardiac proarrhythmic cardiac safety, for reasons explained in more detail in the following chapter discussing cardiac pathophysiology and diseases. For now, simply recall the discussion in Section 2.17: drugs can affect the function of ion channels and a given drug may exert a harmful effect via its interaction with a given ion channel only if the ion channel protein is differently formed as a result of a gene mutation. Such interaction can cause a decrease in the I_{Kr} repolarizing current. Such occurrences are discussed in the following chapter, but first, in this chapter focusing on (healthy) cardiac structure and function, it is appropriate to discuss the normal generation and functioning of the I_{Kr} repolarizing current.

3.10.1   The hERG Cardiac Potassium Ion Channel and the hERG Ionic Current

It was noted in Chapter 2 that genetic studies in other species are very informative concerning the human condition since many genes are conserved across species to a remarkable extent. A *Drosophila* gene of relevance to the world of cardiac conduction research is called *eag,* and the related human gene of interest is called hERG. hERG's full name is the human ether-a-go-go related gene. The derivation of the name hERG has to do with the identification of a mutant *Drosophila* gene that induces twitching legs in flies carrying this mutant form when anesthetized with ether. The *Drosophila* researchers believed that these leg movements resembled those of a go-go dancer, and the gene name ether-a-go-go, represented as *eag*, was coined. Despite a name that may well seem flippant to some, consequences of mutations in the related human gene are serious and potentially fatal.

hERG is expressed in tissues throughout the body, including neurons, smooth muscle, and the cardiac muscle cells (cardiomyocytes). While the exact role of the channels hERG is responsible for forming in some tissues is unknown, it has been elucidated for hERG channels found in the heart. Because its role is known in this context, and because alterations in the hERG channels in heart tissues can lead to lethal cardiac sequelae, within this field this gene has somewhat attained the status that DNA has attained much more widely: the full name is not usually provided before the acronym is used.

In the heart, hERG encodes a protein that forms a particular subunit, the α-subunit, of a certain potassium ion channel. Since there are many potassium ion channels (and other ion channels) in the heart, the acronym hERG is also used to refer to the particular potassium channel that it encodes. Hence, in this book the term hERG channel specifies the potassium ion channel that hERG encodes, and the term hERG current specifies the potassium (K^+) ionic current that flows through the hERG channel. The hERG current is formally called I_{Kr}.

An introduction to the structure of ion channels was provided in Section 2.13. The ion channel discussed there was the sodium (Na^+) ion channel. Sodium and potassium channels belong to the same superfamily of ion channels, and attention now turns to the hERG cardiac potassium channel. The structure of the sodium channel was introduced in Section 2.13 (i.e., before discussing the structure of the hERG channel in this section) for two reasons. First, in the cardiac cycle, sodium channels are responsible for the initiation of activity, i.e., for depolarization. It therefore makes some sense to introduce it first. The more important reason is that the structures of sodium and hERG channels are different in a relatively subtle but meaningful manner.

As described in Section 2.13.1 and schematically represented in Figure 2.2, the voltage-gated sodium channel is monomeric. Each channel comprises four homologous domains, each having six transmembrane helices, resulting in a total of 24 transmembrane helices. The hERG channel also has a total of 24 transmembrane helices, but the fundamental composition of the channel is different. The hERG channel is tetrameric: each of the four subunits (four α-subunits) comprising the channel consists of six transmembrane (S1–S6) regions, and together the four α-subunits combine to make a functional channel. This difference in fundamental structure, i.e., the hERG channel is formed from four separate α-subunits, means that, theoretically, the tetrameric channel can be homomeric, i.e., comprised of four identical α-subunits, or heteromeric. There is strong evidence for heteromeric hERG channels from *in vivo* animal models, but it is not known whether all channels are heteromeric (see Robertson et al., 2005). (With regard to potassium channels in general, there are some 40 different voltage-gated channels that can be classified into 12 distinct subfamilies. α-Subunits can assemble into both homomeric and heteromeric channels—homotetramers and heterotetramers—leading to a wide variety of different channel complexes; see Catterall, 2006.)

Four of the transmembrane helices, S1–S4, in each of the α-subunits comprise the channel's voltage sensor (with S4 being by far the most important part). A pore loop connects transmembrane helices S5 and S6, and the region between S5 and S6 comprises the ion-conducting pore, or channel, through which potassium ions are translocated from one side of the membrane to the other. Figure 3.3 presents a schematic representation of the components of the hERG channel.

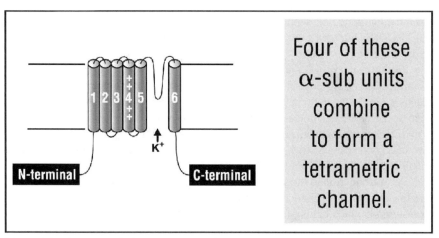

Figure 3.3. The tetrameric hERG potassium ion channel.

As noted, the hERG channel operates in a voltage-gated manner. Certain positively charged amino acids in the S4 helices enable the helices to function as voltage sensors, detecting voltage changes in the transmembrane potential. Detection of depolarization leads to a depolarization-triggered movement within the helices, possibly a helical twist or rotation (Piper et al., 2005). The S4–S5 linkers play a role in conveying this information to the S5 helices. Communication leads to conformational changes in the S5 and S6 helices that result in the activation (opening) of the pore and hence the flow of ions through the pore. This process generates the I_{Kr} current. Inactivation is achieved by other conformational changes that prevent ion flow through the pore and hence terminate the current. Instructions to terminate the current are also possibly communicated to the pore helices by other movements within the S4 helices (Piper et al., 2005).

3.11   PROTEIN TRAFFICKING

hERG cardiac potassium ion channels are comprised of proteins encoded by the hERG gene. A question of interest is: once proteins have been made from the genetic information within a cardiomyocyte's DNA, specifically the hERG gene, how do they end up in the proper location, i.e., as transmembrane proteins located in the cell's plasma membrane? This takes us into the realm of protein trafficking.

Protein trafficking is a process that delivers manufactured proteins to their target location within a cell, i.e., it describes "the intracellular conveyance of proteins" (Pasternak, 1999, p. 273). Protein trafficking is important for some of our discussions within the domain of proarrhythmic cardiac safety, and it is therefore appropriate to introduce cellular organelles that are involved in this process. These are the endoplasmic reticulum and the Golgi apparatus. Since our current focus is on hERG channel proteins, the role of these organelles in hERG protein trafficking is highlighted.

The endoplasmic reticulum is a network of interconnected tubules, vesicles, and sacs. The rough endoplasmic reticulum (there is also a smooth endoplasmic reticulum) is the site of mRNA translation and protein synthesis. The hERG protein is processed into a core-glycosylated protein in the endoplasmic reticulum. To ensure that the protein folds correctly into its tertiary structure (recall the discussions in Section 2.9.1), it forms a complex with one of several proteins called cytosolic chaperones that help it fold into its native (correct) conformation. Once the protein has folded correctly, the first stage of protein trafficking occurs: it is transported in a vesicle to the Golgi apparatus.

The Golgi apparatus is divided into distinct regions (e.g., regions where phosphorylation or glycosylation occurs). In the glycosylation region, complex sugar chains are added to the core-glycosylated hERG in the process of posttranslational modification to produce the fully glycosylated form (recall the discussions in Section 2.16). Once this processing has been completed, the fully glycosylated hERG is packaged into a transport vesicle and taken to its final destination, the plasma membrane. During this transport process, it is important that the orientation of hERG, a transmembrane protein, is maintained so that, when it is incorporated into the membrane, the regions destined to project outside the cell end up in that orientation, as do the regions destined to project inside the cell (we noted in Section 2.12 that transmembrane proteins are embedded in membranes in a specific maner).

4

CARDIAC PATHOPHYSIOLOGY AND DISEASE

4.1 INTRODUCTION

This chapter provides an overview of some cardiac pathophysiologies and diseases relevant to discussions in this book. While each of the events of interest can occur for non-drug-related reasons, our interest lies with their occurrence as drug-induced adverse events.

The first condition discussed falls within the realm of proarrhythmic cardiac safety. Under certain conditions, the QT interval (introduced in Section 3.7) can be prolonged, and QT interval prolongation has been linked to cardiac arrhythmias, particularly a potentially lethal form of ventricular arrhythmia called torsades de pointes (TdP). TdP is introduced in Section 4.2 to familiarize you with this cardiac event before discussing how QT interval prolongation and other electrophysiological phenomena have been hypothesized to play a role in its generation. Attention then turns at the end of the chapter to two cardiac diseases of particular interest in generalized cardiac safety, myocardial infarction and heart failure.

4.2 ARRHYTHMIAS

Disorders of cardiac impulse generation or propagation affect over 2 million individuals in the United States and account for as many as 40,000 deaths each year. These impulse disorders lead to abnormal rhythms called arrhythmias. Arrhythmias can occur in the atria or the ventricles. While arrhythmias include slower patterns of heartbeats than usual (bradycardias), this text focuses on tachycardias, patterns of heartbeats that are faster than usual.

Investigations leading to a better understanding of the mechanisms governing the development and maintenance of the cardiac conduction system may provide greater insight into the pathogenesis of cardiac disease and may provide novel targets for appropriate pharmacotherapy (Rentschler et al., 2003). In addition, they facilitate our understanding of cardiac adverse drug events, and therefore assist in avoiding prescribing certain pharmaceutical agents to susceptible individuals.

Integrated Cardiac Safety: Assessment Methodologies for Noncardiac Drugs in Discovery, Development, and Postmarketing Surveillance. By J. Rick Turner and Todd A. Durham
Copyright © 2009 John Wiley & Sons, Inc.

4.2.1   Atrial Arrhythmias

There are two main types of atrial arrhythmias:

> ➢ Atrial flutter.
> ➢ Atrial fibrillation.

During atrial flutter, the atria contract in a regular but very rapid pattern of about 270 to 330 bpm. During atrial fibrillation, the number of beats per minute is even higher and the pattern is irregular. Atrial arrhythmias often have only a slight affect on heart function. However, these conditions can lead to the formation of blood clots in the atria. An embolus can then travel to the brain and cause a stroke.

4.2.2   Ventricular Arrhythmias

There are several types of ventricular arrhythmias, including:

> ➢ Premature ventricular contractions.
> ➢ Ventricular tachycardia.
> ➢ Ventricular fibrillation.

Premature ventricular contractions occur when the ventricles occasionally contract earlier than usual. This can often be felt as a skipped heartbeat. This condition is very common and usually is not dangerous. However, two or more of these occurring together can be a warning sign of more serious arrhythmias.

Ventricular tachycardia can be caused by myocardial cell irritation, which can occur as a result of a myocardial infarction. These cells cause a regular but rapid heart rate that often leads to inefficient blood pumping. Ventricular tachycardia can lead to ventricular fibrillation, the most serious ventricular arrhythmia. Ventricular fibrillation occurs when myocardial cells contract in a totally disorganized fashion. This lack of coordination means that the heart stops pumping blood. Because the brain can live only for a few minutes without oxygen, ventricular fibrillation leads rapidly to death unless it is treated very quickly. Ventricular fibrillation is often the actual cause of death following a heart attack.

4.2.3   Torsades de Pointes

Torsades de pointes is the characteristic arrhythmia resulting from long QT syndrome (LQTS). It is a particular form of ventricular tachycardia that has three defining characteristics on an ECG recording:

> ➤ It is associated with QT interval prolongation.
> ➤ The shape of the QRS complex, i.e., the QRS morphology, twists around an imaginary axis. There may also be a change in the amplitude of the waveform.
> ➤ The QRS complex takes on many shapes (morphologies) as it twists around this imaginary axis, leading to use of the descriptor polymorphic.

The term torsades de pointes, then, is reserved for polymorphic ventricular tachycardia associated with QT prolongation: without QT prolongation, the term used should simply be polymorphic ventricular tachycardia.

Additional information concerning TdP can be accessed via www.torsades.org. This address takes you to the web site of the Arizona Center for Education and Research on Therapeutics (ArizonaCERT). This is one of 11 such centers funded across the nation by the U.S. Agency for Healthcare Research and Quality. The mission of these centers is to advance the optimal use of drugs, biological products, and medical devices.

4.3   CARDIAC CHANNELOPATHIES: INHERITED LQTS

Various inherited pathologies of cardiac ion channels, called cardiac channelopathies, are possible. The term channelopathy is normally reserved for inherited conditions, as opposed to the functionally similar drug-induced conditions that are of particular interest in this book, and the term heritable arrhythmia syndrome is seen in some sources in this context. Some of these channelopathies lead to inherited LQTS.

As Bunch and Ackerman (2007, p. 335) observed, "The discipline of cardiac channelopathies formally began in 1995 with the discovery of mutations in genes encoding critical ion channels of the heart as the pathogenic basis for congenital LQTS." Schwartz (2005, p.186) commented as follows:

> The identification at the end of March 1995 (Wang et al., 1995; Curran et al., 1995) of the first two long QT syndrome (LQTS) genes represented a major breakthrough not only for cardiac electrophysiology but also for cardiology as a whole, and paved the way for the understanding of how tight the relationship between molecular and clinical cardiology can be. Indeed, the impressive correlation between specific mutations and critical alterations in the ionic control of ventricular repolarization has made LQTS the best example to date for the specificity and value of the correlation between genotype and phenotype.

Inherited LQTS is characterized by abnormal cardiac repolarization that results in QT interval prolongation. It is due to genetic mutations that lead to the production of abnormal variant potassium and sodium ion channel proteins, which then result in abnormal Na^+ or K^+ ionic currents flowing through these channels. This results in the prolongation of cardiac repolarization, represented on the ECG by QT interval prolongation. Inspection of an ECG recording by a trained electrophysiologist/ clinician can reveal the presence of LQTS (it is possible in some cases that an individual's propensity for prolonged QT intervals may not reveal itself for many years). If the syndrome has not been detected by inspection of ECGs, it can reveal itself more dramatically and very dangerously: LQTS can present clinically as abrupt-onset syncope (loss of consciousness), seizures, or sudden death due to TdP (sudden cardiac death is addressed in Section 4.12). Estimates indicate that up to half of the sudden deaths that stem from a cardiac channelopathy may have been preceded by warning signs that went unrecognized. Two examples of such signs include:

> ➢ Syncope brought on by physical exertion.
> ➢ A family history of premature sudden death where the cause was not identified.

As noted earlier, this book does not address clinical diagnosis of QT prolongation on the ECG, nor does it discuss clinical therapy. It is of interest, however, to note that identification of nonlethal QT prolongation in an individual that is caused by noncardiac drugs (i.e., drug-induced QT prolongation) can be the sentinel event leading to the serendipitous identification of an inherited disorder that can benefit from clinical intervention. It has been estimated that 10% of patients who experience drug-induced TdP actually have a quiescent genetic susceptibility for one kind of LQTS, known as LQT2.

4.3.1   Various Forms of LQTS

Several forms of LQTS have now been identified: Bunch and Ackerman (2007) listed nine forms, named LQT1 through LQT9. Each of these LQTSs is the result of a specific genetic mutation. There are both autosomal dominant and autosomal recessive LQTSs (recall the discussions in Section 2.3.6). Except for two rare subtypes (LQT4 and LQT9), LQTS "is a pure channelopathy stemming from mutations in cardiac channel alpha and beta subunits" (Bunch and Ackerman, 2007, p. 336). Hundreds of mutations in nine distinct susceptibility genes have been identified at this point. These mutations generally involve either loss-of-function potassium (K^+) channel mutations or gain-of-function sodium (Na^+) channel mutations, as illustrated in the following section. Each of these syndromes can precipitate potentially lethal forms of ventricular arrhythmia and are therefore of considerable clinical concern.

4.3.2   LQTSs LQT1, LQT2, and LQT3

Inherited LQTSs, then, represent cases where simple genetic mutations can have profound effects and can cause life-threatening physiological states. Table 4.1 lists three of these inherited forms: LQT1, LQT2, and LQT3. In each case, the gene in which the mutation occurs, the protein that is impacted, the ionic current that is impacted, and the consequences of the genetic mutation are listed.

Table 4.1 LQTSs LQT1, LQT2, and LQT3

Channelopathy	Gene in Which Mutation Occurs	Ionic Current	Consequence of Mutation
LQT1	KCNQ1. Encodes a 676-amino acid protein comprising the pore-forming α-subunit of the I_{Ks} potassium channel.	I_{Ks}	Decrease of function in the I_{Ks} potassium current during repolarization: net repolarizing influence is lessened.
LQT2	KCNH2. Encodes a 1,159-amino acid protein comprising the pore forming α-subunit of the I_{Kr} potassium channel.	I_{Kr}	Decrease of function in the I_{Kr} potassium current during repolarization: net repolarizing influence is lessened.
LQT3	SCN5A. Encodes a 2,016-amino acid protein comprising the α-subunit of the I_{Na} sodium channel.	I_{Na}	Gain of function in (or persistence of) the I_{Na} sodium current, a depolarizing influence: net repolarizing influence is lessened.

In the case of LQT1, the KCNQ1 gene encodes for the protein comprising the pore-forming α-subunit of the I_{Ks} potassium channel, the channel through which the K^+ current I_{Ks} flows: this current is the "slow" component of the repolarizing I_K current. The mutation that occurs in the KCNQ1 gene results in a singe amino acid residue substitution in the protein, known as a missense mutation. This results in a decrease in function in the I_{Ks} potassium channel and therefore a decrease in the I_{Ks} current. Since I_{Ks} current is a repolarizing current, less of this current means that net repolarizing influence is lessened, resulting in QT interval prolongation.

The mutation responsible for LQT2 occurs in KCNH2 (also known as hERG, as noted in Section 3.10.1). This gene encodes the α-subunit of the I_{Kr} potassium channel, the channel through which the K^+ current I_{Kr} flows: this current is the "rapid" component of the repolarizing I_K current. This mutation results in decrease in function in the I_{Kr} channel. Since the I_{Kr} current is a repolarizing current, less of this current means that net repolarizing influence is lessened, resulting in QT interval prolongation.

The syndrome LQT3 results from a mutation in SCN5A, a gene that encodes the protein comprising the α-subunit of the cardiac I_{Na} current. This mutation is a single amino acid residue substitution. The mutation results in a gain of function in the I_{Na} channel and therefore an increase in I_{Na} current. Since I_{Na} is a depolarizing current, more of this current also means that net repolarizing influence is lessened, resulting in QT prolongation.

Nomenclature Considerations. As noted in Section 3.10.1 and discussed in more detail here, the gene KCNH2 is also referred to in the literature as hERG, the human ether-a-go-go related gene. It was also noted in Section 3.10.1 that, while the exact role of the ion channels hERG is responsible for forming in some tissues is unknown, it has been elucidated for hERG channels found in the heart.

At this point, a comment on nomenclature is appropriate. One of this book's goals is to provide a self-contained introduction to integrated cardiac safety, including proarrhythmic cardiac safety. A second goal is to prepare you for further study of topics covered in the book that are of particular interest to you. Therefore, in addition to using a system of nomenclature and acronyms that is internally consistent, it appropriate to introduce you to nomenclature that you will encounter in the literature. Hence, the following strategy is employed in this chapter from this point onwards:

➢ The double-barreled term KCNH2/hERG is used to refer to the gene KCNH2, the gene that encodes the protein that forms the α-subunit of the cardiac potassium channel through which the ionic current I_{Kr} flows. This double-barreled strategy is also used for genes related to two other LQTSs discussed in the following section.

➢ The term hERG protein is used for the protein encoded by KCNH2/hERG.

➢ In a slight extension of the policy outlined in Section 3.10.1, the term hERG channel specifies the cardiac potassium ion channel that KCNH2/hERG encodes.

➢ In a slight extension of the policy outlined in Section 3.10.1, the term hERG current specifies the ionic current, I_{Kr}, that flows through the hERG channel that KCNH2/hERG encodes.

4.3.3   LQTSs LQT5 and LQT6

It is instructive at this point to consider two other LQTSs, LQT5 and LQT6. Voltage-gated potassium ion channels can have accessory β-subunits in addition to their α-subunits. Syndromes LQT5 and LQT6 result from mutations in such ion channel β-subunits. Syndrome LQT5 results from a mutation in the KCNE1 gene (also known as MinK). In Table 4.1, it can be seen that the three genes encoding α-subunits range in size from 676 to 2,016 constituent amino acid residues. Accessory β-subunits are physically smaller proteins than α-subunits. KCNE1/MinK encodes a 130-amino acid accessory β-subunit that is a single transmembrane segment. Since it encodes an accessory subunit, KCNE1/MinK does not produce a functional channel when it is expressed alone. It appears to co-assemble in heterologous systems with α-subunits encoded by the KCNQ1 gene to form functional channels for I_{Ks}, and it may co-assemble with α-subunits encoded by KCNH2/hERG and play a role in the generation of I_{Kr}.

Another gene encoding for an accessory subunit is the KCNE2 gene, also known as MiRP1, a KCNE1/MinK homolog. Syndrome LQT6 results from a mutation in KCNE2/MiRP1, which encodes a 123-amino acid β-subunit. This subunit may function as an accessory subunit in the generation of I_{Kr} current (Nerbonne and Kass, 2005; Anantharam and Abbott, 2005).

Less is known about accessory β-subunits in potassium ion channels (and sodium channels) than is known about their α-subunits. Elucidation of the operation of these ion channels is far from simple, and involves *in vitro* research and *in vivo* research in many species. Additionally, while the structure of a channel remains constant across species, its expression and role can vary considerably in different tissues and at different stages in biological development (i.e., across the life span from conception to death). Anantharam and Abbott (2005, p. 110) reviewed the evidence for the co-assembly of KCNE1/MinK- and KCNE2/MiRP1-encoded accessory β-subunits with KCNH2/hERG-encoded α-subunits in various species and concluded the following:

> We conclude that the amassed evidence supports a role for both MinK and MiRP1 in human cardiac physiology and pathophysiology, and a role for regulation of I_{Kr} in some myocytes in some species, but that there is no conclusive evidence for or against their role in human I_{Kr}.

If the subunits encoded by KCNE1/MinK and KCNE2/MiRP1 are found to be involved in ion channel activity, their roles are likely to be supportive roles rather than leading roles. Hence, mutations in them may have less of an overall impact on the ionic current than mutations in α-subunits. While the α-subunit serves as the principal binding site for a wide range of channel modulators, including drugs, Gopalakrishnan et al. (2006, p. 199) noted that, in many cases, the auxiliary subunits that co-associate with the pore-forming α-subunits "could modulate expression, biophysical or pharmacological properties of the α-subunit complex." It is possible that all voltage-gated potassium channels associate with KCNE1/MinK-related subunits (Catterall, 2006).

4.3.4   Our Interest in LQT2

The choice of LQTSs presented in Table 4.1 was driven by two observations:

> ➢ LQT1, LQT2, and LQT3 represent around 60–75% of the total occurrence of LQTS (see Bunch and Ackerman, 2007, p. 337). Additionally, they illustrate how genetic mutations in both potassium and sodium ion channels can lead to LQTS, and do so via different mechanisms (i.e., loss-of-function potassium channel mutations and gain-of-function sodium channel mutations).
> ➢ Drug-induced TdP, a central event of interest in proarrhythmic cardiac safety, is closely related to (inherited) LQT2, and LQT2 is therefore of interest too. Drug-induced TdP and LQT2 "are partially phenocopies stemming from either pharmacologically or genetically mediated perturbations in the I_{Kr} potassium channel" (Bunch and Ackerman, 2007, p. 341).

The second observation is particularly relevant here. Given the association of heritable LQTS with TdP and the fact that certain noncardiac drugs lead to drug-induced QT interval prolongation, investigation of the association between drug-induced QT interval prolongation and TdP is of considerable interest in proarrhythmic cardiac safety. While interest in proarrhythmic cardiac safety lies with drug-induced QT interval prolongation rather than inherited LQTSs *per se*, the study of similarities and associations between drug-induced QT interval prolongation and inherited LQTS can be instructive.

The mechanism of action for the vast majority of drugs that cause QT interval prolongation is inhibition of the hERG current. Hence, the focus of our attention is the hERG current, i.e., the I_{Kr} current, the rapid component of the repolarizing I_K current; the slow component of the repolarizing I_K current, I_{Ks}, is not as sensitive to drug effects. The hERG channel and the hERG current are therefore of particular interest in proarrhythmic cardiac safety for two reasons:

> ➢ The hERG current is considered essential for (human) ventricular repolarization.
> ➢ The hERG channel, through which the hERG current flows, is blocked by noncardiac drugs in preference to any of the many other cardiac potassium ion channels.

4.4   DRUG-INDUCED QT INTERVAL PROLONGATION AND TdP: THE CAUSAL LINK

Action potential prolongation/QT interval prolongation *per se* is not harmful, and it does not adversely affect myocardial pump function (Lagrutta and Salata, 2006; Shah, 2005a). As Hondeghem (2005, p. 235) observed, "Eating, sleeping, getting up, exercise and other pleasurable activities can prolong the QT interval." Thus, while physiological QT prolongation appears not to be torsadogenic, "numerous pathological conditions exist where QT prolongation is frequently associated with TdP" (Hondeghem, 2005, p. 235). These pathological conditions include inherited LQTSs and drug-induced QT prolongation.

Prolongation of the QT interval has become recognized as one indicator or marker for the risk of drug-induced TdP. Shah (2005a) observed that the relationship between QT interval prolongation as measured via the ECG and the clinical risk of TdP is complex, and commented that QT interval prolongation "is at present the best and the simplest clinical measure that is available" in this regard, but also noted that it is "imperfect" (Shah, 2005a, p. 263). Section 4.6 discusses other indicators of risk, but for now, the hypothesized causal link between drug-induced QT interval prolongation and TdP is considered. Shah (2005a, p. 263) wrote as follows:

> Typically, drug-induced TdP is characterized by a syndrome of prolonged QT interval and the long coupling interval of the initial premature beat [Roden, 2004]. Delayed or prolonged ventricular repolarization in this setting gives rise to the development of early afterdepolarizations (EADs) at the levels of the ventricular midmyocardial M-cells and the Purkinje fibres.

Early afterdepolarization is a phenomenon that occurs before the completion of action potential repolarization (delayed afterdepolarization occurs after the completion of action potential repolarization). It involves oscillations in membrane potential that arise during the repolarization phase of the action potential. Shah (2005a, p. 263) continued:

> When the amplitude of the EADs reaches a critical threshold, the resulting ectopic beat triggers a repetitive burst of electrical activity that forms the basis of TdP.

Hence, EADs and concomitant ectopic beats are regarded as the trigger for TdP (see also Lagrutta and Salata, 2006).

4.5   HOW DO NONCARDIAC DRUGS LEAD TO LOSS OF FUNCTION IN hERG CHANNELS?

Mitcheson et al. (2005, pp. 136–137) commented as follows:

> Unintentional block of hERG channels by quite a large number of medications can cause drug-induced LQTS (LQTS), a cardiac disorder that may induce arrhythmias and sudden death due to abnormal action potential repolarization…The diversity of compounds that block hERG and therefore are at risk of causing LQTS is one of the most extraordinary features of this channel.

As we have seen, KCNH2/hERG encodes pore-forming α-subunits of hERG channels, and hERG channels conduct the hERG current that helps to regulate cardiac action potential repolarization. Pharmacological blockade of the hERG channel leads to reduction in hERG current, and reduction of this repolarizing current is at least in part responsible for action potential prolongation and proarrhythmia. Theoretically, this cardiac adverse drug reaction could result from the inhibition of any potassium ion current that plays a role in repolarization. However, as noted earlier, the hERG current is the most susceptible of the various potassium currents involved in repolarization to pharmacological influence. A question of interest, therefore, is: why do so many drugs that differ in their chemical structures preferentially block hERG channels?

Mitcheson et al. (2005) provided a structural explanation for why this may be so, an explanation that also ties in to one of the hERG channel's functional characteristics. First, the inner cavity of the hERG channel appears to be larger than those of other voltage-gated potassium ion channels. Second, while activation of the hERG channel is much slower than for other channels, it displays "uniquely fast inactivation" (Tseng and Guy, 2005, p. 19). Drug molecules can become trapped within the channel by the particularly quick closure of the activation gate. This trapping of drug molecules (drug trapping) within the inner cavity of the channel "increases the affinity of drugs for hERG by slowing the rate of drug dissociation from its binding site" (Mitcheson et al., 2005, p. 148).

Third, certain amino acid residues within the pore-forming α-subunit helices that line the inner cavity of the hERG channel are unique to the *eag* channel family and are therefore not present in the cavities of other potassium ion channels. Because of the three-dimensional geometry that is a central theme of our discussions, certain amino acid residues within the pore-forming α-subunit helices are particularly available to interact with drug molecules. These amino acid residues are important sites for interactions between the channel and most drugs that block it. Additionally, other amino acid residues at the base of the pore helices are critical in the particularly strong binding that occurs for some drug molecules.

Thus, the larger size and different chemical (amino acid) composition of the hERG channel cavity provides "a structural explanation for the unusual pharmacological properties of hERG channels" (Mitcheson et al., 2005, p. 137).

4.6   Dispersion of Repolarization

The phenomenon of QT interval prolongation has attracted a lot of attention in the literature addressing proarrhythmic safety. It has also assumed additional importance because of its prominence in regulatory guidelines addressing both nonclinical (see Chapter 6) and clinical (see Chapter 7) evaluations of torsadogenic liability, i.e., the propensity of a drug to lead to TdP. However, QT interval prolongation is not the only physiological occurrence that has been hypothesized to play a role in torsadogenesis. Another hypothesis focuses on dispersion of polarization (although it should be noted that these hypotheses are not mutually exclusive).

Drug-induced prolongation of the cardiac action potential duration does not occur uniformly throughout the heart, and Shah (2005a, p. 274) observed that, while mechanisms leading to drug-induced TdP are still not fully understood, "it is likely that the differential effects of the drug on different tissue types within the ventricles play an essential role." Drugs that have differential effects on various myocytes (epicardial cells, midmyocardial or M-cells, and endocardial cells) are particularly prone to inducing TdP since these regional differences can lead to "arrhythmogenic spatial dispersion of repolarization" (Shah, 2005a, p. 275). As for the case of QT interval prolongation, attempts have been made to find a reliable way to quantify intramyocardial dispersion of repolarization using the ECG recording. One of these attempts involved a measure called QT dispersion, but this did not prove successful. In contrast, a measure called transmural dispersion of repolarization (TDR) has proved more fruitful.

4.6.1   Transmural Dispersion of Repolarization

TDR is indexed by measuring the interval between the peak and the end of the T-wave, known as T_{peak} to T_{end}, or TPE. The ventricular wall is relatively thin compared with the ventricular surface area. Increased TDR refers to "an abnormal increase in the differences in action potential duration across the ventricular wall, between the left and right ventricles, or between the base and apex of the heart" (Lagrutta and Salata, 2006, p. 458). We noted in Section 4.4 that early afterdepolarizations and concomitant ectopic beats are regarded as the trigger for TdP. Further, it has been hypothesized that an increase in TDR in the ventricle is the substrate of TdP (see Lagrutta and Salata, 2006). Shah also addressed this issue, commenting similarly that "Increase in TDR is now widely believed to be the principle substrate for induction of TdP," and that a drug-induced increase in TDR "probably predicts better the risk of TdP associated with its use" than QT interval prolongation (Shah, 2005a, p. 278). M-cells "are exquisitely responsive to pharmacological agents that block I_{Kr}" and often lead to drug-induced changes in TDR (Shah, 2005a, p. 278).

Interesting studies have been conducted evaluating TDR in patients with inherited LQTS. Additionally, carefully controlled experiments in canine models have provided support for the role of TDR in torsadogenesis. However, while it has been suggested that the TPE index as measured on the ECG may be a more reliable marker of proarrhythmia than QT interval prolongation in both animal models and humans, Shah (2005a, p. 279) noted that "the relevance of TPE in drug-induced proarrhythmias has not been characterized as thoroughly in humans."

4.6.2   Other Indicators of TdP Risk

Shah (2005b) reviewed several indicators or markers of TdP risk derived from the ECG. One of these that appears to be promising concerns changes in the T-wave morphology and a statistical technique called principal component analysis that quantitatively describes the shape of the T-wave as a sum of several components (Lagrutta and Salata, 2006). Readers are referred to Shah (2005b) for more details. Readers are also referred to Hondeghem (2005) for discussions of TRIaD (triangulation, reverse use dependence, and instability) as a foundation for proarrhythmia.

It will be interesting to follow future developments in this field that search for the best indicator of TdP risk, since it is currently imperative in drug discovery and development that torsadogenic liability is identified as early as possible. Chapters 5–7 describe current investigations in this regard in drug design, nonclinical development, and preapproval clinical development, respectively.

4.7   TRAFFICKING DEFICIENCIES IN INHERITED LQTS

It has been estimated that on the order of 20% of cellular proteins are made incorrectly because of mistakes in transcription or translation (Weaver, 2005, p. 376). Various quality control mechanisms attempt to correct these proteins (often by refolding them into the correct tertiary structure: recall discussions in Section 2.9.1), and these mechanisms are successful in many cases. However, correction is not always possible. Aberrant proteins that cannot be corrected are potentially damaging to the cell and are sent to a cytoplasmic structure called the proteasome. The proteasome contains a collection of protease enzymes that degrade the aberrant proteins upon their arrival.

It is possible that some naturally occurring KCNH2/hERG mutations produce ion channel proteins that are potentially functional but do not make it to the plasma membrane because they are recognized as abnormal variants. This possibility appears to be realized. As Ficker et al. (2005, p. 57) noted, "an ever-expanding group of LQT2 mutations" produce trafficking-deficient hERG channels that are retained in the endoplasmic reticulum, and "are thought of as expressing conformational defects recognized by cellular control mechanisms." Trafficking deficiencies therefore represent a third mechanism for loss of function in hERG current: the other two are kinetic alteration of channel function (a reduced hERG current flow through the channel) and insertion of nonfunctioning hERG channels into the plasma membrane.

4.7.1   The Nature of Cytosolic Quality Control Mechanisms

Ficker et al. (2005) discussed hERG channel trafficking and how certain proteins that carry out cytosolic quality control mechanisms perform two functions:

➤ They aid normal variant hERG proteins to fold correctly in order to be shipped to the Golgi apparatus and on to the plasma membrane.
➤ They recognize and "tag" abnormal variant hERG proteins. These proteins are shipped to the proteasome instead of the Golgi apparatus and degraded there.

The molecules actively responsible for performing quality control in the cytoplasm (cytosol) are called chaperone proteins. These chaperones form complexes with hERG proteins and effectively provide an assessment of hERG protein conformations. Where necessary and where possible, these chaperones help incompletely folded hERG proteins to fold into the normal conformation. When this is achieved successfully, the correctly configured protein can be exported to the Golgi apparatus and on to the plasma membrane. However, this is not always the case.

The complexes formed between cytosolic chaperones and abnormal variant hERG proteins are more long-lasting than those formed with normal variants. During this time, the chaperones keep trying to refold the abnormal variants into the correct (and hence exportable) configuration, but eventually it is recognized that the chaperones will not be successful. These still incorrectly folded abnormal variant hERG proteins are then sent to the proteasome for destruction.

4.7.2   Drug-induced Trafficking Deficiencies

So far in our discussions, drug-induced reductions of hERG current have resulted from drug influence on the activity of hERG channels that are located, as they should be, within the cell's plasma membrane. It has become clear, however, that this is not the only mechanism of action for a drug-induced reduction in hERG current.

Another possible reason for an overall reduction in hERG current is that the drug may lead to a protein trafficking deficiency. If the expected complement of normal variant hERG channels does not arrive at the plasma membrane, i.e., if something causes deficiencies in protein trafficking, the expected total amount of hERG current flowing into the cell will be reduced. Inherited abnormal hERG variants with protein trafficking deficiencies were discussed in the last section. The question of interest in this section is: using our knowledge of the quality control mechanisms discussed in the previous section, how might a drug lead to acquired (drug-induced) deficiencies? One possibility that suggests itself is that a drug might have an effect on the chaperone proteins, such that they are no longer able to aid normal variant hERG proteins to fold correctly, and thus to be exported to the Golgi apparatus and on to the plasma membrane. If these chaperones can indeed be nontarget biological structures, drugs interacting with them and inhibiting their processing of normal variant hERG proteins would lead to a protein trafficking deficiency, a reduction in cell surface expression of KCNH2/hERG (a reduction in plasma membrane hERG channels), a reduction in hERG current, and ultimately a novel form of acquired LQTS (Ficker et al., 2005).

This possibility has been realized. Arsenic trioxide (As_2O_3) is used in the treatment of one form of leukemia, and it was the first identified example of a therapeutic drug that causes acquired LQTS not by direct blockade of hERG channels but by inhibition of hERG protein maturation. Productive folding and maturation of hERG proteins are controlled by a cytosolic chaperone called Hsp90. It appears that Hsp90 is a nontarget biological structure for arsenic trioxide, which interferes with its ability to form a complex with hERG proteins. This leads to a reduction in productively folded and matured hERG proteins and to the cascade of events described at the end of the previous paragraph.

The occurrence of a torsadogenic liability that results not from blockade of hERG channels but from a hERG protein trafficking deficiency is both illuminating and concerning. Chapter 6 discusses research performed in nonclinical development to (attempt to) identify torsadogenic liability. Because the near-exclusive mechanism of action of drugs known to cause drug-induced TdP has been drug-induced hERG channel blockade, the safety-testing assays currently used for identification of torsadogenic liability are designed to identify drug molecules that are likely to lead to such a blockade. In contrast, the experimental methodology used to identify this drug-induced trafficking deficiency involved other sophisticated procedures developed for this purpose. It is not known whether the gold standard assay for identifying blockade-driven torsadogenic liability (the patch clamp assay: see Chapter 6) would have identified this trafficking deficiency-driven liability. As Ficker et al. (2005, p. 68) rather disconcertingly concluded their chapter:

> Thus, the important question arises at to whether we would have identified the "true" cardiac liability of As_2O_3 using common hERG safety assays. And, even more importantly, how many other drugs are right now being developed or are already on the market that impair hERG trafficking? Given current safety testing standards, we just cannot know!

4.8   CARDIAC AND CARDIOVASCULAR DISEASES

This section is the beginning of the second part of this chapter, which is considerably shorter than the first part. Up to this point, we have focused on proarrhythmic cardiac safety and discussed cardiac pathophysiology related to torsadogenic liability in some detail. This strategy was employed since readers may be relatively unfamiliar with this material. In contrast, the cardiac diseases discussed next, diseases that fall within the realm of generalized cardiac safety, are likely more familiar to readers, and so they have been addressed more succinctly.

4.9   HYPERTENSION

Hypertension is the most common cardiovascular disease in the United States and many other industrialized countries: it affects approximately 1 billion individuals worldwide (JNC 7, 2004). A recent estimate is that 72 million individuals in the United States have hypertension (American Heart Association/American Stroke Association, 2007).

Two characteristics make hypertension particularly dangerous. First, it has no direct symptoms: an individual can have high blood pressure for years without being aware of this condition (hypertension is often discovered while visiting the doctor for another complaint). Second, it contributes strongly to the etiology of several other cardiovascular diseases. Together, these characteristics mean that considerable organ damage can occur during the time that hypertension remains undetected. Therefore, while relatively few people die from hypertension *per se*, it is nonetheless a very serious condition.

The Seventh Report of the Joint National Committee on Prevention, Detection, Evaluation, and Treatment of High Blood Pressure (JNC 7: National Institutes of Health, 2004) is a definitive publication concerning the treatment (behavioral and pharmacological) of high blood pressure. It provides the following blood pressure classifications for adult blood pressures:

➢ Normal: SBP <120 mmHg and DBP <80 mmHg.
➢ Prehypertension: SBP 120–139 mmHg or DBP 80–89 mmHg.
➢ Stage 1 Hypertension: SBP 140–159 mmHg or DBP 90–99 mmHg.
➢ Stage 2 Hypertension: SBP ≥160 mmHg or DBP ≥100 mmHg.

These classifications are related to management strategies for high blood pressure. This report is the first of the committee's series of reports to use the term prehypertension, a term introduced to signal the need for increased awareness among and education of health care professionals and the general public to reduce blood pressure before it reaches the levels in the hypertensive categories. The relationship between blood pressure and the risk of cardiovascular disease events is "continuous, consistent, and independent of other risk factors. The higher the BP, the greater is the chance of heart attack, heart failure, stroke, and kidney disease" (JNC 7 Express, 2003, p. 2). (Note: the Express version was published in 2003, ahead of the "Full" version in 2004.) Thus, while the classifications provided are useful for directing the management of blood pressure by clinicians who have to make a "treat/do not treat" decision for each patient, it should be recognized that while a blood pressure of 135/85 mmHg falls in the prehypertensive classification, and therefore does not reach the Stage 1 Hypertension classification, it carries a higher risk than lower pressures within the same classification.

There is a simple and straightforward relationship between blood pressure and life expectancy: as blood pressure increases, life expectancy decreases. The simple rule is, therefore, the lower your blood pressure the better.

4.9.1   Hypertension and Organ Damage

The JNC 7 (2004) reviewed the association of hypertension and organ damage. Ischemic heart disease is the most common form of target organ damage associated with hypertension (JNC 7, 2004). Heart failure (see Section 4.11), in the form of systolic or diastolic ventricular dysfunction, results primarily from systolic hypertension (a condition in which SBP is considerably elevated while DBP is relatively normal) and ischemic heart disease.

4.10   CORONARY HEART DISEASE

Coronary heart disease, also called coronary artery disease, typically occurs when the supply of blood to the heart muscle is reduced or completely stopped by the process of atherosclerosis.

Histological examination reveals concentric regions in arteries: the intima, media, and adventitia. Atherosclerosis is "a disease primarily involving pathologic changes in the intima, with reactive changes in media and adventitia" (Blackshear and Kantor, 2007, p. 699). The coronary arteries are among those in which the prevalence of atherosclerotic lesions is highest. Major independent risk factors for the development of atherosclerosis include hypertension, advancing age, smoking, low plasma high-density lipoprotein cholesterol (HDLc), and elevated plasma total and low-density lipoprotein cholesterol (LDLc) (Blackshear and Kantor, 2007).

The buildup of deposits of fatty substances (plaques) within an artery can cause partial blockage. Additionally, plaques can burst, tear, or rupture, leading to the formation of a blood clot that can fully block the artery. The small diameter of coronary arteries means that these vessels can be relatively easily blocked by atherosclerotic and thrombotic events. This can result in angina and myocardial infarction.

4.10.1   Angina Pectoris

Angina refers to chest pains caused when the myocardium does not receive enough blood and oxygen. When a muscle does not receive enough oxygen a condition called ischemia occurs. Ischemia can be very painful, and chest pain is common during myocardial ischemia. The full medical term for angina is angina pectoris, which literally means pain in the chest. This pain is often described as a heavy, crushing pain in the chest, but it can also extend to the shoulders, neck, jaw, back, and arms, especially the left arm.

Chronic stable angina can occur during physical activity and can be precipitated by cold temperatures or carbohydrate-rich meals. The pain of chronic stable angina usually develops over a period of about 10 to 30 seconds and usually is relieved over a period of about 5 to 15 minutes. Levels of angina are defined by duration and intensity as graded by the Canadian Cardiovascular Society classification system, a modification of the New York Heart Association functional classification (see Chen and Brozovich, 2007, p. 796).

Myocardial ischemia can result from an increased myocardial oxygen demand or a decreased myocardial oxygen supply. Angina resulting from an increased oxygen requirement can be termed demand or fixed-threshold angina. Angina resulting from a transiently decreased oxygen supply can be termed supply or variable-threshold angina (Chen and Brozovich, 2007).

4.10.2   Myocardial Infarction

Myocardial infarctions (heart attacks, also known as coronary occlusions) are the single biggest killer of both men and women in the United States. About 1.5 million heart attacks occur each year, and about 500,000 of these are fatal. The term infarct refers to an area of tissue that has suffered permanent injury and died because it did not get enough blood (and hence oxygen). This occurs if the oxygen supply is cut off for more than a few minutes (American Heart Association/American Stroke Association, 2007). The area of myocardium damaged by a heart attack depends on which coronary artery was blocked.

The typical pain from a heart attack may feel like angina at first, but usually becomes more widespread, more severe, and lasts longer. Heart attack victims often experience weakness, sweating, and a fear of dying in addition to their chest pain. However, if only a small area of myocardium dies, it may cause relatively little chest pain that may be mistaken for heartburn. Other people can have a small heart attack without experiencing any pain. People who survive a heart attack are at risk for developing several complications, including arrhythmias and heart failure.

4.11   HEART FAILURE

Rodeheffer and Redfield (2007, p. 1101) commented as follows concerning heart failure:

> Classically, heart failure has been defined as the pathophysiological state in which an abnormality of cardiac function is responsible for failure of the heart to pump blood at a rate commensurate with the requirements of the metabolizing tissues [recall discussions in Section 3.1], or to do so only when filling pressures are excessively increased.

However, it is now recognized that ventricular dysfunction is continuous and progressive in nature, which means that not all patients with ventricular dysfunction have the clinical syndrome of heart failure. Accordingly, heart failure is now categorized into four stages that are associated with increasing morbidity and mortality:

➤ Stage A: Patients have risk factors associated with heart failure (hypertension, coronary heart disease, diabetes, obesity), but they do not have ventricular dysfunction or heart failure symptoms.
➤ Stage B: Patients have structural abnormalities, but still no heart failure symptoms.
➤ Stage C: Patients have ventricular dysfunction accompanied by symptoms of inadequate cardiac output (exercise intolerance) and/or fluid overload (congestion).
➤ Stage D: Patients have advanced symptoms and severe disability.

Mortality rates from acute coronary heart diseases have decreased in recent years due to better management. This means that individuals are surviving with chronic coronary disease and ventricular dysfunction. Coupled with the aging of the population, the decrease in mortality from myocardial infarction has led to an increased prevalence of heart failure, and this trend is likely to continue.

More than 400,000 new cases of heart failure a year are diagnosed in the United States. There are estimated to be around 3 to 5 million individuals with Stage B heart failure and 2 to 3 million with Stage C heart failure. Heart failure results in some 200,000 deaths a year (Rodeheffer and Redfield, 2007).

Heart failure dramatically impairs a person's quality of life as well as shortening their life: most people with this condition will die within five years of being diagnosed. Heart failure commonly causes several symptoms. The heart's output of blood is less than usual, so the body does not get enough oxygen. Patients with this disease typically feel tired and unable to do physical work or exercise. (See also Bock and Goode, 2006.)

4.12   Sudden Cardiac Death

Sudden cardiac death (SCD) has been defined as follows (Kanagala, 2007, p. 493):

> SCD refers to the acute and natural death from cardiac causes within a short period (often within an hour of the onset of symptoms). The time and mode of death are unexpected, and often death occurs in patients without any prior potentially fatal conditions.

The mechanisms that lead to SCD are varied and complex. Most cases of SCD are associated with underlying cardiac arrhythmias, but other causes have been identified. The following list presents various causes (Kanagala, 2007):

➢ Electrophysiological abnormalities (including abnormalities and idiopathic ventricular fibrillation).
➢ Coronary artery disease (including atherosclerotic disease).
➢ Valvular heart disease.
➢ Pulmonary hypertension.
➢ Hypertensive heart disease.
➢ Congenital heart disease.

Atherosclerotic coronary artery disease is the leading cause of SCD, which leads to an estimated 300,000 to 400,000 deaths per year. Eighty percent of fatal arrhythmias associated with SCD are caused by structural coronary arterial abnormalities and their consequences.

4.13   Further Reading

Epstein, R.J., 2003, *Human molecular biology: An introduction to the molecular basis of health and disease.* Cambridge, UK: Cambridge University Press.

American Heart Association/American Stroke Association, 2007, *Heart disease and stroke statistics: 2007 update at-a-glance.* http://www.americanheart.org/downloadable/heart/1166711577754HS_StatsInsideText.pdf, accessed November 19, 2007.

Lee, H-C., 2007, Cardiac cellular electrophysiology. In Murphy, J.G. and Lloyd, M.A. (Eds.), *Mayo Clinic cardiology: Concise textbook,* 3rd edition, Rochester, MN: Mayo Clinic Scientific Press/Informa Healthcare, 295–308.

Thygesen, K., Alpert, J.S., and White, H.D., on behalf of the Joint ESC/ACCF/AHA/WHF Task Force for the Redefinition of Myocardial Infarction, 2007, Universal definition of myocardial infarction, *Circulation.* http://circ.ahajournals.org/cgi/reprint/CIRCULATIONAHA.107.187397, accessed November 19, 2007.

Tom, C.W. and Simari, R.D., 2007, Essential molecular biology of cardiovascular diseases. In Murphy, J.G. and Lloyd, M.A. (Eds.), *Mayo Clinic cardiology: Concise textbook,* 3rd edition, Rochester, MN: Mayo Clinic Scientific Press/Informa Healthcare.

5

DRUG DISCOVERY AND DRUG DESIGN

5.1 INTRODUCTION

The goal of traditional drug discovery is to identify a lead compound, a drug molecule that is a promising candidate for progression to nonclinical testing, and then to develop the molecule into a modified molecule that has the potential to become a useful drug. This process is called lead optimization. The lead compound may be defined along the following lines: it is "a chemical entity that has known structure; high purity that reproducibly and predictably causes the desired biological effect; belongs to a chemical series that shows evidence of a structure-activity relationship (i.e., systematic structural changes lead to significant changes in activity); and has optimizable pharmacokinetics" (Rabinowitz and Shankley, 2006, pp. 61–62). The process of lead identification involves searching vast libraries of closely related molecules using high-throughput screening for time efficiency (see Homon and Nelson, 2006). However, despite the advantages of high-throughput screening, this search could be very laborious since it involves systematically evaluating thousands of potential drug candidate molecules. Historically, generating lead compounds has been more successful than lead optimization, which can be a "rate-limiting step" in drug development (Rabinowitz and Shankley, 2006, p. 63).

The more recent discipline of drug design offers the possibility of creating the optimized molecule by chemically engineering specific desirable modifications into the lead compound molecule. This chapter discusses the computer simulation research, termed *in silico* research, conducted to predict the chemical structure of the optimized molecule (it does not address the chemical processes required to create the molecule), and discussions focus on chemically "engineering safety" into small-molecule drugs.

As was the case in our discussions of the biological basis of adverse drug reactions in Chapter 2, the material in this chapter is presented from a pragmatic perspective and written for readers who are not familiar with the fundamentals of drug design. Readers who are already well versed in this field may prefer to move on to Chapter 6.

Integrated Cardiac Safety: Assessment Methodologies for Noncardiac Drugs in Discovery, Development, and Postmarketing Surveillance. By J. Rick Turner and Todd A. Durham
Copyright © 2009 John Wiley & Sons, Inc.

5.2   MEDICINAL CHEMISTRY

Norgrady and Weaver (2005, p. 6) noted that the science of medicinal chemistry provides "a molecular bridge between the basic science of biology and the clinical science of medicine." Important desired characteristics when designing or optimizing a lead molecule include the following:

> ➤ It is safe.
> ➤ It is efficacious.
> ➤ It can be manufactured in sufficiently large quantities that are financially viable (largescale manufacturing has challenges quite different from those of the relatively smallscale manufacturing that is required for nonclinical research and clinical trials).

As Breckenridge (2004, p. xi) observed, "Medicinal chemists who design drug molecules appreciate the toxicity potential of various chemical groupings in a molecule, and are increasingly able to design out the offending entity without impairing efficacy."

5.2.1   Nomenclature Considerations

Before commencing this section, a comment on our use of nomenclature is appropriate (a similar strategy was taken in Section 4.3.2 to describe this book's use of the terms KCNH2/hERG, hERG protein, hERG channel, and hERG current). Drugs can interact with many biological macromolecules. These biological macromolecules include (but are not limited to) nucleic acids, lipids, and proteins. This chapter focuses on proteins, including transmembrane receptors, ion channels, and enzymes. We will consider the identification of functional groups of a drug molecule that define three potential consequences of these interactions:

> ➤ One set of functional groups interacts with (binds with) the target drug receptor, leading to the desired therapeutic effect.
> ➤ One set may interact with nontarget macromolecules to produce an undesired effect. Proarrhythmic cardiac safety focuses on interactions with the hERG channel, an identified antitarget in this context. Generalized cardiac safety focuses on other undesired interactions that lead to cardiac adverse events.
> ➤ One set may interact with metabolic enzymes that influence the molecule's pharmacokinetic profile.

It should be noted that these functional groups are not necessarily unique in that the groups responsible for the desired therapeutic effect may also be responsible for the nontarget effects or metabolism.

To make your reading of the following material as straightforward as possible, from this point on we use the term receptor to refer to each of the biological macromolecules discussed—drug receptors, ion channels, and metabolic enzymes—with which drugs' functional groups can interact. That is, we operationally define a receptor as one of various proteins with which a drug molecule interacts. While the consequences in each case are different, each interaction is similar in that it involves the binding of a set of the drug's structural features to a macromolecule.

5.3   DRUG DESIGN: STRUCTURAL MOLECULAR ENGINEERING

An ongoing theme in this book is that knowledge of structure facilitates an understanding of function, a concept that is particularly well exemplified in the field of drug design. The starting point in contemporary small-molecule drug development is often knowledge of the molecular structure of the drug's target receptor. This knowledge facilitates attempts to maximize efficacy. Another consideration, and one that is a primary focus in our discussions of proarrhythmic cardiac safety, is to acquire and use knowledge of the structure of the hERG channel to minimize the likelihood of cardiac adverse events, i.e., to enhance safety. While our focus is on such safety considerations, it should be noted that, in reality, both of these considerations are addressed simultaneously: the goal is to engineer safety into the molecule while not decreasing its efficacy.

Given knowledge of target and nontarget receptors, knowledge of the drug molecule's chemical (molecular) structure is also needed. A drug molecule consists of many components that can have several functional groups potentially interacting with a target receptor and one or more nontarget receptors. The terms pharmacophore and toxicophore have become widely used in this regard. The term pharmacophore does not represent an actual molecule or an actual association of functional groups: rather, it is a purely abstract concept that accounts for the common molecular interaction capacities of a group of compounds towards their target receptor. It can be considered the "highest common denominator" of a group of molecules (often molecules in the same class, but not necessarily so) that are recognized by the same receptor and that therefore exhibit a similar pharmacological profile. It describes the essential (steric and electronic: see Section 5.3.2) function-determining areas that produce the greatest biological signal via an optimally energetically favorable interaction with the target receptor.

The term toxicophore is conceptualized similarly, with the important differentiation that the biological signal elicited in this case leads to an unwanted response, i.e., an adverse drug reaction. It is important to note that a drug molecule may have more than one toxicophore by virtue of interaction with several nontarget receptors. It should also be noted here that separation of the pharmacophore and toxicophore may be difficult if there are similarities between the target and nontarget receptors.

The goal in structural molecular engineering is to maintain the structural integrity of the pharmacophore and make appropriate molecular modifications to the toxicophore(s). In some instances, it may be beneficial to synthesize a related new molecule that has the structural characteristics of particular interest rather than trying to modify an existing molecule.

5.3.1   The (Conceptual) Structure of Drug Molecules

This book does not discuss interactions between drugs and receptors in chemical detail. Rather, this topic is addressed from a conceptual perspective that provides (just) enough information to allow you to follow discussion of drug design research addressing the potential for proarrhythmic cardiac adverse drug reactions. In this light, a conceptual definition provided by Norgrady and Weaver (2005, p. 10) is useful: a drug molecule "possesses one or more functional groups positioned in three-dimensional space on a structural framework that holds the functional groups in a defined geometrical array that allows the molecule to bind specifically to a targeted biological molecule." Like receptors, drug molecules are three-dimensional, and interactions between drug molecules and receptors occur in three-dimensional space. The structural arrangement of atoms within the molecule influences the "geometry of approach" as the drug molecule enters the microenvironment of the receptor (Norgrady and Weaver, 2005, p. 23).

Given our focus on small-molecule drugs, the following characteristics are noteworthy. Small-molecule drugs are composed of the following components:

> ➤ A relatively rigid structural framework or backbone, typically an organic (carbon-based) backbone. The relative rigidity of the backbone ensures that the three-dimensional geometry of the molecule does not alter too much.
> ➤ One or more functional groups that are held together on a backbone. These functional groups determine the chemical and physical properties of molecules.

These characteristics are important in facilitating the possible interactions between drug molecules and receptors. The relative rigidity of the backbone ensures that the molecule's functional groups are positioned in three-dimensional space in a specific geometrical array. The ability of a drug molecule to dock with a receptor is facilitated when the molecular geometries of the drug's functional groups and the receptor's functional groups are complementary. This docking, also known as binding, allows the electrons of the drug's functional groups to interact with the electrons of the receptor's functional groups in an energetically favorable manner. When the drug has an energetically favorable interaction with a target receptor, the consequent biological signals result in the drug's desired effects, i.e., its efficacy. When the drug has an energetically favorable interaction with a nontarget receptor, the consequent biological signals result in adverse drug reactions.

5.3.2   Properties of Drug Molecules

Drug molecules have several properties that are of relevance in beneficial pharmaceutical therapy and in their elicitation of adverse drug reactions. Turner (2007) summarized these properties as discussed by Norgrady and Weaver (2005):

> ➤ Physiochemical. Physiochemical properties impact a drug's solubility and pharmacokinetic characteristics, influencing the drug's ability to reach the microenvironment of the receptor.
> ➤ Shape and stereochemical. These properties describe the relative structural arrangement of the drug molecule's constituent atoms, and influence the molecule's final approach toward and interactions with the receptor.
> ➤ Electronic. Electronic properties also affect the drug molecule's interaction with the receptors. The electronic properties of a molecule are governed by the distribution of electrons within the molecule. These properties determine the exact nature of the binding interaction that occurs between the drug molecule and the receptor and the degree to which the interaction is energetically favorable. The energetic exchange that occurs between the drug molecule and the receptor determines the strength of the biological signal that is generated. It is this signal that initiates (in the case of agonists) or inhibits (in the case of antagonists) a cascade of biological signals that result in the physiological (pharmacological) effects of the drug.

Consideration of these properties makes it apparent that the basic scientific disciplines of physics, chemistry, and biology can all contribute considerably to an understanding of drug responses. The contributions of some newer scientific disciplines to drug design are discussed in Sections 5.4 and 5.5.

5.3.3   Removing Toxicophores

The concept of engineering safety into a drug molecule was discussed earlier when describing the molecular design aspects of lessening a drug molecule's adverse effects. An alternative phrase that suggests itself in the context of present discussions is "engineering toxicophores out of a drug molecule." The concept of engineering out toxicophores appears to fit well with the intent of safety-related drug molecule design, i.e., removing (or functionally disabling) an arrangement of atoms and electronic forces within a molecule that lead to unwanted effects while maintaining the molecule's ability to reach the vicinity of its target receptor and to present its pharmacophore to the receptor in the necessary three-dimensional geometric array.

5.3.4   Consideration of Drug Absorption and Metabolism

While our focus in this chapter lies with removing toxicophores to prevent adverse drug reactions, it is instructive to consider two other aspects of successful drug therapy that also relate directly to the molecular structure of the drug. These are drug absorption and drug metabolism.

Rolan and Molnar (2006) noted that poor absorption is still frequently encountered in clinical drug development since the traditional drug discovery processes that led to the investigational drugs in question were chosen more for *in vitro* potency and selectivity characteristics than favorable absorption characteristics. This strategy can result in compounds that perform very well in these *in vitro* environments during early drug development but result in major bioavailability or formulation problems later in the process. More recently, as noted by Rolan and Molnar (2006, p. 125), "some companies have been successful in reducing the proportion of poorly absorbed candidates progressing from the discovery stage to preclinical development by the use of *in silico* and *in vitro* technologies that aim to predict the absorption of drugs in humans."

In the case of orally administered drugs (the preferred method of drug administration, when possible, and the most common form), the drug molecule must be absorbed through the intestinal wall and then successfully survive the first-pass metabolism that attempts to neutralize this xenobiotic invader, where "successfully" means that at least an adequate percentage of the drug administered actually reaches the target receptor in a chemical state that is able to elicit the desired biological response. Therefore, in addition to engineering out toxicophores and maintaining pharmacophores, the drug design engineers must also preserve the drug molecule's ability to reach its target receptor intact or without metabolic changes to the pharmacophore.

With regard to a potential drug molecule's absorption, it would be useful if absorption could be predicted via *in silico* modeling during drug design: as Li and Hidalgo (2006, p. 178) noted, "the labor involved in generating experimental data to estimate drug absorption potential is substantial. Therefore, the possibility of developing computer programs capable of predicting drug absorption is very attractive." An initial strategy here is to rule out or at least identify compounds that are likely to present absorption problems. The application of Lipinski's "rule of 5" is usefully employed here as a first screen to remove from consideration molecules that have a high probably of not being successfully absorbed based on generalizations about drug structure and properties described in Section 5.3.2. (This methodology is beyond the scope of this chapter, and readers are referred to Lipinski et al., 2001, for further information.)

However, while this initial strategy can work well, progress from that point on can be slow, since "permeability and absorption are not basic properties of the molecules determined by the chemical structure, and therefore predictable by using chemical predictors alone" (Li and Hidalgo, 2006, p. 178). Permeability and absorption are influenced by several factors, including pH levels and the precise nature of a drug's formulation. Despite these challenges, however, some progress has been made in this area, and several molecular descriptors have proved useful to a certain extent in predicting permeability and absorption parameters.

The term metabophore is used to describe the three-dimensional arrangement of atoms within the molecule that is responsible for the molecule's metabolic properties or potential once it is absorbed. The metabophore defines the substrate specificity of the xenobiotic metabolizing enzyme that may prevent a drug from reaching its target or nontarget receptor(s). Drug-metabolizing enzymes can be considered nontarget receptors that bind and metabolize a drug based upon its enzyme-specific metabophore. Having a successful metabolic profile with regard to its desired pharmacodynamic effect is therefore an important characteristic of the lead molecule.

Optimal drug design is therefore extremely complex: attempting to predict the absorption, metabolism, efficacy, and safety of a drug-like molecule is not a trivial undertaking. The following sections address the basics of *in silico* modeling, but it is appropriate here to note that knowledge of pharmaceutics (the formulation of a drug such that it is absorbed successfully) and pharmacokinetics (what the body does to the drug) is useful in addition to considerations relating to the drug's pharmacodynamic and/or toxicodynamic activity. Research scientists involved in drug design and development are aware that understanding pharmacokinetic and concentration-response relationships is extremely beneficial, and knowledge from these areas is now being applied extensively in this area (Tozer and Rowland, 2006).

5.4   BIOINFORMATICS

In vitro and nonhuman *in vivo* testing have long been the traditional means of evaluating responses to a drug molecule before considering the commencement of clinical trials. As noted in Section 5.1, however, the traditional drug discovery process is particularly arduous. Contemporary drug design is quite different thanks to two disciplines that have converged in pharmaceutical research, namely, molecular biology and computer-based information technology. An ever-increasing knowledge of the chemical structure of molecules of interest (including small-molecule drugs and their receptors) facilitates the study of the molecule's function and action. However, the sheer volume of the information necessary to begin to understand and eventually to predict the likely interaction between a drug molecule and a receptor is daunting.

The advent of powerful computing systems has proved invaluable in this regard. The discipline of bioinformatics is essentially a biological field with massive data sets that require enormous computing power to analyze. The importance of bioinformatics was addressed by Bader and Enright (2005, p. 254):

> Bioinformatics will play a vital role in overcoming this data integration and modeling challenge, because databases, visualization software, and analysis software must be built to enable data assimilation and to make the results accessible and useful for answering biological questions.

The phenomenal growth in information from molecular biological studies includes detailed knowledge of many functional aspects of biology: how genetic material codes for the production of proteins; knowledge of the structure and function of proteins; how proteins create metabolic pathways; and how environmental factors affect the phenotypic expression of a person's genotype to create a unique individual human being with a unique set of metabolic pathways. The combination of detailed biological and chemical data and the advancement in computing systems (often sophisticated networks of relatively small computers rather than very powerful individual machines) has facilitated the development of bioinformatics as a powerful interpretational tool.

High-quality structural models can reveal an enormous amount of biologically important information concerning the function of a protein, how it is related to other proteins, and with what receptor a drug molecule may or may not interact. Going one step further, it may provide information relevant to identifying the actual site on the receptor with which the drug molecule binds. Bioinformatics is therefore of considerable benefit in proteomic and pharmacoproteomic research.

Structural bioinformatics and functional bioinformatics are powerful allies in deciphering the information coded in a protein's primary sequence of amino acid residues and thus predicting, or modeling, the protein's structure and function. Since so many drug receptors are proteins, greater knowledge of the structure of the proteins will improve our ability to design drug candidates that may interact with these receptors in a beneficial therapeutic manner. While still far from perfect, *in silico* methods of predicting secondary structure and solvent accessibility using only a protein's primary sequence have matured considerably in recent years (Ofran and Rost, 2005). The ability to predict tertiary structure is currently less well developed but is improving.

5.5   COMPUTER-ASSISTED MOLECULAR DESIGN

One application of this knowledge base and computing power is computer-aided molecular design. Models of particular cellular structures such as drug target and nontarget receptors can be generated and used in hypothesis testing using *in silico* approaches. *In silico* development focuses on many aspects of the molecule, including its ability to reach the region of the drug receptor, its ability to approach and bind with the receptor, and, in particular, with the precise nature of the binding interaction with the target receptor. Therefore, before drug molecule synthesis, extensive computer modeling takes place in an attempt to identify a molecule that has a high probability of achieving the desired interaction with a target receptor and a low probability of leading to adverse drug reactions. The results of such simulation experiments can potentially identify a novel drug molecule that is safe and efficacious relatively more easily, cheaply, and quickly than other approaches in drug discovery.

It should be noted here that engineering out toxicophores can be considerably harder than engineering in pharmacophores, especially at the beginning of the process. While the single target receptor is known, there is an enormous range of nontarget receptors. Some functional groups on a drug molecule may be known to comprise a toxicophore that should be avoided when designing any new drug. In contrast, there is always the possibility that a functional group on a new molecule will react with a known nontarget receptor in an unexpected and undesirable manner, or that it will interact in an undesirable manner with a previously unidentified receptor. Engineering out toxicodynamic groups can perhaps be more readily achieved when the mechanism of action of a given adverse drug reaction is known and separable from the mechanism of action of the desired response. This may be achieved either by limiting drug access to the location of the nontarget receptor or by increasing the drug specificity for the target versus nontarget receptor.

5.5.1   Future Advancements in *in Silico* Methodologies

Gallion et al. (2005, p. 155) noted that "The ability to extrapolate from *in silico* experimentation to human trials remains a formidable challenge." Additionally, these authors commented that "one of the greatest challenges in research will be facilitating a cultural acceptance of *in silico* optimization schemes" (Gallion et al., 2005, p. 141). To fulfill their potential, *in silico* modeling and other computational approaches used in predicting the characteristics of drug-like molecules will require the development of extremely large databases of high quality and diverse information. Nonetheless, despite these challenges, *in silico* modeling may be extremely informative in the future. As Gallion et al. (2005, p. 155) observed, "As the science evolves, it is hoped that future lead optimization activities will be guided less by intuition and more by information."

5.6   *IN SILICO* MODELING AND THE hERG CHANNEL

The previous sections in this chapter have outlined in general terms the *in silico* approach to drug development, with a focus on drug safety. Attention now turns to drug cardiac safety and specifically to proarrhythmic cardiac safety. As it happens, computational evaluation and prediction has been used more in cardiotoxicity than in other areas of safety pharmacology. For the remainder of this chapter, we focus on *in silico* modeling conducted in one specific area of cardiotoxicity: torsadogenic liability. This research attempts to predict whether a new drug molecule is likely to interact with the hERG cardiac potassium ion channel in a torsadogenic manner.

Mitcheson et al. (2005, p. 137) commented as follows:

> The diversity of compounds that block hERG and therefore are at risk of causing LQTS is one of the most extraordinary features of this channel. To date, based on chemical structure alone, it has not been possible to predict whether new compounds have the potential to block hERG...Clearly, a detailed understanding of the structural basis for the binding of compounds to hERG could facilitate the development of an *in silico* screening tool.

The crystallographic structure of the (human) hERG channel is not yet known, so currently available x-ray solved structures from other species can be useful. Examples of these include the bacterial MthK and KcsA potassium channels from *Methanobacterium thermoautotrophicum* and *Streptomyces lividans*, respectively (see Recanatini et al., 2005). These potassium channels belong to the 2TM family. This nomenclature refers to the fact that 2TM channels have two transmembrane segments, called M1 and M2. As described in Section 3.10.1, the hERG channel is a tetrameric structure comprised of four α-subunits, each of which has six transmembrane segments. MthK and KcsA are also tetrameric structures, with each tetramer containing an M1 and an M2 transmembrane segment that has a membrane-reentrant pore loop between them. These segments function very much as the S5 and S6 transmembrane segments do in hERG, forming the pore through which the K^+ ions flow. Segments M1 and M2 have a linker between them, as do hERG channel S5 and S6 segments. The M1-linker-pore-M2 region of MthK and KcsA is therefore (somewhat) similar to the S5-linker-pore-S6 region of the hERG channel. Our knowledge of the structure of bacterial ion channels in developing *in silico* models for the human potassium channel of interest is discussed further in Section 5.6.2.

Recanatini et al. (2005) provided a useful summary of *in silico* modeling pertaining to the hERG channel's structure and functioning, its drug-binding abilities, and its torsadogenic liability. This current overview is based largely on their chapter, with additional material from Triggle et al. (2006). The overview discusses two modelling strategies in computational drug design: the ligand-based approach and the target-based approach.

5.6.1   The Ligand-based Approach

If researchers have information about molecules that display the biological property of interest (in this case, hERG channel block and hence a reduction in hERG current) but not about the receptor with which it interacts (in this case, the antitarget hERG channel), the ligand-based approach is employed. The ligand-based modeling strategy focuses on the drug molecule, or more precisely the molecule's pharmacophore, or toxicophore as the case may be, that leads to the energetic interaction between the molecule and the receptor. This is most simply done by identifying the required functional groups for a particular biological response. These observations are collectively known as structure-activity relationships (SARs) for a particular biological response. These SARs can be further defined by mathematical models that are derived from a known set of compounds with known physicochemical properties (the test set) that produce a measurable biological response in quantitative structure-activity relationship (QSAR) studies. Such QSAR studies utilize regression analysis to identify shared characteristics of the test set of compounds and mathematically relate these characteristics to the measured biological response. This is particularly valuable in developing an understanding of the required receptor interactions without specific knowledge of the receptor's structure. Ideally, QSAR equations facilitate the identification of novel compounds of interest that should be evaluated for the desired biological response. Unlike QSAR, which relates physicochemical properties to biological activity, three-dimensional QSAR (3D-QSAR) is a newer method that relates three-dimensional properties of a compound to biological activity. Three-dimensional QSAR is useful in pharmacophore identification. (See Recanatini and Cavalli, 2008).

A QT/hERG toxicophore (sometimes called a QT/hERG pharmacophore in the literature, since a toxicophore is simply a pharmacophore that leads to an undesired response) can be conceptualized as a three-dimensional arrangement of functional groups that interacts with the hERG channel and leads to QT interval prolongation. In Section 5.3 we noted that a pharmacophore can be considered as the highest common denominator of a group of molecules that are recognized by the same receptor and that therefore exhibit a similar pharmacological profile. We also noted that such molecules are often molecules in the same class but that this is not necessarily so. As we subsequently saw in the previous section, the phenomenon of hERG channel block and the accompanying torsadogenic risk is one where many chemically diverse compounds have a similar effect.

Researchers have derived *in silico* models that attempt to identify a pharmacophore and then quantitatively predict hERG channel block. Three-dimensional QSAR models for hERG current inhibition have been created based on different sets of drugs that are known to lead to QT prolongation via hERG channel blockade. Elkins et al. (2002; see Recanatini et al., 2005, p. 174) built a model of the General hERG Pharmacophore. This pharmacophore model consisted of one positively ionizable feature (likely the basic nitrogen component common to all the drugs upon which the model was based) that forms the central functional group, and four hydrophobic centers, not all of which were necessarily present in all of the drugs upon which the model was built. Another model containing very similar features was built independently by Cavalli et al. (2002; see Recanatini et al., 2005, p. 174). This model consisted of a protonated (positively charged) nitrogen functional group and three aromatic (hydrophobic) moieties. The notable difference between the two models is the position of the central cationic functional group in relation to the surrounding hydrophobic moieties. Recanatini et al. (2005) speculated that this difference may arise because the pharmacophores may originate from a different three-dimensional orientation due to a folded molecular conformation in one case and an extended conformation in the other (as noted previously, drug molecules, like biological structures, are three-dimensional structures).

5.6.2   The Target-based Approach

If researchers also have information about the three-dimensional receptor upon which a drug acts, the target-based approach can employed. This approach allows ligand-docking models to be constructed.

Since experimental determination of the hERG channel's complete three-dimensional structure has proved so difficult, computer modeling procedures have been used in attempts to obtain a three-dimensional model of the protein complex that constitutes the hERG channel, i.e., a "3D description of this important pharmacological anti-target" (Recanatini et al., 2005, p. 175). Some of these approaches start with the known structures of the bacterial potassium channels MthK and KcsA. These structures act as the starting template in homology modeling, and useful templates are those that possess as much similarity to the expected structure of hERG as possible. This similarity extends both to aspects of the overall architecture of the channel and to similarities in amino acid residue sequences in the respective protein components of the channels.

When discussing the conceptual structure of small-molecule drugs in Section 5.3.1, we noted the following properties. First, they have a relatively rigid structural framework or backbone, the relative rigidity of which ensures that the three-dimensional geometry of the molecule does not alter too much. Second, they have one or more functional groups that are held together on the backbone, and these functional groups determine the properties of the molecule. An analogous conceptual approach can be useful when thinking about creating an *in silico* representation of hERG. First, attention needs to be paid to building (deriving) a backbone comprised of protein subunits and their assembly into a tetrameric system. This attention can lead to a preliminary structure that then requires considerable refinement. One issue concerns just how well the M1-linker-pore-M2 regions of MthK and KcsA channels model the S5-linker-pore-S6 region of the hERG channel. There is certainly a functional similarity in that these regions form the respective central pores through which K^+ ions flow. However, the S5-S6 linker in the hERG channel is longer than related linkers in other potassium channels, and its sequence of amino acid residues also differs. This makes modeling the electrostatic characteristics and properties of the critical pore region particularly difficult. The amino acid composition and orientation of the actual central pore cavity then need attention.

Another important issue that needs addressing in simulation models is the role played by, and hence the influence of, transmembrane segments S1-S4 in hERG: these segments are not present in members of the 2TM family of ion channels such as the MthK and KcsA channels. We saw in Section 3.10.1 that transmembrane segments S1-S4 (and particularly segment S4) function as the voltage sensor for hERG. While the hERG channel binding with drugs occurs in the pore region, it is therefore critical to incorporate influences of transmembrane segments S1-S4 in the overall *in silico* simulation model, perhaps with particular attention being paid to their role in the structural stability of the channel. As we noted earlier for small-molecule drugs, maintaining their three-dimensional structure and orientation is crucial to their functional performance.

Finally, as if there were not enough complexity already, attention also needs to be paid to potential influences from the plasma membrane, a "hydrated phospholipid bilayer" in which the hERG channel is embedded (Recanatini et al., 2005, p. 180). Thus, while reductionism is certainly informative, allowing detailed focus on specific parts of the overall puzzle, a holistic approach is ultimately needed. Recanatini and colleagues' conclusion to their chapter deserves to be quoted directly (Recanatini et al., 2005, p. 180):

> Computational ligand- and target-based methods are emerging as useful tools to interpret at the physicochemical and atomic level the characteristics of the hERG K^+ channel and the hERG-blocking drugs. It has been shown that the integration of computational, electrophysiological and mutagenic studies can be truly synergistic in providing clues as to the behaviour of this complex system. It might be advanced that, through some more deepened methodological and computational efforts, modelling studies on hERG will lead to accurate predictions of both channel-functioning and drug-binding ability, which are the final goals of any investigation on this K^+ channel.

5.7   FURTHER READING

The items in this Further Reading section are listed chronologically rather than alphabetically to chronicle the development of the various specialties discussed. Representative articles from an array of journals have been included to indicate the range of sources of such information.

5.7.1   Books

Baxevanis, A.D. and Ouellette, B.F.F. (Eds.), 2005, *Bioinformatics: A practical guide to the analysis of genes and proteins,* 3rd edition, Hoboken, NJ: John Wiley & Sons.

Handen, J.S. (Ed.), 2005, *Industrialization of drug discovery: From target selection through lead optimization*, Boca Raton, FL: CRC Press/Taylor & Francis.

Fischer, J. and Ganellin, C.R. (Eds.), 2006, *Analogue-based drug discovery*, Weinheim, Germany: Wiley-VCH.

Florence, A.T. and Attwood, D., 2006, *Physiochemical principles of pharmacy*, 4th edition, London: Pharmaceutical Press.

Langer, T. and Hoffmann, R.D. (Eds.), 2006, *Pharmacophores and pharmacophore searches*, Weinheim, Germany: Wiley-VCH.

Rang, H.P. (Ed.), 2006, *Drug discovery and development: Technology in transition*, Philadelphia: Churchill Livingstone/Elsevier.

Smith, C.G. and O'Donnell, J.T. (Eds.), 2006, *The process of new drug discovery and development,* 2nd edition, New York: Informa Healthcare.

Tsai, C.S., 2006, *Biomacromolecules: Introduction to structure, function, and informatics*, Hoboken, NJ: John Wiley & Sons.

Hu, X. and Pan, Y. (Eds.), 2007, *Knowledge discovery in bioinformatics: Techniques, methods, and applications*, Hoboken, NJ: John Wiley & Sons.

Huang, Z., 2007, *Drug discovery research: New frontiers in the post-genomic era*, Hoboken, NJ: John Wiley & Sons.

van Eyk, J.E. and Dunn, M.J. (Eds.), 2007, *Clinical proteomics: From diagnosis to therapy*, Weinheim, Germany: Wiley-VCH.

Walsh, G., 2007, *Pharmaceutical biotechnology: Concepts and applications*, Chichester, UK: John Wiley & Sons.

Dale, J.W. and von Schantz, M., 2008, *From genes to genomes: Concepts and applications of DNA technology,* 2nd edition, Hoboken, NJ: John Wiley & Sons.

Ye, S.Q. (Ed.), 2008, *Bioinformatics: A practical approach*, Boca Raton, FL: Chapman & Hall/CRC.

5.7.2 Journal Articles

Elkins, S., Crumb, W.J., Sarazan, R.D., Wikel, J.H., and Wrighton, S.A., 2002, Three-dimensional quantitative structure-activity relationship for inhibition of human ether-a-go-go-related gene potassium channel, *Journal of Pharmacology and Experimental Therapeutics*, 301:427–434.

van der Waterbeemd, H. and Gifford, E., 2003, ADMET *in silico* modelling: Towards prediction paradise? *Nature Reviews Drug Discovery*, 2:192–204.

Contrera, J.F., Matthews, E.J., Kruhlak, N.L., and Benz, D.R., 2004, Estimating the safe starting dose in phase I clinical trials and no observed effect level based on QSAR modeling of the human maximum recommended daily dose, *Regulatory Toxicology and Pharmacology*, 3:185–206.

Egan, W.J., Zlokarnik, G., and Grootenhuis, P.D.J., 2004, *In silico* prediction of drug safety: Despite progress there is abundant room for improvement, *Drug Discovery Today: Technologies*, 1:381–387.

ten Tusscher, K.H., Noble, D., Nobel, P.J., and Panfilov, A.V., 2004, A model for human ventricular tissue, *American Journal of Physiology: Heart and Circulatory Physiology,* 286:H1573–H1589.

Bergstrom, C.A., 2005, Computational models to predict aqueous drug solubility, permeability and intestinal absorption, *Expert Opinion on Drug Metabolism and Toxicity,* 1:613–627.

Delaney, J.S., 2005, Predicting aqueous solubility from structure, *Drug Discovery Today*, 10:289–295.

Magna, N., Duffy, J.C., Rowe, P.H., and Cronin, M.T., 2005, Structure-based methods for the prediction of the dominant P450 enzyme in human drug transformation: Consideration of CYP3A4, CYP2C9, and CYP2D6, *SAR and QSAR in Environmental Research,* 16:43–61.

Marrero-Ponce, Y., Iyarreta-Veitia, M., Montero-Torres, A., et al., 2005, Ligand-based virtual screening and *in silico* design of new antimalarial compounds using nonstochastic and stochastic total and atom-type quadratic maps, *Chemical Information and Modeling,* 45:1082–1100.

Vedani, A., Dobler, M., and Lill, M.A., 2005, *In silico* prediction of harmful effects triggered by drugs and chemicals, *Toxicology and Applied Pharmacology*, 207: 398–407.

Balakin, K.V., Savchuk, N.P., and Tetko, I.V., 2006, *In silico* approaches to prediction of aqueous and DMSO solubility of drug-like compounds: Trends, problems, and solutions, *Current Medicinal Chemistry*, 13:223–241.

Brown, H.S., Galetin, A., Hallifax, D., and Houston, J.B., 2006, Prediction of *in vivo* drug-drug interactions from *in vitro* data: Factors affecting prototypic drug-drug interactions involving CYP2C9, CYP2D6, and CYP3A4, *Clinical Pharmacokinetics*, 45:1035–1050.

Jalaie, M. and Shanmugasundaram, V., 2006, Virtual screening: Are we there yet? *Mini Reviews in Medicinal Chemistry*, 6:1159–1167.

Ji, Z.L., Wang, Y., Yu, L., et al., 2006, *In silico* search of putative adverse drug reaction related proteins as a potential tool for facilitating drug adverse effect prediction, *Toxicology Letters*, 164:104–112.

Michelson, S., Sehgal, A., and Friedrich, C., 2006, *In silico* prediction of clinical efficacy, *Current Opinion in Biotechnology*, 17:666–670.

Rodriguez, B., Trayanova, N., and Noble, D., 2006, Modeling cardiac ischemia, *Annals of the New York Academy of Sciences*, 1080:395–414.

Sarai, N., Matsuoka, S., and Noma, A., 2006, simBio: A Java package for the development of detailed cell models, *Progress in Biophysics and Molecular Biology*, 90:360–377.

Vedani, A., Dobler, M., and Lill, M.A., 2006, The challenge of predicting drug toxicity *in silico*, *Basic and Clinical Pharmacology and Toxicology*, 99: 195–208.

Bender, A., Scheiber, J., Glick, M., et al., 2007, Analysis of pharmacology data and the prediction of adverse drug reactions and off-target effects from chemical structure, *ChemMedChem*, 2:861–873.

Cavero, I., 2007, Using pharmacokinetic/pharmacodynamic modelling in safety pharmacology to better define safety margins: A regional workshop of the Safety Pharmacology Society, *Expert Opinion on Drug Safety*, 6:465–471.

Dokoumetzidis, A., Kalantzi, L., and Fotaki, N., 2007, Predictive models for oral drug absorption: From *in silico* methods to integrated dynamical models, *Expert Opinion on Drug Metabolism and Toxicology*, 3:491–505.

Du, L., Li, M., You, Q., and Xia, L., 2007, A novel structure-based virtual screening model for the hERG channel blockers, *Biochemical and Biophysical Research Communications,* 355:889–894.

Elkins, S., Mestres, J., and Testa, B., 2007, *In silico* pharmacology for drug discovery: Applications to targets and beyond, *British Journal of Pharmacology,* 152:21–37.

Gaither, L.A., 2007, Chemogenomics approaches to novel target discovery, *Expert Reviews of Proteomics,* 4:411–419.

Ghasemi, J. and Saaidpour, S., 2007, QSPR prediction of aqueous solubility of drug-like organic compounds, *Chemical and Pharmaceutical Bulletin,* 55: 669–674.

Jacobson-Kram, D. and Contrera, J.F., 2007, Genetic toxicity assessment: Employing the best science for human safety evaluation. Part I: Early screening for potential human mutagens, *Toxicological Sciences,* 96:16–20.

Leong, M.K., 2007, A novel approach using pharmacophore ensemble/support vector machine (PhE/SVM) for prediction of hERG liability, *Chemical Research in Toxicology,* 20:217–226.

Loging, W., Harland, L., and Williams-Jones, B., 2007, High-throughput electronic biology: Mining information for drug discovery, *Nature Reviews Drug Discovery,* 6:220–230.

Materi, W. and Wishart, D.S., 2007, Computational systems biology in drug discovery and development: Methods and applications, *Drug Discovery Today,* 12:295–303

Ohno, Y., Hisaka, A., and Suzuki, H., 2007, General framework for the quantitative prediction of CYP3A4-mediated oral drug interactions based on the AUC increase by coadministration of standard drugs, *Clinical Pharmacokinetics,* 46: 681–696.

Quackenbush, J., 2007, Extracting biology from high-dimensional biological data, *Journal of Experimental Biology,* 210:1507–1517.

Stansfeld, P.J., Gedeck, P., Gosling, M., et al., 2007, Drug block of the hERG potassium channel: Insight from modeling, *Proteins,* 68:568–580.

Tseng, G.N., Sonawane, K.D., Korolkova, Y.V., et al., 2007, Probing the outer mouth structure of the hERG channel with peptide toxin footprinting and molecular modeling, *Biophysical Journal*, 92:3524–3540.

Vedani, A., Descloux, A.V., Spreafico, M., and Ernst, B., 2007, Predicting the toxic potential of drugs and chemicals *in silico*: A model for the peroxisome proliferator-activated receptor gamma (PPAR gamma), *Toxicology Letters*, 173: 17–23.

Yi, H., Cao, Z., Yin, S., et al., 2007, Interaction simulation of hERG K$^+$ channel with its specific BeKm-1 peptide: Insights into the selectivity of molecular recognition, *Journal of Proteome Research*, 6:611–620.

5.7.3   Book Chapter

Dalibalta, S. and Mitcheson, J.S., 2008, hERG channel physiology and drug-binding structure—activity relationships. In Vaz, R.J. and Klabunde, T. (Eds.), *Antitargets: Prediction and prevention of drug side effects,* Weinheim: Wiley-LISS, 89–108.

6

NONCLINICAL DEVELOPMENT

6.1 INTRODUCTION

At the end of the drug discovery/design phase of lifecycle drug development, sponsors need to make a go/no-go decision concerning possible progression of the drug molecule to the next phase. If the sponsor decides to move forward at this point, the molecule moves into a nonclinical development program. This chapter provides a brief overview of nonclinical research in general (see Rogge and Taft, 2005; Gad, 2006; Greaves, 2007, for more detailed information) before turning specifically to studies relevant to proarrhythmic cardiac safety. It has become important to identify compounds with the potential to induce QT prolongation as early as possible in lifecycle drug development, and such investigations are now a central part of nonclinical research.

The ICH guidance S7A (2001), *Safety Pharmacology Studies for Human Pharmaceuticals*, provided general guidance for nonclinical investigation. This information has been supplemented by ICH Guidance S7B (2005), *Nonclinical Evaluation of the Potential for Delayed Ventricular Repolarization (QT Interval Prolongation) by Human Pharmaceuticals*, which presented proposed standard tests for QT interval prolongation in nonclinical studies. These assays include testing for inhibition in hERG channel currents, assessment of action potentials in myocardial cells, and examination of QT intervals via ECG recordings in various animal models. These models include larger mammalian species in which the control of ventricular repolarization is influenced by hERG-like channels.

6.2 THE NEED FOR NONCLINICAL RESEARCH

As Turner (2007) noted, the use of animals in laboratory studies is an emotional topic for many people, but the importance of safety information gained from animal studies in the development of medicines for humans cannot be overstated. While the strategies discussed in the previous chapter are informative, and may become even more so in time, it is necessary to test safety and efficacy in living tissues and organisms. This is first done in nonclinical research before possible progression to human (clinical) studies. The *in vitro* and *in vivo* testing conducted during a nonclinical development program is invaluable for identifying and screening out compounds that are undoubtedly toxic, but these methodologies cannot fully predict

Integrated Cardiac Safety: Assessment Methodologies for Noncardiac Drugs in Discovery, Development, and Postmarketing Surveillance. By J. Rick Turner and Todd A. Durham
Copyright © 2009 John Wiley & Sons, Inc.

how humans will respond to candidate compounds that appear safe on the basis of the nonclinical testing performed. Nevertheless, regulatory authorities currently require a certain amount of nonclinical information.

6.2.1   The 3Rs

A set of standards known as the 3Rs—reduction, refinement, and replacement of laboratory studies wherever possible—addresses these issues and attempts to optimize "the balance between the needs of society and the welfare of animals" (Folb, 2006, p. 48). Folb (2006) described the 3Rs as follows:

> ➤ Reduction. The number of animals should be reduced to the absolute minimum that will achieve the necessary result by placing greater focus on the objectives of the study, achieving better experimental design, and minimizing the need for repeat studies. One example is to promote greater sharing and dissemination of test data worldwide to contribute to a reduction in animal testing.
> ➤ Refinement. Adjustments to study designs and methodologies have led to a reduction in the number of animals used, and in many cases have made testing more humane, without reducing the scientific validity of the testing, and indeed in some cases improving it.
> ➤ Replacement. Significant progress is being made in developing *in vitro* replacement models for some tests, including target organ toxicity.

Animal models are used in clinical research, when there is currently no alternative: researchers have an ethical duty to determine if there is an alternative way of acquiring the information that would be gained from an animal study. Future innovations may reduce the need for some animal studies, and such innovation would be welcomed by the pharmaceutical industry.

6.3   THE STRENGTHS AND LIMITATIONS OF NONCLINICAL DATA

A fundamental strength of nonclinical data is that they constitute meaningful quantitative information that improves the likelihood of moving safely to subsequent human studies. It is useful to gain information about the biological effects of various levels of exposure to the drug and, in the present context, to establish a safe clinical starting dose and safety margins if and when the drug moves forward into clinical research.

However, animal responses to drugs are not perfectly predictive of human responses. As Greaves (2007, p. vii) noted, "The outstanding difficulty in this area of drug development remains the prediction of likely adverse effects in patients based on findings in laboratory animals." The choice of animal species for nonclinical studies is not easy, since there can be (sometimes marked) differences in the metabolic fate of a drug in various nonhuman species and in humans.

6.4   PHARMACOKINETICS

Dhillon and Gill (2006, p. 1) defined pharmacokinetics as "a fundamental scientific discipline that underpins applied therapeutics" and noted that this discipline "provides a mathematical basis to assess the time course of drugs and their effects in the body." Four pharmacokinetic processes of importance are:

➤ Absorption.
➤ Distribution.
➤ Metabolism.
➤ Elimination.

These are reviewed briefly in the following sections.

6.4.1   Absorption

Absorption addresses the transfer of the drug compound from the site of administration into the bloodstream. When investigating drug absorption, studies are typically conducted in the same animal species that is used in later pharmacological and toxicological studies, and (wherever possible) the route of drug administration is the route intended for eventual clinical administration. Several quantitative pharmacokinetic terms are used to describe the plasma or blood concentration-time profile of an administered drug (and/or its metabolites, which may or may not be pharmacologically active themselves). These include:

➤ C_{max}: The maximum concentration or maximum systemic exposure.
➤ T_{max}: The time of maximum concentration or time of maximum exposure.
➤ $t_{1/2}$, Half-life: The time required to reduce the plasma concentration to one-half of its initial value.
➤ AUC, area under the plasma-concentration curve over all time: A measure of total systemic exposure. The expression $AUC_{(0-t)}$ denotes the area under the curve from zero to any time point t.

6.4.2   Distribution

Distribution addresses the transfer of the drug compound from the site of administration to the systemic circulation and then to bodily tissues. Both *in vitro* and *in vivo* studies are informative. *In vitro* studies, for example, examine plasma protein binding. *In vivo* studies may use whole body autoradiography to display visually how much drug-related material has reached different parts of the body over time. The term drug-related material is used here since this technique generally cannot distinguish between the administered (parent) drug and its metabolites.

6.4.3   Metabolism

Metabolism addresses the biochemical transformation of a drug with the basic intent of eliminating it from the body. Section 2.15 discussed enzymes, with a focus on metabolic enzymes and metabolism. A radiolabeled drug may be used to help determine its metabolic fate, in particular the quantity and identity of the metabolites formed.

6.4.4   Elimination

Elimination concerns the removal of the drug compound from the body. The parent drug compound and its metabolites can be eliminated into urine and feces. Drug-related material in the feces may result from unabsorbed drug or material secreted via the bile. The primary mode of investigation here is elimination balance studies. A radiolabeled drug compound is administered, and radioactivity is then measured from elimination sites (e.g., urine, feces, expired air). These studies provide information concerning which organs are involved in elimination of the drug and its metabolites and the time course of this elimination.

6.5   PHARMACOLOGY STUDIES

Van der Laan (2006, p. 217) noted that animal studies are conducted to examine the pharmacological and toxicological effects of the investigational drug "first in relation to each other, and later in relation to the effects in humans." The former objective is more straightforward than the latter.

Research pharmacology studies can be classified into primary and secondary studies. Primary research pharmacology studies are directly relevant to the proposed therapeutic use of the drug compound. Our interest here lies with secondary research pharmacology studies, which focus on any effects that are unrelated to the proposed therapeutic use.

6.5.1 Secondary Research Pharmacology Studies

Secondary research pharmacology studies investigate the overall pharmacological activity of the drug compound, with a particular focus on activity that may occur that is not directly related to the drug's proposed therapeutic use. These studies can be conducted *in vitro* and/or *in vivo*. Studies conducted *in vitro* include the drug molecule's likely binding with nontarget receptors. Studies conducted *in vivo* investigate the general pharmacological action of the drug in animal models. It should be noted that some unintended pharmacological effects may turn out to be serendipitous discoveries of therapeutically beneficial biological activity. However, our primary interest in this book is on unintended effects that are of concern from a cardiotoxicity perspective.

6.5.2 Safety Pharmacology Studies

Safety pharmacology studies investigate potentially undesirable effects of the drug compound. They are typically conducted in the rat and the dog, but primate models can also be used. Typically, studies employ a single-dose design using the intended therapeutic dose. These studies focus on functional changes in major organ systems within the body: later studies focus on structural changes. Issues of function and structure can be meaningfully separated for discussion, but it must be remembered that they may be connected. Functional changes can occur in the absence of structural change, they can precede structural change, and they can potentially contribute to structural change. Safety pharmacology evaluations include (Gad, 2002):

- ➢ Cardiovascular system: assessment of blood pressure, heart rate, and basic cardiac electrophysiology. Additional investigation of QT prolongation is called for in certain cases.
- ➢ Respiratory system: assessment of the rate and depth of breathing, and pulmonary function.
- ➢ Central nervous system: assessment of skeletal muscle tone, locomotion, reflexes, body temperature, autonomic function, learning and memory.
- ➢ Renal system: renal function and renal dynamics.
- ➢ Gastrointestinal system: gastric acid secretion, gastric emptying, nausea, vomiting.
- ➢ Immune system: passive cutaneous anaphylaxis (PCA) test for potential antigenicity.

6.6   Toxicological Studies

Toxicology studies provide descriptions of adverse effects and address their mechanisms of action. Drugs can be categorized into chemical classes, and different drugs belonging to the same class often have some toxicological effects in common: that is, some side effects can be reasonably expected from all novel drugs in that class. However, and very importantly in the context of torsadogenic liability, it is also likely that each drug will have a unique overall toxicology profile, largely influenced by the drug's physicochemical properties (Hellman, 2006). Therefore, a given drug may not display the typical side effects seen for other drugs in the same class, and/or it may display unique side effects that have not been seen for previous drugs in the same class.

Most compounds that exert toxicological influences (toxicants) induce their effects by interacting with normal cellular processes (Hellman, 2006). The ultimate result of many toxic responses is cell death leading to loss of important organ function. Other toxicological effects are the result of interactions with various biochemical and physiological processes that do not affect the survival of the cells. Common mechanisms of toxic action include:

> Interference with cellular membrane functions.
> Disturbed calcium homeostasis.
> Disrupted cellular energy production.
> Reversible or nonreversible binding to various proteins, nucleic acids, and other macromolecules.

Toxicological studies are conducted in a progression. First, exploratory toxicology studies help to target the main organs and physiological systems involved, and provide a quantitative estimation of the drug's toxicity when administered, in single or repeated doses, for a relatively short period of time. Second, initial regulatory toxicology studies are required before the drug is administered to humans for the first time, and therefore support these first-time-in-human (FTIH) studies. These pre-FTIH studies typically include 14- or 28-day repeated-dose toxicology studies in two species. Third, post-FTIH regulatory toxicology studies are conducted to support more complex clinical investigations. These additional studies, conducted in parallel with clinical trials, are expensive and are typically done only if sponsor believes that the drug has a good chance of receiving marketing approval. They include:

> Toxicological studies in two or more species lasting for up to one year.
> Carcinogenicity tests and reproductive toxicology studies lasting for up to two years.
> Interaction studies that examine possible interactions with other drugs.

6.7   INVESTIGATION OF TORSADOGENIC LIABILITY

Attention now turns to nonclinical investigation concerning torsadogenic liability. This section reviews *in vitro* and *in vivo* screening approaches. The need for this research is captured well by using part of the quote from Mitcheson et al. (2005, p.137) used previously in Section 5.6 and adding an additional sentence:

> The diversity of compounds that block hERG and therefore are at risk of causing LQTS is one of the most extraordinary features of this channel. To date, based on chemical structure alone, it has not been possible to predict whether new compounds have the potential to block hERG. Therefore it has become necessary to use relatively expensive and time consuming *in vitro* and *in vivo* screening approaches to identify compounds with the potential to induce QT prolongation as early as possible in the drug development process.

6.7.1   ICH Guidance on Nonclinical Evaluation of Torsadogenic Liability

The ICH Guidance S7B provides a testing strategy for nonclinical assessment of the potential for a drug to delay ventricular repolarization, and information from this guidance is summarized here. The first section provides a succinct recap of relevant material discussed in earlier chapters of this book, and it may be useful to note some of the main points again here:

- ➢ The QT interval is timed from the onset of the QRS complex to the offset of the T-wave as seen on the ECG.
- ➢ This time interval is a measure of the duration of ventricular depolarization and subsequent repolarization.
- ➢ Delayed repolarization increases the time interval (length) of the QT interval in both inherited long QT syndromes and drug-induced QT interval prolongation.
- ➢ When ventricular repolarization is delayed and the QT interval is prolonged, there is an increased risk of ventricular tachyarrhythmia, including TdP. This is particularly so when it occurs in combination with other risk factors such as structural heart disease. (See Section 14.2.)
- ➢ Ventricular repolarization is the net result of the activities of many ion channels and ion transporters, and is influenced by the flow of sodium, calcium, and potassium ionic currents through the plasma membrane. As noted in Section 3.9, discussions in this book focus on the KCNH2/hERG (I_{Kr}) current that flows through the KCNH2/hERG cardiac potassium channel.

> Potassium ionic currents I_{Kr} and I_{Ks} (the rapid and slow components of the I_K current) occur during phase 3 of the action potential. They are responsible for the sustained downward slope of the action potential following phase 2 (the plateau phase) and seem to have the most influence in determining the duration of the action potential, and thus the QT interval.
> The KCNH2/hERG gene encodes the hERG protein, the pore-forming α-subunit of the hERG channel.
> KCNH2/hERG channels are tetrameric structures (four α-subunits) and can be homotetrameric or heterotetrameric.
> These α-subunit proteins can form hetero-oligomeric complexes with KCNE1/MinK- and KCNE2/MiRP1-encoded accessory β-subunits. These β-subunits may modulate the gating properties of the channels.
> The most common mechanism of action in drug-induced QT interval prolongation is inhibition of KCNH2/hERG current via drug block of the KCNH2/hERG channel.

This ICH guidance listed the following objectives for its studies:

> Identify the potential of a drug molecule (and its metabolites) to delay ventricular repolarization.
> Relate the extent of the delayed ventricular repolarization to the concentrations of the drug molecule and its metabolites.
> Elucidate the mechanism of action of the delayed ventricular repolarization.
> In conjunction with other relevant information, estimate the risk of delayed ventricular repolarization and QT interval prolongation in humans.

The last bullet point contains two noteworthy elements. First, the word estimate is meaningfully employed in the guidance since any information obtained from nonclinical studies can only estimate any effects of the drug molecule in humans. Second, and relatedly, the purpose of nonclinical studies is to provide information that forms the rational basis for making another go/no-go decision: should the sponsor proceed to a clinical development program? If the decision is to proceed, the nonclinical data will guide subsequent clinical development.

Both *in vitro* KCNH2/hERG current assays (assessment methodologies, or tests) and *in vivo* QT assays can be usefully employed here, and they provide complementary information. These methodologies can obtain information at the following four functional levels:

> Ionic currents measured in isolated animal or human cardiac myocytes, cultured cardiac cell lines, or heterologous expression systems for cloned human ion channels.
> Action potential parameters in isolated cardiac preparations or specific electrophysiology parameters indicative of action potential duration in anesthetized animals.

➤ Proarrhythmic effects measured in isolated cardiac preparations or animals.
➤ ECG parameters measured in conscious or anesthetized animals.

6.8   METHODOLOGIES FOR THE NONCLINICAL INVESTIGATION OF QT INTERVAL PROLONGATION

Before describing various assays that are available for the nonclinical investigation of delayed ventricular repolarization it is appropriate to make a general point about nonclinical research that is particularly applicable to this specific arena: as in all experimental research, care must be taken to choose the most appropriate study design and methodology. Gad (2006, p. 6) made the following observation:

> In all areas of biological research, optimal design and appropriate interpretation of experiments require that the researcher understand both the biological and technological underpinnings of the system being studied and of the data being generated. From the point of view of the statistician, it is vitally important that the experimenter both know and be able to communicate the nature of the data and understand its limitations.

Optimum quality experimental methodology is as critical in nonclinical research as in clinical studies. As in other instances of the use of the prefix "non" (e.g., nonparametric statistical analysis, nonexperimental studies) the prefix is not pejorative and does not indicate a relative lack of importance: it simply distinguishes between different aspects of lifecycle drug development.

6.8.1   *In Vitro* Electrophysiology Studies

In vitro electrophysiology studies can provide information concerning a drug molecule's effect on action potential duration and/or cardiac ionic currents. This can help elucidate cellular mechanisms affecting repolarization, and these studies can employ either single-cell or multicellular preparations. Human ion channel proteins expressed in noncardiac cells (heterologous expression systems) can be used to assess the drug molecule's effects on specific individual ion channels. Multicellular test systems allow study of the duration of the action potential resulting from the net influence of more than one ionic current.

    The choice of animal species to use in (any) nonclinical research is always challenging. Some species may be particularly useful in some cases and less so in others. An additional level of complexity is the fact that *in vitro* and *in vivo* tests using the same species can differ in value. In the case of torsadogenic liability, one of the challenges in understanding KCNH2/hERG channel SARs is to determine which *in vitro* biological activity best measures the interaction of the drug compound with the channel (Li et al., 2006), i.e., the degree of reduction in KCNH2/hERG current that will result. Attention must be paid to both the biological system in which KCNH2/hERG is expressed and the methodology used for measuring the biological activity. The typical *in vitro* choices of biological systems are KCNH2/hERG channels expressed in stably transfected Chinese hamster ovary cells or human embryonic kidney cells. Expression of KCNH2/hERG channels in these heterologous cell systems permits their study in isolation from other proteins (Leishman and Waldron, 2006). The patch clamp technique, and particularly the whole-cell patch clamp (e.g., see Leishman and Waldron, 2006, pp.39–50), is a mainstay of drug screening paradigms.

An important consideration with regard to assays is their throughput, i.e., how many assays can be conducted in a certain time. The manual patch clamp offers large amounts of quality data but has a low throughput. However, these low-throughput techniques can be useful once selectivity screening has identified compounds of interest. This more limited set of candidate compounds can then be investigated more thoroughly and their mechanisms of action clarified (Leishman and Waldron, 2006).

6.8.2   Integrative Tissue Assays

We noted in Section 5.6.2 that reductionistic strategies have the advantage of allowing attention to focus on a particular influence of interest and to examine this in the absence of extraneous influences. However, it is also informative to see how drug compounds interact with the KCNH2/hERG channel in the presence of the other ion channels present in the complete physiological system. Integrative tissue assays provide this opportunity. Electrophysiological integrative tissue assays are typically extracellular recordings of electrical activity, and "the cardiac Purkinje fiber assay is recommended as an assay to be considered as part of an integrated risk assessment for the propensity of novel pharmaceutical agents to cause cardiac arrhythmias due to block of the hERG channel" (Leishman and Waldron, 2006, p. 59). Like the assays discussed in the previous section, this assay is not a high-throughput assay, but it can be of considerable use in investigating promising compounds identified by earlier screening. Leishman and Waldron (2006, p. 59) noted that the Purkinje fiber assay can be used "as a stepping stone between *in vitro* and *in vivo* experiments," being conducted between KCNH2/hERG patch clamp and *in vivo* dog studies.

6.8.3   *In Vivo* Electrophysiology Studies

In vivo animal models can provide additional understanding of any electrophysiological effects of parent drugs and metabolites prior to screening human participants for any drug-induced effects on ventricular repolarization in clinical trials (these clinical trials are discussed in the following chapter). Greaves (2007, p. 271) noted that the dog has been "the model of choice for the pharmacological characterization of new cardiovascular drugs and has made major contributions to the study of hypertension over many decades." In this specific context, he also noted the following (Greaves 2007, p. 271):

> The beagle dog probably represents the best model for drug-induced electrocardiographic effects in humans, particularly if electrocardiographic investigation is conducted carefully with consideration of peak plasma drug concentration...This sensitivity of the beagle dog may be related to the ease of electrocardiographic monitoring in this species compared with rodents, or even monkeys.

Useful discussions of the use of radio telemetry in the beagle dog and the assessment of ECG and hemodynamic parameters are provided by Gauvin et al. (2006) and Soloviev et al. (2006).

6.9   "CORRECTING" QT INTERVAL MEASUREMENTS FOR THE CONCURRENT HEART RATE

As noted in the preface, we have employed a planned and progressive strategy in writing this book. On several occasions material is introduced at one point, elaborated on at a later point, and then integrated with other material in due course. We hope that this strategy will assist the reader to progressively assimilate both detail and context. This is one of those occasions.

The QT interval as seen on the surface ECG was introduced in Section 3.7. In our discussions so far, we have focused on the QT interval, its potential drug-acquired prolongation, and the potential consequences of this prolongation. However, the QT interval is impacted by heart rate, which adds a considerable degree of complexity to its meaningful interpretation across various circumstances. The ICH S7B guidance (p. 8) introduced and commented on this issue as follows:

> The QT interval and heart rate have an inverse, nonlinear relationship, which varies among species and between animals within a species. Thus, a change in heart rate exerts an effect on [the] QT interval, which can confound the assessment of the effect of the test substance on ventricular repolarization and the QT interval...Therefore, the interpretation of data from *in vivo* test systems should take into account the effect of coincident changes in heart rate...When the effects [on heart rate] are due to a test substance, the most common approach is to correct the QT interval for heart rate (QTc) using formulae such as Bazett or

Fridericia. The choice of heart rate correction formula should be justified with data from the test system.

As noted in Section 3.7, the time interval between the onset of the QRS complex and the offset of the T-wave as seen on the ECG is defined as the QT interval. It is now appropriate to consider the inverse relationship between heart rate and the QT interval. Consider the case of a heart rate of 60 beats per minute (bpm), a number chosen to make the math easy in this example. This represents one heartbeat per second, so the total length, in the time domain, of all ECG segments during one beat would add up to one second. Given that we are interested in subcomponents that fall within the time interval of one second, this period of time is represented in this research field as 1,000 milliseconds (msec). Each component of the ECG can therefore be assigned a length, or duration, in milliseconds. The length of the QT interval can be obtained by measurement from inspecting the ECG and identifying the QRS onset and the T-wave offset.

As the heart beats faster, i.e., as heart rate increases, the duration of an individual cardiac cycle decreases, since more cardiac cycles now occur in the same time. At a heart rate of 120 bpm, therefore, the cardiac cycle has been reduced to 500 msec. Given this sizable decrease in the overall duration of the cardiac cycle, it is not surprising that each of the components of the cardiac cycle also decrease in duration, i.e., shortens. However, as well as being inverse, this relationship is also nonlinear, as noted in the previous quote from ICH S7B. Therefore, we cannot simply say that the QT interval at a heart rate of 120 bpm will be precisely half of that at 60 bpm, even given the precise 50% reduction in the length of the overall cardiac cycle.

Since it is of interest to examine the QT interval at various heart rates, the interval can be "corrected" for heart rate, a process that leads to the term QT corrected for heart rate, abbreviated as QTc. This correction can be accomplished in various ways according to various formulae. As noted in the previous quote from ICH S7B, two common methods of obtaining QTc in nonclinical studies are those of Bazett and Fridericia. While it is important to note here that such corrections are appropriate in nonclinical studies, these correction methods are discussed in more detail in the following chapter in relation to their use in calculating QTc data from QT interval data collected from humans in preapproval clinical trials.

6.10   QT PROLONGATION IS NOT THE ONLY PARAMETER OF INTEREST

As the name of ICH Guidance S7B suggests, it focuses on QT interval prolongation as an index of torsadogenic liability. However, as we saw in Chapter 4, QT prolongation is not the only index of interest in the prediction of TdP. It is important to note that such guidances can take several years to go through preparation and an extensive review process. The authors and reviewers of this guidance were well aware of potential further developments and refinements in assessing torsadogenic liability from nonclinical models: the final section of this ICH guidance makes it clear that other indices can also be important, and encourages further research to develop additional models and to "test their usefulness in predicting risk in humans" (ICH Guidance S7B, 2005, p. 10).

6.11 ADDITIONAL NONCLINICAL CONSIDERATIONS AND INVESTIGATIONS

Several circumstances can lead to retrospective evaluation of results from the initial nonclinical studies and/or additional follow-up *in vitro* and/or *in vivo* studies:

> ➤ The results of the original nonclinical studies are inconsistent.
> ➤ Results from subsequent preapproval clinical studies are inconsistent with the (consistent) results obtained from nonclinical studies. This occurrence exemplifies van der Laan's observation (2006, pp. 215–216) that "Safety assessment is an iterative process carried out during development in close cooperation between pharmacologists, toxicologists and clinicians."
> ➤ Unexpected adverse drug reactions are identified once the marketed drug has been taken by a large number of patients.

Once a drug has received marketing approval and is being used by many patients, it is possible that additional and unexpected risks may be identified (see Chapters 10–12). Identification of additional risk may mean that the benefit-risk balance that was deemed favorable at marketing approval now tips in the unfavorable direction. Various actions—including voluntary market withdrawal by the sponsor, additional labeling specified by regulatory authorities, and mandatory market withdrawal—can result from this change in the benefit-risk balance. If the drug is not withdrawn, the sponsor will likely conduct more toxicological experiments to investigate the product's safety in more detail. Therefore, toxicologists can contribute at various stages of lifecycle drug development. Identification of an unexpected toxicity after marketing authorization will likely lead the sponsor to review the toxicological experiment to search for a mechanism of action. The integrated risk assessment model presented on page 4 of ICH S7B succinctly captures the contribution of *in vitro* I_{Kr} assays, *in vivo* QT assays, clinical information, and follow-up studies to the overall evaluation of evidence of risk.

6.12 ATTEMPTING TO EXTRAPOLATE FROM NONCLINICAL DATA TO HUMAN RESPONSES

While nonclinical studies are informative, there are many nontrivial limitations of nonclinical development programs with regard to predicting the effects (desirable and undesirable) of the drug should it subsequently be administered in clinical trials. Two factors that are important in assessing the risks of human drug exposure on the basis of animal toxicity data are the extent of exposure that will occur in humans and the likely similarity between animals and humans in the effects caused by the drug: as Faich and Stemhagen (2005, p. 230) noted, "Differing effects in animals and humans may occur because of differences in drug action including differences in absorption, distribution, and receptor distribution and function."

Consider the last factor first. The degree of similarity between nonhuman and human target and nontarget receptors, and their degree of affinity for the drug molecule, is one consideration. In Section 2.6.2 we noted that the genomes of various animals are remarkably similar to the human genome, and some of the genes of particular relevance to our discussions of proarrhythmic cardiac safety are preserved to a great degree across different species. However, even similar biological structures will potentially be surrounded by different physiological milieus in different species, and the distribution, density, and precise function of these structures may also vary.

Martinez (2005) provided another discussion of the interspecies differences in physiology and pharmacology. Two quotes are provided here, one from the beginning of her chapter and one from the end. The quote from the beginning of her chapter (Martinez, 2005, p.11) provides a succinct summary of our discussions in this chapter:

> Preclinical animal data are an integral component of the product development process, being used for predicting the potential for drug toxicity and for estimating first-time doses in humans. These extrapolations are based upon an assumption of a correlation between the exposure-response relationship in animals and man. Unfortunately, there is no single animal species that can serve as the "perfect" surrogate for human subjects, and the appropriate surrogate species needs to be evaluated for each situation.

The quote from the end of her chapter (Martinez, 2005, pp. 55–56) then takes nonclinical deliberations to a whole other level:

> While [the Martinez] chapter focused on animal models, comparative anatomy and physiology, and the extrapolation of preclinical data to humans, a far more complex question is whether or not preclinical data can also predict toxicities that may be associated with a specific patient population. Numerous physiological changes can occur during disease conditions, and these changes can impact drug distribution, protein binding, clearance, drug metabolism, and tissue sensitivity. While we raise this question, we recognize that this point in and of itself can be the subject of an entire textbook. Nevertheless, it is a point worth considering as we use preclinical data to predict appropriate drug dosages in humans.

6.13   STEM CELL RESEARCH AND ITS IMPLICATIONS FOR CARDIOTOXICITY RESEARCH

Stevens and Roberts (2007) discussed the use of stem cells in cardiotoxicity research. Stem cells, whether embryonic or tissue-derived, can undergo self-renewal since they have a higher capacity to proliferate than specialized tissue cells. They can also differentiate into other cell types such as more functionally specialized mature cells. In addition to their use in other fields such as regenerative medicine, stem cells offer promise within the drug development process. Stem cells can facilitate the development of disease models and allow more effective screening of drug molecules. Human cardiomyocytes can provide a useful *in vitro* model system, but high-throughput safety screening procedures are hindered by a lack of healthy donors. Given their ability to self-renew and differentiate into cardiomyocytes, human stem cells may provide a larger number of cells for *in vitro* safety tests (see also Meyer et al., 2007).

It should also be noted here that this use of stem cells is not limited to cardiotoxicity. Human cells may also generate suitable models for hepatoxicity, genotoxicity, and reproductive toxicology screens, among others, as well as help improve the selection of lead candidates and reduce drug failures in later stages of drug development.

6.14   INVESTIGATION OF TORSADOGENIC LIABILITY FOR BIOLOGICALS

As noted in Section 5.3.1, the primary focus throughout this book's discussions to date has been on evaluating the QT liability (and torsadogenic liability) of small-molecule drugs, drugs that are now often designed and then synthesized and manufactured. However, with the growing number of biologicals that have been approved, and more relevantly from the point of view of current discussions, the large number of biologicals that are now in development, assessing their QT liability is also of importance. However, at the time of writing, the regulatory guidance for QT liability assessment of biologicals is not as clear as it is for small-molecule drugs. Therefore, it is important to emphasize that our discussions of biologicals should be thought of as highlighting relevant issues rather than providing reports of assessment strategies issued by regulatory agencies. A relevant article by Vargas et al. (2008) is discussed shortly.

Small-molecule drugs have a relatively rigid structural backbone, typically carbon-based, that ensures that the three-dimensional geometry of the molecule does not alter too much. One or more functional groups, which determine the chemical and physical properties of the drug molecule, are held together on this backbone, and the rigidity of the backbone ensures that these functional groups are presented to receptors in order to achieve energetically favorable interactions with them (recall the discussions in Chapter 5). Not surprisingly, "small-molecule drugs" have a small molecular size and molecular weight: a typical definition would be molecules with a molecular weight less than 700 daltons (d) (e.g., see Ghose et al., 1999). For example, choosing two drugs that are discussed in Chapter 11, the molecular weight of terfenadine is 476 d and the molecular weight of cisapride is 483 d. In contrast, biologics are macromolecules characterized by much greater size and molecular weight. As one example of a category of large-molecule drugs discussed later in this chapter, monoclonal antibodies can have molecular weights greater than 140,000 d, some 300 times greater than cisapride. Fusion proteins can be in the range of 100,000 to 200,000 d, and recombinant proteins can be in the order of 30,000 d. The implications for QT liability assessment of these large-molecule drugs are considered shortly, following a brief introduction to biologics.

Walsh (2007) noted that the terms biological, biopharmaceutical, products of pharmaceutical biotechnology, and biotechnology medicines have become an accepted part of the pharmaceutical literature, but that they can mean different things to different people. He commented that the term biological generally refers to medicinal products derived from blood, as well as vaccines, toxins, and allergen products. The term biotechnology has a broader meaning, referring to "the use of biological systems (e.g., cells or tissues) or biological molecules (e.g., enzymes or antibodies) for/in the manufacture of commercial products" (Walsh, 2007, p. 2). The term biopharmaceutical originated in the 1980s and came to describe a class of therapeutic proteins produced by modern biotechnological techniques. Specifically, these techniques are genetic engineering or, in the case of monoclonal antibodies, hybridoma technology.

In this chapter, and in subsequent discussions, the term biological is used synonymously with the term large-molecule drug: the terminology of other authors when cited is respected.

6.14.1 Genetic Engineering

Walsh (2007, p. 37) defined genetic engineering as follows:

> [Genetic engineering] describes the process of manipulating genes (outside of a cell's/organism's normal reproductive process). It generally involves the isolation, manipulation and subsequent reintroduction of stretches of DNA into cells and is usually undertaken in order to confer on the recipient cell the ability to produce a specific protein, such as a biopharmaceutical.

The term recombinant DNA (rDNA) technology is used interchangeably with genetic engineering. Recombinant DNA is "a piece of DNA artificially created *in vitro* which contains DNA (natural or synthetic) obtained from two or more sources" (Walsh, 2007, p. 37). The majority of currently approved biologicals are proteins produced in engineered cell lines by recombinant means. One example is the production of insulin in recombinant *Escherichia coli* and recombinant *Saccharomyces cerevisiae* for use in the treatment of diabetes mellitus (insulin is discussed in more detail in Chapter 12). In addition to these proteins, biologicals now encompasses nucleic acid-based (both RNA-based and DNA-based) products and whole cell-based products (Walsh, 2007).

6.14.2   Hybridoma Technology

As Walsh (2007, p. 371) noted, "Polyclonal antibody preparations have been used for several decades to induce passive immunization against infectious diseases and other harmful agents, particularly toxins." There are two ways to obtain antibody preparations used to induce passive immunity. One is from animals, and such preparations are generally termed antisera. The other is from humans, and such preparations are called immunoglobulin preparations or simply immunoglobulins. The antibody IgG is the predominant antibody type present.

While their therapeutic benefits are considerable and invaluable, antisera can induce adverse drug reactions, often in the form of hypersensitivity reactions. Some of these, e.g., anaphylaxis, can be life-threatening. Adverse drug reactions to immunoglobulins, purified from the serum or plasma of human donors, are far less frequent. Most immunoglobulins are capable of binding to a specific target that is usually an infectious microorganism or virus. In the terminology introduced for use in our discussions in Chapter 5, we can think of these microorganisms or viruses as the target receptors for the immunoglobulins.

In the past two decades or so, nonspecific or monoclonal antibodies have been the main focus of medical application of antibody-based therapy. Walsh (2007, p. 374) noted that monoclonal antibody technology was first developed in the mid-1970s by fusing certain "immortal" cells with antibody-producing β-lymphocytes. Some of the resultant hybrids, or hybridoma cells, were stable antibody-producing cells that can be cultured long-term to effectively provide an inexhaustible supply of monoclonal antibody. Hybridoma technology thus facilitates "the relatively straightforward production of monospecific antibodies against virtually any desired antigen" (Walsh, 2007, p. 374). Walsh (2007, Table 13.2, pp. 380–381) listed almost 30 monoclonal antibodies that have been approved for medical use, along with their therapeutic indications. While a good proportion of these are related to the oncology therapeutic area, this is certainly not the only actual/potential use of monoclonal antibodies and their derivatives: others include the detection and treatment of cardiovascular disease and the reversal of acute transplant rejection (Walsh, 2007).

Brief accounts of the manufacturing of biologicals are provided by Turner (2007, pp. 41–45 and 197–199, respectively). Detailed discussions can be found in Ho and Gibaldi (2003) and Walsh (2003, 2007).

6.15   WHAT NONCLINICAL QT LIABILITY ASSESSMENTS ARE APPROPRIATE FOR BIOLOGICALS?

ICH Guidance S6, *Preclinical Safety Evaluation of Biotechnology-derived Pharmaceuticals*, was published in 1997. The following text is taken from Section 1.3 (p. 2):

> This guidance is intended primarily to recommend a basic framework for the preclinical safety evaluation of biotechnology-derived pharmaceuticals. It applies to products derived from characterized cells through the use of a variety of expression systems including bacteria, yeast, insect, plant, and mammalian cells....The active substances include proteins and peptides, their derivatives, and products of which they are components; they could be derived from cell cultures or produced using recombinant deoxyribonucleic acid (DNA) technology, including production by transgenic plants and animals.

Examples of such products include cytokines, plasminogen activators, recombinant plasma factors, growth factors, fusion proteins, enzymes, receptors, hormones, and monoclonal antibodies. The guidance notes that its principles may also be applicable to rDNA protein vaccines, chemically synthesized peptides, plasma-derived products, endogenous proteins extracted from human tissue, and oligonucleotide drugs.

Parts of ICH S6 parallel the contents of ICH S7A. For example, safety pharmacology studies should be done to reveal functional effects on major physiological systems, including the cardiovascular system. However, ICH S7A went further by including KCNH2/hERG channel testing for all systemically available compounds. However, it did note exceptions (p. 6–7):

> For biotechnology-derived products that achieve highly specific receptor targeting, it is often sufficient to evaluate safety pharmacology endpoints as part of toxicology and/or pharmacodynamic studies, and therefore safety pharmacology studies can be reduced or eliminated for these products.

The ICH S7B guidance addressed the nonclinical evaluation of QT liability. While this guidance stated that it applies to new chemical entities, i.e., small-molecule drugs for human use, there is no explicit statement on the evaluation of QT liability for biologicals. However, given the statement just quoted from ICH S7A, it would not be unreasonable for the general reader to think that the studies required for small-molecule investigational drugs are not required for biopharmaceutical investigational drugs. However, this interpretation on the part of a sponsor may be dangerous. Two questions that suggest themselves in this context are:

> Why is this exception just cited noted in ICH Guidance S7A?
> If it does apply to the studies detailed in ICH Guidance S7B, is granting this exception fully justified in light of current knowledge?

As an initial step in considering what an appropriate strategy for biologicals might be, it is helpful to briefly remind ourselves of some earlier discussions in Chapters 4 and 5. Quite a large number of small-drug molecules have the propensity to cause unintentional block of the KCNH2/hERG channel, and hence the KCNH2/hERG current, leading to delayed cardiac repolarization. As noted in Section 4.5, Michelson et al. (2005, p. 137) observed, "The diversity of compounds that block hERG and therefore are at risk of causing LQTS is one of the most extraordinary features of this channel." The mechanism of this channel block depends on small-molecule drugs passing into the cell through the plasma membrane and therefore having access to the inner cavity of the KCNH2/hERG from the inner side of the plasma membrane. These small-molecule drugs can then bind with certain aromatic amino acid residues in the inner cavity of the KCNH2/hERG channel pore and lead to loss of function of the channel.

However, when we move into the realm of large-molecule drugs, i.e., biologicals, circumstances change considerably. Because of their size, biologicals cannot pass through the plasma membrane into the cell. Therefore, they cannot gain access to the inner cavity of the KCNH2/hERG channel, and cannot lead to channel loss of function in the same manner as small-molecule drugs. A question of interest therefore becomes: are there other mechanisms of action by which biologicals could impact KCNH2/hERG channel function? There are two possibilities here, considered in turn.

6.15.1 Potential Interactions at the Outer Mouth of the KCNH2/hERG Channel

Given that KCNH2/hERG is a transmembrane protein, it has an external pore region as well as an internal one: indeed, as we have seen, KCNH2/hERG current passes through this pore. It is therefore of interest to consider whether biologicals could bind with the external pore region and hence influence, possibly block, KCNH2/hERG channel activity. One example of such binding was described by Zhang et al. (2003). The scorpion toxin BeKm-1 binds selectively to a "toxin binding site" on KCNH2/hERG's external pore and causes loss of function of the channel (see also Korolkova et al., 2004; Yi et al., 2007). However, from the present perspective, the salient point here is the high specificity of this toxin-KCNH2/hERG binding. It is due to dynamic changes in reduction of binding free energy and conformational rearrangement at the interface between BeKm-1 and KCNH2/hERG: that is, both energetic and structural features contribute to this toxin-receptor interaction (Yi et al., 2007).

Consider now the case of biologicals, using monoclonal antibodies as an example. It is theoretically possible that such biologicals could bind to nontarget receptors, including KCNH2/hERG. However, available scientific evidence suggests that this is unlikely. First, the requirements for toxin-KCNH2/hERG binding are very specific. Second, it was noted in Section 6.14.2 that hybridoma technology facilitates the relatively straightforward production of monoclonal antibodies against virtually any desired antigen. The very high specificity and selectivity of these therapeutic proteins, and of fusion proteins, means that these biologicals are associated with a very high potential for on-target activity and a very low potential for interaction with nontarget receptors.

From a scientific perspective, this evidence could be taken to suggest that standard (small-molecule) nonclinical assays for KCNH2/hERG liability may not be needed for biologicals. (See Section 6.15.3 for further discussion.)

6.15.2 Potential Impact of Biologicals on hERG Protein Trafficking

Drug-induced trafficking deficiencies were discussed in Section 4.7.2. It was noted that arsenic trioxide prolongs the QT interval, i.e., produces drug-induced LQTS, not by direct blockade of hERG channels but by inhibition of hERG protein maturation (e.g., see Barbey et al., 2003; Ohnishi et al., 2000). An increasing awareness of QT liability from this mechanism of action in small-molecule drugs prompts consideration of the following question, raised during a Webinar entitled *Cardiac Safety in Large Molecules: New Regulatory Expectations, New Strategies*, held on February 26, 2008: Might biologicals have such an impact on KCNH2/hERG protein trafficking?

Before attempting to answer this question, it is necessary to bear in mind the following:

➢ Small-molecule drugs exert their influence on protein trafficking deficiency from inside the cell (recall the discussions in Section 4.7.2).
➢ In contrast to small-molecule drugs, biologicals do not penetrate the cell membrane and so do not enter the cell.

The question of interest can therefore be made more specific: Might biologicals be able to exert an influence on KCNH2/hERG protein trafficking from outside the cell? The best answer to this question at this time is probably that this is a possibility, but we have no knowledge of how precisely this might happen. It is certainly true that ligands can bind to receptors on the plasma membrane and generate biological signals that impact intracellular workings without entering the cell. However, in this specific case, there are no definitive answers at this time.

6.15.3   What Approach Seems Appropriate Here?

In a presentation given during the Webinar mentioned in the previous section, Vargas (2008) discussed monoclonal antibodies and concluded by providing the following personal comments regarding nonclinical cardiovascular safety testing strategies for biologicals:

> ➤ There is no scientific rationale to perform a KCNH2/hERG assay on a biological as a routine study. It should be viewed as a secondary assay and could be used to assess the mechanism of action for any indication of concern regarding QT interval prolongation observed in animal or clinical studies.
> ➤ Appropriate cardiovascular safety endpoints can be integrated into toxicology studies. Dedicated *in vivo* cardiovascular safety pharmacology studies are therefore not required, but may be pursued if there is a mechanistic (target) basis of concern.
> ➤ The same [general] approach can be applied to biologicals other than monoclonal antibodies, but the approach should be tailored on a case-by-case basis.

As noted at the start of Section 6.14, the present discussions should not be regarded as providing reports of assessment strategies issued by regulatory agencies. Nonetheless, a recent publication by Vargas et al. (2008) is noteworthy as it provided a scientific review of the literature with regard to the hERG liability and QTc risk of large biological therapeutics. Various types of biologicals are already approved, and many types are currently in clinical development (see Leader et al., 2008). Vargas et al. (2008) focused in particular on monoclonoal antibodies (mAbs), concluding that they, and other types of biological therapeutics that have very high target selectivity, have low risk for blocking the hERG channel (Vargas et al., 2008). As they commented:

> Consequently, we recommend that it is not appropriate to conduct an *in vitro* hERG assay as part of a preclinical strategy for assessing the QTc prolongation risk of mAbs and other types of biologicals. It is more appropriate to assess QTc risk by integrating cardiovascular endpoints into repeat-dose general toxicology studies performed in an appropriate non-rodent species.

It will be interesting to follow future regulatory develpments in this arena. In the meantime, it is highly recommended that sponsors start a dialog with regulatory agencies as soon as possible in the development of biologicals.

6.16 FURTHER READING

Antzelevitch, C., 2006, Cellular basis for the repolarization waves of the ECG, *Annals of the New York Academy of Sciences,* 1080:268–281.

Arrigoni, C. and Crivori, P., 2007, Assessment of QT liabilities in drug development, *Cell Biology and Toxicology*, 23:1–13.

Chaves, A.A., Zingaro, G.J., Yordy, M.A., et al., 2007, A highly sensitive canine telemetry model for detection of QT interval prolongation: Studies with moxifloxacin, haloperidol and MK-499, *Journal of Pharmacological and Toxicological Methods*, 56:103–114.

Davie, C., Valentin, J.P., Pollard, C., et al., 2004, Comparative pharmacology of guinea pig cardiac myocyte and cloned hERG (I_{Kr}) channel, *Journal of Cardiovascular Electrophysiology*, 15:1302–1309.

Dumotier, B.M. and Georgieva, A.V., 2007, Preclinical cardio-safety assessment of torsadogenic risk and alternative methods to animal experimentation: The inseparable twins, *Cell Biology and Toxicology*, 23:293–302.

Guo, J., Massaeli, H., Xu, J., et al., 2007, Identification of I_{Kr} and its trafficking disruption induced by probucol in cultured neonatal rat cardiomyocytes, *Journal of Pharmacology and Experimental Therapeutics*, 321: 911–920.

Hanson, L.A., Bass, A.S., Gintant, G., et al., 2006, ILSI-HESI cardiovascular safety subcommittee initiative: Evaluation of three non-clinical models of QT prolongation. *Journal of Pharmacological and Toxicological Methods*, 54: 116–129. [ILSI-HESI: The Health and Environmental Sciences Institute of the International Life Sciences Institute]

Hanton, G., 2007, Preclinical cardiac safety assessment of drugs, *Drugs Research and Development*, 8:213–218.

Hanton, G., Yvon, A., Provost, J.P., Racaud, A., and Doubovetzky, M., 2007, Quantitative relationship between plasma potassium levels and QT interval in beagle dogs, *Laboratory Animals*, 41:204–217.

Holzgrefe, H.H., Cavero, I., Buchanan, L.V., Gill, M.W., and Durham, S.K., 2007, Application of a probabilistic method for the determination of drug-induced QT prolongation in telemetered cynomolgus monkeys: Effects of moxifloxacin, *Journal of Pharmacological and Toxicological Methods*, 55:227–237. [This article also appears in the Further Reading section in Chapter 7, where the role of moxifloxacin in the "Thorough QT/QTc Study" is discussed.]

Holzgrefe, H.H., Cavero, I., Gleason, C.R., et al., 2007, Novel probabilistic method for precisely correcting the QT interval for heart rate in telemetered dogs and cynomolgus monkeys, *Journal of Pharmacological and Toxicological Methods*, 55:159–175.

Lawrence, C.L., Bridgland-Taylor, M.H., Pollard, C.E., Hammond, T.G., and Valentin, J.P., 2006, A rabbit Langendorff heart proarrhythmia model: Predictive value for clinical identification of Torsades de Pointes, *British Journal of Pharmacology*, 149:845–860.

Lawrence, C.L., Pollard, C.E., Hammond, T.G., and Valentin, J.P., 2005, Nonclinical proarrhythmia models: Predicting Torsades de Pointes, *Journal of Pharmacological and Toxicological Methods*, 52:46–59.

Mank-Seymour, A.R., Richmond, J.L., Wood, L.S., et al., 2006, Association of torsades de pointes with novel and known single nucleotide polymorphisms in long QT syndrome genes, *American Heart Journal*, 152:1116–1122.

Nahas, K. and Geffray, B., 2004, QT interval measurement in the dog: Chest leads versus limb leads, *Journal of Pharmacological and Toxicological Methods*, 50:201–207.

Nolan, E.R., Feng, M.R., Koup, J.R., et al., 2006, A novel predictive pharmacokinetic/pharmacodynamic model of repolarization prolongation derived from the effects of terfenadine, cisapride and E-4031 in the conscious chronic av node-ablated, His bundle-paced dog, *Journal of Pharmacological and Toxicological Methods*, 53:1–10.

Ollerstam, A., Persson, A.H., Visser, S.A., et al., 2007, A novel approach to data processing of the QT interval response in the conscious telemetered beagle dog, *Journal of Pharmacological and Toxicological Methods*, 55:35–48.

Pugsley, M.K. and Curtis, M.J., 2006, Safety pharmacology in focus: New methods developed in the light of the ICH S7B guidance document, *Journal of Pharmacological and Toxicological Methods*, 54:94–98.

Rajamani, S., Eckhardt, L.L., Valdivia, C.R., et al., 2006, Drug-induced long QT syndrome: hERG K^+ channel block and disruption of protein trafficking by fluoxetine and norfluoxetine, *British Journal of Pharmacology*, 149:481–489.

Schwoerer, A.P., Blutner, C., Brandt, S., et al., 2007, Molecular interaction of droperidol with human ether-a-go-go-related gene channels: Prolongation of action potential duration without inducing early afterdepolarization, *Anesthesiology*, 106:967–976.

Siebrands, C.C. and Friederich, P., 2007, Structural requirements of human ether-a-go-go-related gene channels for block by bupivacaine, *Anesthesiology*, 106: 523–531.

Stravopodis, D.J., Margaritis, L.H., and Voutsinas, G.E., 2007, Drug-mediated targeted disruption of multiple protein activities through functional inhibition of the hsp90 chaperone complex, *Current Medicinal Chemistry*, 14:3122–3138.

Tattersall, M.L., Dymond, M., Hammond, T., and Valentin, J.P., 2006, Correction of QT values to allow for increases in heart rate in conscious beagle dogs in toxicology assessment, *Journal of Pharmacological and Toxicological Methods*, 53:11–19.

Testai, L., Breschi, M.C., Martinotti, E., and Calderone, V., 2007, QT prolongation in guinea pigs for preliminary screening of torsadogenicity of drugs and drug-candidates, *Journal of Applied Toxicology*, 27:270–275.

Thomsen, M.B., 2007, Double pharmacological challenge on repolarization opens new avenues for drug safety research, *British Journal of Pharmacology*, 151: 909–911.

Valentin, J.P., Hoffman, P., De Clerk, F., Hammond, T.G., and Hondeghem, L., 2004, Review of the predictive value of the Langendorff heart model (Screenit system) in assessing the proarrhythmic potential of drugs, *Journal of Pharmacological and Toxicological Methods*, 49:171–181.

Wang, L., Wible, B.A., Wan, X., and Ficker, E., 2007, Cardiac glycosides as novel inhibitors of human ether-a-go-go-related gene channel trafficking, *Journal of Pharmacology and Experimental Therapeutics*, 320:525–534.

7

THE THOROUGH QT/QTc STUDY

7.1   INTRODUCTION

We have now reached the point where attention turns to studies conducted during preapproval clinical development programs. This chapter discusses one particular study that has assumed considerable importance in proarrhythmic cardiac safety, the "Thorough QT/QTc Study," abbreviated here as the TQT study. Chapter 8 then discusses a wide array of safety assessments typically conducted in preapproval clinical development. As noted in Chapter 6, while nonclinical studies can certainly provide valuable safety information, it is imperative that additional (and complementary) investigations of drug safety are conducted in human participants.

As Turner (2007) noted, the commencement of human pharmacology trials, also referred to as first-time-in-human (FTIH) and first-time-in-man (FTIM) trials, can lead to a range of emotions for clinical researchers. It is a time of excitement since the drug has reached this milestone and a time of anticipation and hopeful expectation. Additionally, and perhaps more so, it is a time of trepidation and anxiety. The discussions in the previous chapter emphasized that no animal model is a perfect predictor of the precise effects, on-target or off-target, of the drug when administered to humans. Differing drug effects in animals and humans may occur because of differences in pharmacokinetic characteristics such as absorption and distribution, and in receptor distribution and function (Morganroth, 2005). This reality means that, at the commencement of human pharmacology trials, there is the ever-present possibility that serious safety issues may arise. On relatively rare occasions, life-threatening drug-induced conditions have occurred in participants during these trials. The disastrous events that occurred in March 2006 are an all-too-painful example of this. In a placebo-controlled trial of compound TGN1412, eight healthy participants were randomized to the test drug or placebo in a 3:1 ratio (such a ratio maintains randomization but allows more safety data to be collected for the test drug). As Senn (2007, p. 402) noted, the six participants given the test drug "suffered extremely serious rapidly developing side effects with, in come cases, long-term consequences for their health" (see also Nada and Somberg, 2007; Dayan and Wraith, 2008).

Human pharmacology trials are typically conducted in the clinical pharmacology units of residential or in-patient medical centers, where 24-hour supervision and extensive monitoring of participants' health status is possible.

Integrated Cardiac Safety: Assessment Methodologies for Noncardiac Drugs in Discovery, Development, and Postmarketing Surveillance. By J. Rick Turner and Todd A. Durham
Copyright © 2009 John Wiley & Sons, Inc.

(An exception to this is oncology drug development, where these trials are often performed in sick, hospitalized patients.) Human pharmacology studies are pharmacologically oriented trials that typically look for the best range of doses of the investigational drug to employ. These trials typically involve healthy adult participants, and they provide essential initial information about the pharmacokinetics and pharmacodynamics of the investigational drug as well as its safety. Typically, between 20 and 80 healthy adults participate in these relatively short studies, and participants are often recruited from university medical school settings where trials are being conducted. The participants' health status is carefully documented at the start of the study via physical examinations, clinical laboratory tests, and medical histories. Limiting early studies to healthy participants allows the sponsor to attribute any untoward findings to the drug, or to a particular dose of the drug, since significant background diseases are all but absent in the healthy study participants.

These early clinical studies can involve the use of a placebo control group. The incorporation of a placebo group in human pharmacology study designs is not for comparative purposes—as is the case in the TQT study and later therapeutic exploratory and therapeutic confirmatory trials—but because some of the study procedures in these trials can be somewhat invasive, performed many times, and associated with some adverse effects themselves: frequent blood draws, for example, often result in a lowering of hematocrit. Without a placebo control group in the study, it would not be possible to rule out a drug effect when observing such occurrences, which are expected, easily explained, and not drug related (Durham and Turner, 2008).

7.1.1 Full Disclosure Statement

We noted in the preface that this book is intended to be a self-contained introduction to the field of integrated cardiac safety, with an emphasis on the word introduction. Our goal is to provide you with the underpinnings of, and the vocabulary used in, the various branches of cardiac safety, thereby providing you with the tools that will enable you to get the maximum benefit from reading the work of acknowledged experts in these fields and from hearing them speak at meetings.

Before commencing our discussions in this chapter, we would like to emphasize a point that pertains to any sponsors who may be reading the book. This chapter discusses the regulatory guidance on conducting a TQT study provided in ICH Guidance E14. As will be seen in following sections of the chapter, the guidance provided is not always crystal clear, and a number of differing interpretations of sections of the guidance are likely equally reasonable. Therefore, while the EMEA, FDA, and Health Canada have all implemented ICH E14, it is possible that they may interpret some of the sections in subtly different ways. At the time of writing (March 2008), Health Canada has released additional documents describing how they are likely to interpret parts of ICH E14 in relation to study protocols and study reports received by them (see Section 11.4 for more details), and it is likely that other regulatory agencies, including the FDA, will do the same (see Sager et al., 2005). Sager et al. (2005) also noted that the conduct of the TQT, while required for almost all drugs seeking registration in North America, "may be required somewhat less frequently in Europe and Japan because of the view held by many regulators in those regions that the results of preclinical testing can, in some cases, obviate the need for the thorough QT study." With continued development of nonclinical models, and with advancing time, it is possible that these various regions may become more similar in their overall approach to preapproval QT liability testing.

As well as providing some direct quotes from ICH E14, we have also expressed some personal viewpoints concerning the interpretation of some sections of the guidance. We wish to make it absolutely clear that these viewpoints are perspectives that may or may not be shared by others. We claim neither infallibility nor authoritativeness and emphasize that these viewpoints are in no way sanctioned or endorsed by any regulatory agency. We hope that our discussions may alert sponsors planning to conduct a TQT study for the first time to the complexities of this process, and we strongly encourage you to contact experts at a company that specializes in conducting such studies and, with their help, to establish a study-specific dialog with the respective regulatory agency very early in your planning.

7.2   BENEFIT-RISK ASSESSMENTS IN THE CONTEXT OF THE TQT STUDY

A drug molecule identified in the drug discovery/design phase that has progressed satisfactorily through its nonclinical development program enters its clinical development program as an investigational drug. If the investigational drug surmounts all of the obstacles in this clinical development program, an occurrence that is far from guaranteed at the outset, the sponsor will request marketing permission from a regulatory agency (or multiple agencies if it wishes to market the drug widely). The regulatory standard for the approval of a new drug for marketing can be framed succinctly as follows:

> ➤ The overall benefit-risk profile of the investigational drug must be judged by the regulatory agency considering its approvability to be acceptable from a public health perspective.

This short statement may initially seem relatively straightforward, but its succinctness, while useful in summary form, belies the extent and intricacy of the necessary considerations and deliberations needed to reach a positive risk-balance judgment. The statement does, however, capture two fundamental aspects of regulatory decisions:

> ➤ The decisions are judgments that must be made by the regulatory agency on the basis of evidence that is available at the time.

> Regulatory decisions are made from a public health perspective, and from this perspective the estimated overall benefits to the population for whom the drug will be prescribed if approved must be judged to be greater than the estimated harm.

With regard to the second bullet point, it is an unfortunate reality that no drug is immune from the possibility of unwanted responses in certain individuals. Therefore, for a given investigational drug to be approved for marketing, the regulatory agency needs to be presented with compelling evidence that the likely benefits to the target population with the disease or condition of interest outweigh the likely risks to the target population. Judgments about the benefit-risk balance of an investigational drug require, by definition, consideration of both benefit and risk. This means that the therapeutic benefit of the investigational drug needs to be estimated quantitatively and considered in conjunction with quantitative estimations of risk. Given this book's focus on evaluations of drug safety, operationalized as assessments of risk, readers are referred to Durham and Turner (2008), Kay (2007), and Piantadosi (2005) for more detailed discussions of benefit estimations.

7.3   NOMENCLATURE CONSIDERATIONS

The last sentence in the previous paragraph noted that, in this book, the evaluation of drug safety is operationalized as the assessment of risk, and it is appropriate to expand on this comment. As in all of the "Nomenclature Considerations" that occur near the beginning of various chapters, our intent is not to be dogmatic but rather to explain the reasons for our choice of certain terms rather than others. It is ultimately the sentiment and not the actual term that is important in communications, but the sentiment intended to be conveyed by a particular term can sometimes be uncertain. Therefore, defining the intended meaning to be conveyed by a particular term can be useful. It is also appropriate to note that exactly the same intended meaning can be conveyed by other authors using different terminology.

The discipline of drug safety does not assess the safety of a drug *per se*, but assesses the harm done by a drug. In nonclinical research many aspects of a drug compound's potential toxicity are evaluated, including genotoxicity (mutagenicity), carcinogenicity, and reproductive toxicity (see the previous chapter). As Durham and Turner (2008, pp. 14–15) noted, "Relatively less evidence of toxicity is considered as relatively greater evidence of the safety of the drug." In preapproval clinical trials, the risk of harm to patients who would be prescribed the drug if approved is generally evaluated via adverse event data collected during the trials, and in postmarketing surveillance it is evaluated via the collection of data concerning adverse drug reactions. Safety, then, is effectively operationalized as the absence of evidence of harm. Evaluating something by noting the lack of something else may appear to be a less than optimum state of affairs, but there is

NOMENCLATURE CONSIDERATIONS

no immediately evident replacement. In an environment where various groups are monitoring the pharmaceutical industry very carefully, ready to seize upon any items or occurrences perceived as untoward, the alternative term drug harm may bring additional emotional fuel to situations that already have more than enough, especially since the term drug safety is functionally synonymous. In general, we will therefore continue with the term drug safety.

7.3.1 The Terms Volunteer, Participant, and Patient

Two comments on nomenclature are appropriate as we move to the consideration of preapproval clinical trials in this part of the book. In the previous section we used the term healthy adult participants to describe the participants typically employed in human pharmacology trials. In this context, readers are likely to encounter the term normal volunteers in many sources in the literature, so an explanation for our choice of terminology should be provided. We have found during classroom teaching that the term volunteer, typically only seen in connection with human pharmacology trials, can prove confusing to students, particularly when discussing the ethics of clinical trials: It can mistakenly (but readily and reasonably) be taken to imply that participants in other trials are not volunteers. Similarly, the term normal may mistakenly imply that participants in other trials are abnormal in ways not related to having or not having the disease or condition of interest. The term healthy adult participant circumvents such misperceptions.

Second, the term participant is itself deserving of comment. The term subject is commonly seen in the context of clinical trials and is perfectly acceptable, as is the more austere term experimental unit of analysis. We have chosen the term participant in the context of clinical trials since it is a softer and more palatable term to many readers. The term patient is also commonly seen in this context, but from a research methodological perspective the term participant is, respectfully, more appropriate. One defining difference between a clinical trial and clinical practice is that the former is an experimental study conducted for the greater good, and the latter is conducted for the good of specific individuals being treated by a physician on a case-by-case basis.

By definition, preapproval clinical trials are conducted to evaluate an investigational drug on the assumptions that it is not definitively known whether the drug has a therapeutic benefit or whether it poses a risk to participants. If it were known that the drug had a therapeutic benefit, it would be unethical to deprive those participants randomized to the placebo treatment of the therapeutic benefit. Similarly, if it were known that the drug posed a risk to participants, it would be unethical to administer it. Participants in preapproval clinical trials do not take part in the trial for their immediate personal good. If a participant is randomized to the placebo treatment group the participant cannot gain any therapeutic benefit, but is also not able to suffer any side effects directly caused by the investigational drug. Conversely, if the participant is randomized to the investigational drug treatment group, the participant may or may not experience a therapeutic benefit: The drug may or may not convey a therapeutic benefit, and even if it does so in general, there may be reasons why that particular participant does not benefit from this particular drug compound.

It is certainly true that some participants in clinical trials are under the care of a personal physician at the time that they are recruited into the trial and that they are certainly patients in that sense. It is also true that individuals who participated in clinical trials for the greater good—to allow the assessment of an investigational drug's benefit-risk balance—may later be prescribed the drug should it be approved, whether or not they were in the drug treatment group or the placebo group during the trial. Therefore, they would benefit from their participation (and the participation of all other individuals in the drug's preapproval trials) at a later time as patients receiving the drug in a clinical practice setting under the care of their personal physician. Nonetheless, during the time of participation in the trial, when they are not receiving individualized clinical care but are being treated exactly the same as all other individuals in the trial, the term participant is more suited from a purely experimental methodological perspective than the term patient.

This distinction may become less clear in certain cases, such as clinical trials involving individuals with a very serious disease such as a life-threatening cancer. Individuals in such trials would be under personal clinical care during their participation in the trial. Additionally, for ethical reasons, it is not appropriate to randomize some individuals to a placebo treatment in such cases. An active control treatment is therefore used (a placebo treatment is also a control treatment, but a nonactive one). It such cases, the control treatment chosen is typically the best approved treatment available at the time of the trial, referred to as the gold standard treatment. These trials are thus designed to investigate whether the investigational drug provides an advantage over and above the existing gold standard treatment. (The issues surrounding the conduct of a TQT study in such situations are discussed later in the chapter in Section 7.16.1.)

As in all instances in this book when we introduce nomenclature considerations, our intention is not to be dogmatic: It is simply to explain why we have chosen to use certain terminology.

7.4   A BRIEF RECAP OF ACQUIRED QT INTERVAL PROLONGATION AND TdP

The topic of acquired QT interval and its putative role in the genesis of TdP was discussed in Chapter 4 (Section 4.4). Since we have covered a lot of ground since then, a brief recap of these topics, which are of central importance in our discussions of proarrhythmic cardiac safety, may be helpful here.

As noted in Section 4.2.3, TdP is the characteristic arrhythmia that can result from QT interval prolongation—an increase in the time interval between the onset of the QRS complex and the offset of the T-wave—in the case of both inherited LQTS and acquired QT prolongation. It is a particular form of ventricular arrhythmia that has three defining characteristics on an ECG recording:

> It is associated with QT interval prolongation.
> The QRS morphology twists around an imaginary axis, and there may be a change in the amplitude of the waveform.
> The QRS takes on many morphologies as it twists around this axis, leading to the use of the descriptor polymorphic.

Hence, the term TdP is reserved for polymorphic ventricular arrhythmias that are associated with QT prolongation: without such accompanying prolongation, the term polymorphic ventricular arrhythmia is appropriate.

Drug-induced QT interval prolongation usually occurs in one of two ways. The first of these, which is currently more extensively documented, is loss of function in the KCNH2/hERG channel, i.e., less KCNH2/hERG current (I_{Kr}) flow from the inner side of the plasma membrane to the outer side through the KCNH2/hERG channel. This blockade is the result of drug interactions with amino acid residues in the inner cavity of the channel pore. The second is a drug-induced KCNH2/hERG protein trafficking deficiency. An increasing number of drugs are being identified that have an effect on the chaperone proteins that enable KCNH2/hERG proteins to fold correctly and thus to be exported from the endoplasmic reticulum to the Golgi apparatus and on to the plasma membrane. The chaperone protein Hsp90 normally helps KCNH2/hERG proteins to fold successfully. However, Hsp90 seems to be an off-target receptor for the drug arsenic trioxide. This drug therefore prevents the normal complement of KCNH2/hERG proteins from reaching the plasma membrane and being inserted correctly into the plasma membrane as KCNH2/hERG channels, and therefore causes a decrease in overall KCNH2/hERG current.

A decrease in KCNH2/hERG current plays a role in delayed repolarization of cardiac myocytes and the cascade of events leading to arrhythmias.

7.5   CORRECTION OF THE QT INTERVAL – QTc

As discussed in the previous chapter (Section 6.9), the QT interval is inversely related to heart rate: the QT interval is longer for slower heart rates and shorter for faster heart rates. Given this relationship, the QT intervals measured from the ECG are typically adjusted, or corrected, for heart rate. Once the actual QT intervals measured have been corrected in this manner, the term QTc is used. These QTc data are the data used in the statistical analyses conducted following the completion of a TQT study. The name "Thorough QT/QTc Study" can be thought of as reflecting that both QT data, i.e., the actual measurements made from ECG recordings, and QTc data, i.e., the data used in the statistical analyses conducted, are involved in a TQT study.

As noted in Section 6.9, there are two common corrections for the QT interval: Bazett's and Fridericia's corrections. The "best" correction is a subject of discussion, and, as will be seen in the next section, where ICH Guidance E14 is discussed in some detail, that guidance proposed that several values should be reported from a TQT study, including:

- ➤ The actual (uncorrected) QT interval.
- ➤ Heart rate.
- ➤ QTc according to the Fridericia formula, represented as QTcF.
- ➤ QTc according to the Bazett formula, represented as QTcB.
- ➤ QT corrections of any other type. If any of these is employed, it is particularly important to include an active control to establish assay sensitivity.

When presenting actual data, the designation QTc by itself is not sufficient: It indicates that the data presented have indeed been corrected for heart rate, but it does not define the method. Therefore, while the term QTc can be used as a generality, specific data presentations should indicate which correction method was used by placing the appropriate suffix at the end of the descriptor, i.e., QTcF or QTcB.

Fridericia's and Bazett's corrections essentially try to normalize the QT interval to a heart rate of 60 bpm. Fridericia's correction is calculated as:

$$QTcF = \frac{QT}{RR^{1/3}} = \frac{QT}{\sqrt[3]{RR}}$$

where RR represents resting heart rate, or resting rate. Bazett's correction is calculated as:

$$QTcB = \frac{QT}{RR^{1/2}} = \frac{QT}{\sqrt{RR}}$$

Fridericia's and Bazett's corrections are certainly not the only corrections that have been devised: for example, Camm et al. (2004, p. 44) listed 22 corrections. Writing on the issues surrounding the historical choice of formula, Camm et al. (2004, p. 43) noted the following:

> Of all the formulas used in the past, the most commonly used are Bazett's square-root formula ($QTc = QT/RR^{1/2}$) and Fridericia's cube-root formula ($QTc = QT/RR^{1/3}$). Between the two, Bazett's formula is more commonly used and most reported normal values are given using Bazett's formula, mainly because of its simplicity (most simple calculators have a function for a square root but not for a cube-root computation which gives a practical "advantage" to Bazett's over Fridericia's correction).

It should be noted here that Bazett's correction is still the most commonly used correction formula in clinical practice: most ECG machines used in clinical practice settings automatically provide this correction.

Another correction involves the use of linear regression techniques to normalize the QT interval to a heart rate of 60 bpm. The ICH E14 identifies a particular correction calculated in this manner used in the Framingham study (see Tisdale et al., 2007, for discussion of this correction; see also Kannel and Sorlie, 1975). Regression approaches can be used from other large databases in a similar manner as well. Using pretreatment data from a study, the QT interval is regressed on $(1-RR)$ to obtain estimates of the slope for the following equation:

$$QTc = QT + b(1 - RR)$$

A different correction methodology is called the individual corrected QT, or QTcI. This approach employs linear regressions that are calculated for each individual participant in the study. Pretreatment QT and RR data are used to fit a separate regression for each participant. A slope coefficient is applied to each participant on an individual basis as opposed to using the same coefficient in the population-level regression approaches discussed earlier. Typically, QTcI would be used as the primary endpoint in a TQT study if the investigational drug had a significant effect on the heart rate (HR). This type of correction is most appropriate in TQT studies for which a large number of pretreatment data, including varying heart rates, are available for each subject. Morganroth (2005, p. 11) noted that the "individual QTc has been routinely employed in the Thorough ECG Trial and should be considered the primary endpoint for this trial's determination of the effect of the new drug on cardiac repolarization in such cases." Litwin et al. (2008, p. 716) similarly noted that "Individual correction of the QT (QTcI) is the preferred primary method of analysis," but additionally noted that, when QTcI is used as the primary endpoint, secondary analysis of QTcF and QTcB should also be reported.

It was noted in Section 1.3 that the ICH was formed from a government body and an industry association from the EU, the United States, and Japan. The representatives from the United States were the FDA and the Pharmaceutical Research and Manufacturers of America (PhRMA). The PhRMA formed a QT Statistics Expert Working Group, which published a report of relevance to present discussions. In this report they favored the Fridericia correction, as noted in the following quote (PhRMA, 2005, p. 251):

> No single correction will work for every dataset, and therefore understanding the limitations of each correction is critical. The Bazett and Fridericia corrections are based on simple models and are easy to understand. Both formulas produce similar results when the range of heart rates is not extreme… For most populations, however, Fridericia's formula generally provides a more accurate correction. Although the Fridericia correction is

often designated as the primary correction, it is prudent to present the results using several corrections.

As an indication of another degree of complexity that we discuss in Chapter 14, *Future Directions in Drug Safety*, ICH E14, alerts sponsors to the issues surrounding the application of correction formulae to QT data collected from ECG recordings in which the heart rate has changed rapidly, since the change in the QT interval is not instantaneous. This phenomenon of time-lag between a change in heart rate and the ensuing change in QT interval is called hysteresis, and it is discussed in more detail in Section 14.2.1.

7.6   THE ICH GUIDANCE E14

The ICH Guidance E14, *Clinical Evaluation of QT/QTc Interval Prolongation and Proarrhythmic Potential for Non-Antiarrhythmic Drugs*, was finalized in October 2005. As we write this chapter (February 2008), the guidance has been implemented by the EU, United States, and Canada but not by Japan. The central focus of ICH E14 is the TQT study, a study that "is intended to determine whether the drug has a threshold pharmacologic effect on cardiac repolarization, as detected by QT/QTc prolongation" (ICH E14, 2005, p. 3). This chapter discusses various elements of the TQT study as described in ICH E14, including design, experimental methodology, and analysis.

The preparation of regulatory guidance documents, including ICH documents, is a complicated and lengthy process. Input from various stakeholders is solicited, various perspectives are incorporated in draft documents, and an extensive review and revision process is completed before the release of the final document. While necessary, some of these preparatory steps can lead to guidances that do not, and arguably should not, provide precise and unequivocal formulaic instructions on the conduct of recommended studies. These characteristics are addressed in more detail shortly, but first, the word recommended deserves attention. The following statements appear in the introductory section of ICH E14 (p. 1):

> FDA's guidance documents, including this guidance, do not establish legally enforceable responsibilities. Instead, guidances describe the Agency's current thinking on a topic and should be viewed only as recommendations, unless specific regulatory or statutory requirements are cited. The use of the word *should* in Agency guidances means that something is suggested or recommended, but not required.

In the spirit of this definition, we have used the words recommended and should in subsequent discussions, but, as sponsors are well aware, the ramifications of not following these recommendations can be considerable.

As noted, regulatory guidances, including ICH E14, do not always provide precise and unequivocal formulaic instructions on the conduct of recommended studies. One reason for this in the specific case of ICH E14 is likely to be that the field of proarrhythmic cardiac safety is relatively young and evolving quickly. Since its final release, and even during the final review and publication process, the field progressed in terms of assimilation and interpretation of existing knowledge and the acquisition of new knowledge and related interpretations. A second reason is the appreciation that not every TQT study should (or can) be conducted in precisely the same manner. This realization is captured in the final sentence of the following quote (ICH E14, 2005, p. 1):

> This guidance provides recommendations to sponsors concerning the design, conduct, analysis, and interpretation of clinical studies to assess the potential of a drug to delay cardiac repolarization. This assessment should include testing the effects of new agents on the QT/QTc interval as well as the collection of cardiovascular adverse events. The investigational approach used for a particular drug should be individualized, depending on the pharmacodynamic, pharmacokinetic, and safety characteristics of the product, as well as on its proposed clinical use.

This last sentence is enlightening in several ways. First, it is to be expected that not all TQT studies will be conducted in exactly the same manner. Judicious consideration of the circumstances surrounding each investigational drug is therefore appropriate. It is also beneficial to start a dialog with the regulatory agency as early as possible in this regard: It is invaluable for a sponsor to gain the agency's agreement with and acceptance of the rationale and justification for the TQT study design proposed as early in the preapproval clinical development program as possible. Second, the phrase "as early as possible" in the previous sentence is relevant in terms of the temporal placement of the TQT study within the overall preapproval clinical development program. While the TQT study is a critical one, it is not likely to be the first one conducted. As noted in the previous quote from ICH E14, the investigational approach used for a particular drug should be individualized, depending, in (large) part, on its pharmacokinetic, pharmacodynamic, and safety characteristics. Detailed and extensive pharmacokinetic information is typically, and most effectively, obtained during human pharmacology trials conducted at the very start of the preapproval clinical development program. This information is important in all cases, but especially so in certain cases where a modified approach to evaluating torsadogenic liability is required (discussed in Section 7.16). Typically, the TQT study is conducted in parallel to or after therapeutic exploratory trials but prior to the initiation of therapeutic confirmatory trials. Some regulators consider that the main purpose of the TQT study is to determine the appropriate level of the ECG assessment in confirmatory trials. Third, the proposed clinical use of the investigational drug has an impact on the collection of evidence concerning, and the weight given to, the drug's proarrhythmic liability. If the investigational drug is intended to be used in life-threatening situations where its expected therapeutic benefit is considered extremely high, or to fill an unmet medical need in treating a serious disease, a greater degree of proarrhythmic liability may be considered acceptable by the regulatory agency, since the overall benefit-risk balance may still be acceptable.

Having commented on the flexible nature of ICH E14, however, we believe that the statistical analyses described and recommended for the majority of TQT studies are presented in a way that may be confusing to some readers. Consequently, we have endeavored to provide some clarification of the recommended statistical approaches in two ways. First, the next section introduces the concept of confidence intervals, the use of which is a central aspect of the statistical approaches outlined in ICH E14. Second, we have included additional perspectives on the TQT study from a number of other authors. One source we have cited is PhRMA's QT Statistics Expert Working Group. Given their initial involvement with ICH and their ongoing interest in this area, we believe that the research and perspectives of industry representatives are very relevant here.

7.7   CONFIDENCE INTERVALS AND THEIR EMPLOYMENT IN HYPOTHESIS TESTING

The participants in a clinical trial represent a sample taken from the general population of interest. Analysis of this trial's data provides a precise result for that particular sample. However, and importantly, the sample is likely to be a (very) small percentage of the population from which the sample was chosen. This means that had a different sample of participants been chosen, the chances of the data obtained being identical are so infinitesimally small that we can safely say that they would be different. The question of interest therefore becomes: How different would they likely be? Ideally, we would like the data to be extremely similar, thereby providing a result that is extremely similar to that obtained in the original trial: The more similar the results of a second trial, the more confidence we could reasonably place in the results of the original trial. While the word confidence in the previous sentence was used in its everyday use, the term is also used in the discipline of Statistics in a precise manner, introduced in this section.

In a TQT study we are interested in making several comparisons. One of these is to compare the prolongation of the QT/QTc interval due to the administration of the investigational drug with the prolongation of the QT/QTc interval due to the administration of the placebo. (Even though the placebo is pharmacologically inert it is still the case, as in any trial, that a [very] small response may be seen in subjects receiving the placebo: That is, responses to a placebo will often not be precisely zero.) The treatment effect of an investigational drug can be represented in various ways: for this example, we will regard it as the difference between the adjusted mean of the responses among the sample of participants receiving the investigational drug and the adjusted mean of the responses among the sample of participants receiving the placebo. The term 'adjusted' in the previous sentence refers to a covariate adjustment to the response of interest. In the case of the TQT study, the mean response is adjusted for the baseline QT/QTc value (and often referred to as baseline-adjusted). Readers who are unfamiliar with adjusted means can regard these values in a similar manner as they would the simple mean. Adjusted means are the expected (or typical) response for a particular treatment standardized for the covariate (e.g., baseline). In practical terms, the adjusted mean response to the placebo is subtracted from the adjusted mean response to the investigational drug. In the TQT trial, this calculation of the investigational drug's treatment effect represents the degree of QT/QTc interval prolongation that can be reasonably attributed to the investigational drug.

7.7.1   The Point Estimate

As noted earlier, the treatment effect described in the previous section has been precisely calculated from the sample of participants in one particular study. The question now becomes: how confident can we be that this treatment effect is representative of the true but unknown treatment effect on the general population from which this sample was chosen? This question can be answered by calculating and placing confidence intervals (CIs) around the precise value obtained in this single trial. In this context, the precise value obtained in the trial is termed the point estimate: it is a known value that estimates the true but unknown value for the general population.

If appropriate experimental methodology has been employed in any given trial, the point estimate is likely to be representative of, i.e., similar to, the true but unknown population value, but not to be precisely the same as that value. Therefore, placing CIs around the point estimate provides a more informative representation of the likely location of the true but unknown population value. In many scenarios, a two-sided CI is placed around a point estimate. In others, a one-sided CI is placed on one particular side of the point estimate.

7.7.2   Two-sided Confidence Intervals

When a two-sided CI is employed, the point estimate is enclosed within a range of values defined at its lower end by the lower limit of the CI and at its upper end by the upper limit of the CI. Many statistical analytical strategies involve the calculation and placement of two-sided CIs around a point estimate. In some cases, such as the case of data obtained in a TQT study, the point estimate will lie precisely in the center of the CI, i.e., equidistant from the lower limit and upper limit. This occurs since the lower limit and the upper limit of the CI are calculated by subtracting and adding the same value from and to the point estimate. (The calculation of this value is not of immediate concern here.) In other cases, such as the relative risks discussed in Chapters 8 and 12, this is not so. The point estimate for a relative risk lies towards the center of the CI, but it will be somewhat closer to the lower limit than to the upper limit (discussion of the reason for this can wait until Chapter 8).

The degree of confidence that a given CI will cover the range of the true but unknown population value depends on which CIs are used. While it is possible to meaningfully calculate CIs for any percentage greater than 0 and less than 100, two commonly used values are the 95% CI and the 99% CI. When 95% CIs are placed around a point estimate, we can be 95% confident that the range of values defined by the lower and upper limits of the CI covers the true but unknown population value. If we calculate and place 99% CIs around a point estimate, we can be 99% confident that the range of values encapsulated by the lower and upper limits of the CI cover the true but unknown population value.

Imagine for a moment the scenario of developing an investigational drug for the treatment of high blood pressure, i.e., an antihypertensive drug. For this drug to be clinically useful it must lower blood pressure, and a clinical trial would compare the decrease in blood pressure due to the administration of the investigational drug with that resulting from the placebo, which, as noted, is unlikely to be precisely zero. However, it must be borne in mind that it is theoretically possible that the investigational drug will actually *increase* blood pressure compared with placebo. Therefore, in statistical terminology, we must conduct two-sided tests in this context: we need to examine the possibility that the drug may increase blood pressure as well as the (intended) possibility that it will lower blood pressure. With regard to the placement of CIs around the point estimate, this logic translates into the fact that we need to place intervals on both sides of the point estimate.

If we wish to express a 99% degree of certainty (a higher degree of confidence) rather than a 95% degree of certainty that a given range of values will contain the true but unknown population value, that range of values will be wider than it would be when expressing a 95% degree of certainty. Expressed more succinctly:

> ➤ Two-sided 99% CIs placed around a point estimate are always wider than 95% CIs.

7.7.3   One-sided Confidence Intervals

In contrast to a two-sided CI, where interest lies with both the lower limit and the upper limit of the interval encapsulating the point estimate, a one-sided CI focuses on the placement of a single interval on one particular side of the point estimate.

In the case of the TQT study, we are interested in changes in QT/QTc in one direction only. That is, we are interested in the degree to which an investigational drug may increase the QT/QTc compared with placebo, and not in potential QT/QTc decreases. We are therefore interested in the location of the placement of a limit above the point estimate, i.e., the limit will have a higher numerical value than the point estimate. As for two-sided CIs, it is possible to meaningfully calculate a one-sided CI for any percentage greater than 0 and less than 100, but again, the 95% and 99% levels of confidence are commonly used. In the TQT study the 95% one-sided CI is of particular interest. While the terms lower limit and upper limit are not really applicable since we only have interest in, and hence only calculate, one limit in the case of a one-sided confidence interval, in the setting of the TQT study this limit is typically referred to as the upper bound of the 95% one-sided CI.

It should be clarified and emphasized here that the upper bound of a 95% one-sided CI around a point estimate will not fall at the same place as the upper limit of a 95% two-sided CI calculated for the same point estimate. The statistical reasons for this do not need to be addressed at this point (they are discussed later in the chapter) but the important consequence does need to be noted: The upper bound of the 95% one-sided CI will be closer to the point estimate than the upper limit of the 95% two-sided CI. In fact, the upper bound of a 95% one-sided CI is equivalent to the upper limit of a two-sided 90% CI. It is therefore vital to be clear about precisely which form of CI one calculates and presents when reporting the results from a TQT study. The typical way of presenting results is to report the upper bound of the 95% one-sided CI. However, since the upper limit of the 90% CI is identical in this case to this value, the result can be expressed in that manner too. The interpretation of the upper limit of a two-sided 90% CI is that we are 95% confident that the upper limit is greater than the true unknown value of the population value (e.g., mean change in QTc), meaning that it is not likely that the true mean is greater than the upper limit. This is the same interpretation that can be made using the upper bound of the one-sided 95% CI.

7.8 STUDY DESIGN CONSIDERATIONS

The primary objective of the TQT study is to rule out, with 95% statistical confidence, effects of an investigational new drug on the QTc interval that would be of regulatory concern. The threshold of regulatory concern "is around 5 msec as evidenced by an upper bound of the 95% confidence interval around the mean effect on QTc of 10 msec" (ICH E14, 2005, p. 3). The ICH E14 (p. 4) noted that the TQT study "should be adequate and well-controlled, with mechanisms to deal with potential bias, including use of randomization, appropriate blinding, and concurrent placebo control group."

The TQT study is typically conducted using healthy participants as part of the early preapproval clinical development program. The choice of this participant population seemingly represents a trade-off between practicality and the ability to apply the results to the eventual target population. Morganroth (2005, p. 208) commented as follows:

> From a clinical point of view, it seems more meaningful to conduct the Thorough ECG Trial in the population that is the target of the drug's use; however, selecting patients with clinical diseases or older apparently healthy people will make the ECG results in the Thorough ECG Trial nondefinitive. This is because patients who have multiple degrees of disease intensity often have multiple comorbidities and take different concomitant medications. The balancing of all these factors that can effect the duration of the QTc interval, would require too large a sample size and too difficult a recruitment to make the ECG trial thorough.

It is useful to keep in mind here that the TQT study is really a bioassay: it is used to investigate whether the investigational drug has any effect on QTc and, if so, to estimate that effect in a highly controlled set of participants and a highly controlled setting. The purpose of the study is not to cause marked QT prolongation or TdP. Rather, the importance of identifying that the investigational drug leads to QTc prolongation of greater than 10 msec in a highly controlled setting is that it alerts all concerned that the drug, if approved, is more likely to result in marked QT prolongation when given to thousands of patients, some of whom may have subclinical forms of inherited LQTS.

The results of the TQT study guide the extent of intensive monitoring of QT/QTc effects required in later stages of development, e.g., in therapeutic exploratory and therapeutic confirmatory trials: The greater the QT liability suggested by the results of the TQT study, the greater the need for later ECG monitoring. The TQT study is performed before these later clinical trials are commenced. However, as noted earlier, the TQT study is not likely to be the first study conducted in the preapproval clinical development program. At the time the TQT study is designed, it is appropriate to have collected a certain amount of data regarding the investigational drug's pharmacokinetic profile and the likely doses for use in later trials. This information is then used to plan the timing of ECG monitoring as part of the TQT study. For cost reasons, it may be advantageous to the sponsor to conduct the TQT study only after dose selection studies have narrowed the dose range to a small number of therapeutic doses. However, this strategy may be at odds with the desire to identify, as a result of the TQT study, the extent of intensive cardiac monitoring needed in later stages of development.

7.8.1   Relative Advantages of Parallel and Crossover Designs

The usual strengths and weaknesses of parallel and crossover designs should be considered when designing a TQT study. The primary advantage of crossover studies is that each participant serves as his or her own control, thereby reducing the intersubject variability for estimates of the effect on QT/QTc. A result of this reduction in variability is that a smaller sample size is required for an appropriately powered study. Second, additional data from individuals in a crossover trial may enhance the ability to use regression-based methods to correct the QT interval for heart rate to produce QTc data. Balanced crossover designs, i.e., those for which each treatment is administered prior to every other treatment, are helpful in that any crossover effect is balanced.

However, crossover trials are generally not recommended when the investigational drug has a long half-life (requiring lengthy washout periods) or when multiple doses are being evaluated. In these instances, a parallel-group design may be considered advantageous.

7.8.2   The Role of Experimental Controls

The term experimental control pertains to elements of the study that can be used to eliminate particular sources of variability from the evaluation of interest. As stated in ICH E14 (p. 4):

> An important problem in the measurement of the QT/QTc interval is its intrinsic variability. This variability results from many factors, including activity level, postural changes, circadian patterns, and food ingestion. It is critical to address intrinsic variability in the conduct of the "thorough" QT/QTc study.

In this context, the term intrinsic variability refers to variability within an individual. As noted in Section 4.4, Hondeghem (2005, p. 235) observed that 'Eating, sleeping, getting up, exercise and other pleasurable activities can prolong the QT interval." Morganroth et al. (1991) reported that the QTc interval can vary by as much 75 msec in healthy men over the course of a day. Experimental controls that may be implemented to minimize this intrinsic variability include ensuring that each participant's ECGs are recorded while lying down comfortably following 5–10 minutes of rest, at the same times of day for all observation periods (i.e., baseline and post-baseline for a parallel study or each period of a crossover trial), and with the same meal schedule on each occasion of measurement, ideally one to two hours before ECG recordings. It is also important to avoid televisions, cell phones, iPods, iPhones, and any other electronic devices that can provide distraction (Satin, 2008). When controls such as these are implemented, potentially confounding factors can be removed from consideration (or largely diminished) when interpreting any differences observed in QTc intervals between the investigational drug and the placebo.

7.8.3   Establishing Assay Sensitivity: The Role of the Positive Control

Another source of variability in QT/QTc measures made during a TQT study is due to the sampling process itself. It is possible that, through sampling variation alone, a real effect on the QTc interval may not be detected for the investigational drug relative to the placebo. Given the importance assigned to the TQT study in the overall assessment of QT liability, its ability to detect effects of clinical significance, if they exist, must be established. This ability is termed assay sensitivity. Assay sensitivity in this case is typically provided by using a study design that includes a positive control: If a clinically relevant effect on QTc can be detected for the positive control, a treatment known to increase QTc relative to the placebo control, the study is considered to have assay sensitivity.

The logic here is as follows. Failure of a particular TQT study to detect an increase in QTc during the administration of a compound that is well established to cause such an increase relative to placebo means that there is an absence of assay sensitivity. In such a case, it is not possible to put credence in a lack of a QTc increase relative to placebo during the administration of the investigational drug, since there are two possibilities that cannot be distinguished: either the investigational drug truly does not increase QTc, or it does indeed increase QTc at least as much as the positive control but the absence of assay sensitivity means that this increase cannot be detected. In contrast, if a particular TQT study correctly identifies the expected increase in QTc during the administration of a positive control that is well established to cause such an increase, the study has demonstrated assay sensitivity. In this case, if an increase in QTc interval is not seen during the administration of the investigational drug, the result is more compelling and credible since the role of sampling variability can likely be eliminated as a source of this lack of QTc interval increase.

Considerations for the choice of the positive control were outlined in ICH E14 (p. 4):

> The positive control should have an effect on the mean QT/QTc interval of about 5 msec (i.e., an effect that is close to the QT/QTc effect that represents the threshold of regulatory concern, around 5 msec). Detecting the positive control's effect will establish the ability of the study to detect such an effect of the study drug. Absence of a positive control should be justified and alternative methods to establish assay sensitivity provided. If an

investigational drug belongs to a chemical or pharmacological class that has been associated with QT/QTc prolongation, a positive control selected from other members of the same class should be considered to permit a comparison of effect sizes, preferably at equipotent therapeutic doses.

The Safety of Administering a Positive Control. A potential paradox may have been noted by the reader at this point. The ICH E14 regulatory guidance suggests that, during the TQT study, a positive control—a drug that is known to prolong the QTc interval—should be given to study participants. Given that all of our discussions of proarrhythmic cardiac safety in this book revolve around the potential torsadogenic liability of such increases, why would the administration of a compound known to increase the QTc interval be recommended? This is a perfectly reasonable question.

The answer is that an increase in QTc of 5 msec has been determined to have an extremely small likelihood of causing ventricular arrhythmias of clinical concern. Therefore, the benefits of administering a positive control that leads to a 5 msec increase—the ability to determine the QTc liability of the investigational drug, which may be of considerable clinical concern—are considered to outweigh the risk of its administration. In fact, if a participant in a TQT study developed TdP after a dose of the positive control employed, it would be much better to have identified this in the setting of a clinical pharmacology unit as opposed to an outpatient setting. We noted in Section 7.8 that marked QT prolongation may be identified in patients once the marketed drug has been administered to thousands of patients, some of whom may have subclinical forms of inherited LQTS. It is also possible that a participant in the TQT study may have a subclinical form of inherited LQTS, and that this would be discovered as a result of the drug-induced episode of TdP. In this case, not only would the participant be in a setting that would allow optimal medical care for this particular occurrence of TdP, but the discovery of the inherited LQTS would alert the participant that ongoing clinical consultations would be beneficial.

Use of Moxifloxacin as a Positive Control. While there are several drugs that could potentially serve as a positive control in this context, Morganroth (2005) noted that the antibiotic moxifloxacin has become accepted as the standard positive control since its administration leads to a predictable change in QTc. Moxifloxacin is an 8-methoxyquinolone antibacterial with enhanced potency against important gram-positive pathogens, notable *Streptococcus pneumoniae* (Ball, 2000; see also Culley et al., 2001). Litwin et al. (2008, p. 716) cited an average moxifloxicin effect over multiple time points (time-averaged) of 5–8 msec for the QTc. The use of a marketed positive control may present concerns over the need for appropriate blinding. However, provided that the central reading center is blinded, double blinding of moxifloxicin is not required for the TQT study (Morganroth 2005).

7.8.4   The TQT Four-Arm Study Design

Although not explicitly prescribed in the ICH E14 guidance, a four-arm study design is recommended by Morganroth (2005) and by Litwin et al. (2008): This design includes two doses of the investigational drug, a placebo control, and a positive control, which comprise the four treatment arms. One of the doses of the investigational drug is the anticipated clinical dose and the other is a supratherapeutic dose. There are several advantages of this incorporation of the supratherapeutic dose. First, use of a supratherapeutic dose can help define the magnitude of risk using the steepness of the dose-QTc relationship. Second, the use of such a high dose in healthy participants may mimic the risks of the therapeutic dose in a target population of patients with concurrent diseases, or mimic the consequences of an inappropriately high dose being prescribed and/or administered to a patient. For example, a patient with impaired metabolic capacity would not metabolize the drug as quickly as expected when prescribed a certain dose, and so the patient is likely to experience a higher plasma concentration of the drug, one that may be similar to that produced by a supratherapeutic dose in healthy participants without hepatic impairment. Third, consider a scenario where the eventual therapeutic dose turns out to be much higher than the originally planned therapeutic dose, i.e., the dose included in the TQT study. Without the inclusion of a supratherapeutic dose, the sponsor would not have any data that could be used to estimate the QT liability of the new therapeutic dose. This advantage holds true only if the new therapeutic dose is still below the supratherapeutic dose employed in the study, which argues for the supratherapeutic dose to be considerably higher than the originally intended therapeutic dose. Morganroth (2005, p. 208) commented as follows:

> The individuals in a Thorough ECG Trial should have no variables that will influence the ECG parameters, and thus the study population for the Thorough ECG Trial should be healthy young volunteers. However, to mimic the new drug's interaction with any effect modifiers that might be present in the target population (e.g., heart disease, metabolic abnormalities, concomitant drug metabolic inhibitors, or abnormal metabolism) a supratherapeutic dose treatment arm in the healthy volunteers must be employed. It is anticipated that this supratherapeutic dose given to healthy volunteers will mimic the worst-case effects (save for a frank overdose) of the drug in the target population, allowing the Thorough ECG Trial study to be conducted in healthy volunteers rather than in the target population.

The supratherapeutic dose "should be modeled based on the known pharmacologic properties of the drug and how the extent of exposure will change when it is taken by a patient who has effect modifiers" (Morganroth, 2005, p. 209). As a guideline, Morganroth suggested that "the minimal clinical dose compared to the supratherapeutic dose should be at least 3–5x apart and that certain agents such as antihistamines or antibiotics should be over 10x apart." However, this is often a key point of discussion between sponsors and regulators. The maximum dose of an investigational drug that can be given to healthy participants in a TQT study differs greatly from compound to compound. Sometime the maximum therapeutic dose is the same as the maximum tolerated dose, and a supratherapeutic dose cannot be given.

In summary, the standard TQT study includes a treatment group for the investigational drug at the intended clinical dose, a placebo control group, a positive control group (typically given moxifloxacin), and a treatment group given a supratherapeutic dose of the investigational drug.

7.9   DATA COLLECTION: MEASUREMENT OF QT INTERVALS

Having looked at study design considerations for the TQT study, our attention now turns to the experimental methodologies employed to collect the data. Given that the objective of the TQT study is to rule out potentially harmful cardiac effects of an investigational drug, a number of factors must be considered, including:

➢ Timing of the ECG (QT interval) acquisition.
➢ Accuracy and precision of the QT/QTc interval measurement.
➢ Sources of variability in the QT/QTc interval.

The ECGs used are 12-lead ECGs. They can be stand-alone ECGs or ECGs collected as part of a 12-lead, continuous 24-hour Holter recording. The ECGs should be collected at a number of nominal time points in all observation periods (if continuous 24-hour recordings are used, these time points need to be identified within the total recording). Collection of ECGs at the same time points in all observation periods ensures that the experimental conditions (e.g., diurnal variation) are similar when each treatment is administered. Data obtained in this manner are considered time-matched data, meaning that the QTc effect at the same time can be compared within a participant (in the case of crossover) or between participants (in a parallel group study). Litwin et al. (2008) recommend sampling at 12–15 time points. This is very similar to Morganroth's (2005) recommendation of 12–16 time points.

During a pretreatment (baseline) period, 12-lead ECGs are acquired on a fixed schedule of various nominal time points (e.g., hourly), which are typically dictated by pharmacokinetic characteristics. If the study utilizes a crossover design, there may be a single baseline period or multiple respective baseline periods that precede each treatment period of the crossover sequence. If the latter strategy is employed, only the first baseline will be a long one, but it may not be as long as the observation period when participants are administered study treatment. For each on-treatment period (i.e., one for each participant in a parallel group study or one per participant per treatment arm in a crossover study), ECGs are acquired on the same fixed schedule of time points. Replicates are collected for each nominal time point.

Inherent variability of the QT interval can be managed in a number of ways. First and foremost, the ECGs should be collected in a consistent manner throughout the TQT study (e.g., consistent posture, times of day to account for circadian patterns and food ingestion, as already noted in Section 7.8.2). Second, if the ECGs are collected at multiple centers, study staff should receive training to ensure consistency with respect to placement of the leads and use of the equipment. Acquisition of optimum quality raw data is essential, and no number of corrective strategies can fully reinstitute or replace this quality.

A second variability management strategy is to collect replicate ECGs at each nominal time point in the study (baseline and postbaseline) and use the arithmetic average (the mean) of the replicates to yield a single QT value per nominal time point. Such a strategy can substantially reduce the standard deviation for change from baseline QT/QTc and, therefore, reduce the required sample size for adequate power. Using a simulated dataset, Hollister and Montague (2005) demonstrated that the standard deviation decreases exponentially as the number of replicates increases. In practical terms, the use of two or three replicates has a substantial advantage over a single value with regard to precision, but the additional gain in precision attained by using more than three replicates is relatively modest. Each replicate ECG's collection should be separated by a few minutes (two-minute intervals is common) during the recording window for each nominal time point of data collection, and should occur before blood is drawn for pharmacokinetic assessments.

The timing (or spacing) of ECG acquisition should consider the time concentration profile of the compound and metabolites attained in early pharmacokinetic studies. As described in ICH E14 (p. 4), "an adequate drug development programme should ensure that the dose-response and generally the concentration-response relationship for QT/QTc prolongation have been characterized, including exploration of concentrations that are higher than those achieved following the anticipated therapeutic doses." The doses studied could vary according to the drug under investigation, i.e., a single dose studied might be sufficient for drugs with short half-lives and no (active) metabolites. In all cases, the ECGs should be collected at time points around the C_{max} of the doses studied. Although pharmacokinetic characteristics may dictate lengthy observation periods to evaluate the effect of the test treatment, positive controls need only be used long enough to observe the expected effect.

Study ECGs are usually taken from a resting participant and acquired from 12-lead surface ECGs, optimally from equipment capable of digital signal processing. Like all equipment used in regulatory studies, the ECG equipment should be regularly serviced and calibrated, with sufficient documentation to satisfy regulatory expectations. The digital recordings are then "typically transferred from the collection site to a centralized laboratory with 26CFR Part 11 compliant data management and analysis tools to process the 12-lead digital data" (Mortara, 2005, p. 136). The ICH E14 guidance regards ambulatory monitoring of the ECG as having only "potential value" since its use is not considered fully evaluated and the typical thresholds of regulatory concern (defined using surface ECGs) may not apply to QT/QTc intervals ascertained from ambulatory ECGs. However, on the basis of recent research into the use of Holter monitors for the purpose of identifying drug-induced QT changes, ambulatory monitoring appears to be as useful as resting ECGs while providing more intensive data collection (Sarapa, 2005), and Holter monitoring has become the accepted standard for TQT studies. When using high fidelity Holter monitors (1000 Hz sampling), the study participants are instructed to remain supine for several minutes periodically so that good, quality tracings can be taken.

Measurement of the actual QT intervals from the ECGs recorded in a TQT study would typically involve measurement by a few skilled readers (whether or not assisted by a computer) operating from a single centralized or core ECG laboratory, typically called simply a core ECG lab (see discussions in Section 8.4.1 concerning core labs and local labs). These readers may or may not use semi-automated approaches. In such approaches, algorithms can be programmed into software to make an initial judgment of QTc, and readers can then check and/or correct such readings. Measurements are typically taken using digital onscreen calipers while the ECG is viewed on a screen. As suggested in ICH E14, the most appropriate methodology has not been identified but the precordial leads and lead II are often used to measure the QT interval.

It is recommended in ICH E14 that the readers be blinded to time (e.g., pre-treatment or posttreatment), treatment, and participant. Further, estimates of intra- and interreader variability should be assessed by having the readers reevaluate a subset of the data, including normal and abnormal readings. Consistency throughout a TQT trial is the most important consideration.

7.9.1   A Rationale for the Collection of Replicate ECGs

In the report from the PhRMA QT Statistics Expert Working Group, a number of studies were cited to justify the use of replicates. The group commented as follows (PhRMA, 2005, p. 246):

> A rationale for recording replicate ECGs is that the QT interval is assumed to be a continuous parameter that is measured with error. The clinical assumption is that even under stable conditions, an individual's true QT/QTc interval can vary over several minutes. How much of the variability observed under stable conditions over several minutes is due to natural biological variability and how much is due to measurement error is open to question. Using the mean from several ECGs recorded over a few minutes would be one way to reduce potential measurement error and obtain a more precise estimate of the subject's true response at a nominal time.

Collection of three replicates at each of 12–16 time points results in 36–48 individual ECGs per participant per observation period (e.g., baseline and on-treatment periods for a parallel group or for each treatment period of a crossover study). This quantity of data should be enough to compute individual correction (QTcI, as introduced in Section 7.5) for QTc under most circumstances in the baseline period (in the case of a parallel-group study) or baseline periods (taken all together from a crossover study).

7.9.2   Data Supplied to the Sponsor by the Core ECG Laboratory

Once the core ECG lab has completed its data measurements and interpretation, it supplies the study sponsor with data corresponding to each replicate for each time point of all treatment periods. More specifically, this includes (Morganroth, 2005):

> ➢ Standard ECG intervals and morphological assessments of each ECG recorded in the trial.
> ➢ ECGs submitted to the study sponsor with annotation of the interpretations. These ECGs are supplied as Extensible Markup Language (XML) files, a format that can be transferred across various platforms and that has been agreed to by the FDA. A separate dataset with the ECG measurements (e.g., QT, RR) is also provided to the sponsor.

7.10   ENDPOINTS EVALUATED IN THE TQT STUDY

Attention now turns to the statistical analysis of QT interval data collected during the TQT study and the QTc values derived from these data. First, however, it is appropriate to consider the endpoints that are evaluated at the conclusion of the study.

As we have seen, during a TQT study, ECGs and QT/QTc intervals obtained from them are collected at multiple time points throughout the study. In the case of a parallel-group study, the QTc data acquired include the following:

> ➢ A series of baseline QTc values (in replicate) collected at a number of nominal time points prior to the initiation of any study drug. These data will have been recorded for all participants in the study.
> ➢ QTc values (in replicate) collected on a fixed schedule of nominal time points during the on-treatment period. These data will have been collected for all participants in each of the treatment groups (e.g., therapeutic dose of the investigational drug, supratherapeutic dose of the investigational drug, positive control, and placebo). The time points of ECG collection will be the same for all groups in the study, enabling a comparison between groups of mean response on a time-matched basis.

In the case of a crossover study, the QTc data include the following:

> ➤ A series of baseline QTc values (in replicate) collected at a number of nominal time points prior to the initiation of the study drug. The baseline observations may consist of a single baseline period (prior to the first period of the crossover sequence) or multiple baseline periods (e.g., prior to treatment in each period of the crossover sequence).
> ➤ QTc values (in replicate) collected on a fixed schedule of nominal time points during each of the treatment periods of the crossover sequence. These data will have been collected for all participants in each of the treatment periods (e.g., therapeutic dose of the investigational drug, supratherapeutic dose of the investigational drug, positive control, and placebo). The time points of ECG collection will be the same for all periods in the study, enabling a comparison between treatments of the mean within-participant response on a time-matched basis.

Since the primary objective of the TQT study is to rule out a mean change in QTc of a magnitude of regulatory concern, an important consideration is how to define an outcome, or endpoint, for which the mean effect will be evaluated. Ultimately, the effect of interest is the treatment effect, defined as the between-treatment difference in baseline-adjusted response. With the quantity of data collected and the primary objective in mind, the following questions suggest themselves:

1. How are the replicate QT/QTc measurements handled?
2. From what time point is the change in QTc measured? That is, what is the baseline?
3. What is the endpoint (i.e., response) used to describe the QTc treatment effect of interest? Is it the:
   - QTc at all time points measured?
   - QTc at a single particular time point?
   - QTc at a few specified time points?

Responses to these questions are discussed in order. As a preview of the discussion to come, however, we can note that the answer to each of the questions within Question 3 is "yes." This reflects the notion stated earlier that ICH E14 recommended a general approach, one that has been interpreted in a myriad of ways.

As we have noted, replicate QT values for each time point are typically obtained and averaged, and this mean provides single QT/QTc values that are used in the subsequent statistical analyses. It should be noted here that one use of the replicates described in the literature is not consistent with this description. This exceptional case will be discussed in the response to Question 3 after all of the other points have been discussed in order.

With up to three replicates per nominal time point, the recommended approach is to average the replicate values to obtain a single value per time point. Using this single value per nominal time point, it is possible to calculate, for each treatment, the change from baseline at each time point or to define another summary statistic (e.g., area under the curve, or AUC: recall the discussions in Section 6.4.1). The summary statistic, however it may be defined, is then summarized descriptively using measures of central tendency.

The QT/QTc intervals are obtained at multiple time points in the baseline period (or periods, in the case of a crossover study with period-specific baselines). Hence, the term change from baseline requires a clear definition of what the baseline value represents. The selection of QT/QTc values to analyze should consider the potential of analyses to reflect a regression to the mean. That is, if the highest pretreatment QT values are selected as representative of the baseline, post-treatment values will likely be lower, simply as a result of the selection criteria for baseline values as a comparison. As with other clinical studies, the use of control groups mitigates the potential of inappropriate interpretations due to regression to the mean. Morganroth (2005, p. 211) commented that the use of multiple ECGs to represent the baseline is preferred over a single ECG:

> The recommendation is that baseline ECGs should be computed as the mean of multiple ECGs to enhance the precision of the measurement in light of the large degree of spontaneous variability in QTc duration. Regulatory guidance is to collect drug-free ECGs on two or three different days to help document inter-day variability in the baseline.

One way to define what baseline value should be used is to consider the endpoint of interest. For example, if a sponsor is interested in the mean change in QTc across all time points, a baseline value defined as the mean QTc of all values in the pretreatment period seems to represent a meaningful comparison of like random variables. On the other hand, if the primary interest lies with the mean change from baseline at a particular nominal time point, a baseline value defined as the mean over all pretreatment values does not seem to be a meaningful comparison, since averaging over time points dilutes the effect of any diurnal variation. There are various approaches that may be utilized to define the baseline, but a baseline using a single value is not recommended. In any case, the baseline value is intended to represent the typical QTc value, which is not affected by any study treatment. The baseline value is used as a covariate to adjust for differences in baseline between treatments (e.g., investigational drug and placebo).

The PhRMA QT working group listed six different endpoints by which to measure the mean effect on QTc. The endpoints are listed in Table 7.1 and numbered for later reference. Note that in the Definition column of this table, the terms "changes from baseline" and "differences from baseline" have been used. In the paper from the PhRMA QT working group, these descriptions referred to "time-matched changes from baseline" and "time-matched differences from baseline." If a study included the same nominal time points in the baseline period and the treatment periods, then it would be possible to calculate a time-matched change from baseline for each treatment in the study. However, we have chosen to delete the term time-matched from this description since some studies will not utilize identical ECG collection time points in all periods of the study. The baseline value, however it is defined, plays a critical role in defining the QTc effect of interest.

TABLE 7.1. Endpoints Defined by the PhRMA QT Statistics Expert Working Group (PhRMA, 2005, p. 253)

Endpoint	Definition
1. QT/QTc change from baseline	For each participant and at each time point, compute the differences between QTc intervals on the drug [during the treatment period] and at baseline.
2. QT/QTc change from baseline at participant– specific T_{max}	For each participant, use the first ECG collected at or after the time of peak concentration (T_{max}) of each analyte (parent drug and metabolites) and compute changes from baseline in QT/QTc intervals. The median T_{max} from all subjects who received active drug can be used in the analysis of QT/QTc changes in a placebo period or group.
3. QT/QTc change from baseline at population T_{max}	For each participant, compute QT/QTc changes from baseline at the population T_{max}.
4. Maximum QT/QTc increase from baseline	For each participant, determine the largest increase from baseline.
5. AUC of QT/QTc intervals relative to baseline	For each participant, compute the trapezoidal area under the QT/QTc-time curve from time zero to t hours (this quantity is denoted by QTc AUC_{0-t}).
6. Time-averaged QT/QTc intervals relative to baseline	For each participant, average QT/QTc changes from baseline.

Each of these endpoints has been identified by Hollister and Montague (2005), who also included a discussion of the advantages and disadvantages of each of these approaches. Some of them are discussed in greater detail here, including comments from the PhRMA QT working group.

Endpoint 1, the QT/QTc change from baseline, is calculated on a per-participant basis by computing the difference between the on-treatment QT/QTc and the baseline value. If the same time points were used in the baseline and the on-treatment periods, this change value can be calculated using the time-matched baseline value. The advantages of this method are twofold: It allows for the correction of diurnal effects, and it can be used together with drug concentrations to estimate QT/QTc prolongation as a function of drug concentration (PhRMA, 2005). However, a disadvantage is that examination of all time points can result in inflation of the Type I error due to multiple testing. A Type I error occurs when a statistically significant result is found when it does not really exist. When conducting any single-hypothesis test, there will always be the possibility that a Type I error will occur. However, we can limit this likelihood by structuring our analytical strategy such that we will only declare a result to be statistically significant if the likelihood of a Type I error is sufficiently low.

A common way to do this is to declare a result to be statistically significant only if the probability of such a result (or one more extreme) occurring by chance is less than 5%, i.e., less than 1 in 20. This is the basis for the commonly employed criterion of using a p-value less than 0.05 (i.e., $p<0.05$) to claim a result as statistically significant. In this scenario, we have set our Type I error rate at $\alpha = 0.05$ (or 5%). Our earlier comment that "examination of all time points can result in inflation of the Type I error due to multiple testing" relates to the fact that, as more hypothesis tests are conducted, i.e., more results are examined, the likelihood of finding a statistically significant result by chance alone increases. This occurrence is represented in Table 7.2, which shows how the Type I error becomes progressively inflated as up to 20 independent tests are conducted, each at an α-level (our chosen Type I error rate) of 0.05.

TABLE 7.2. Maximum Probability of Committing a Type I Error When Each Hypothesis Is Tested at $\alpha = 0.05$

Number of Hypotheses Tested at $\alpha = 0.05$	Maximum Probability of Type I Error
1	0.050
2	0.098
3	0.143
4	0.185
5	0.226
6	0.265
7	0.302
8	0.337
9	0.370
10	0.401
15	0.537
20	0.642

As can be seen, when up to 10 tests are conducted, the overall Type I error may be as high as 0.4. This means that if 10 tests are conducted, there is up to a 40% chance that one of the results will be declared statistically significant by chance alone. Even if (only) three hypotheses are each tested at the α-level of 0.05, there is up to a 14% chance that one of the results will be declared statistically significant by chance alone. That is, the probability of committing a Type I error increases almost three-fold. In such cases, a strategy for managing multiple testing, or multiplicity, needs to be specified. That is, a strategy for maintaining the overall (experimentwise) Type I error rate at the traditional α = 0.05 level is needed. The need for a management strategy to maintain the overall Type I is relevant to the analysis of TQT study results and is discussed in Section 7.12.

Endpoint 2, the QT/QTc change from baseline at participant-specific T_{max}, may also be considered. The ICH Guidance E14 recommended this approach if the drug has large between-participant variability in the rate of absorption or metabolism. However, C_{max} and T_{max} are typically the most variable pharmacokinetic parameters, which would contribute to uncertainty about the true QT/QTc effect (Hollister and Montague, 2005). Another disadvantage here is that a PK sample must be collected just prior to every ECG.

In ICH E14 the favored endpoint is Endpoint 4, the largest difference in QTc. The largest difference is defined on a per-participant level by identifying the maximum change from baseline without regard for at which time point it was obtained (Hollister and Montague, 2005), an approach that means that the time at which the maximum difference was obtained could differ among all participants. Again, if the appropriate baseline values are available, the maximum change from baseline could consider the maximum time-matched change from baseline. This difference is then summarized descriptively for each treatment group using measures of central tendency, i.e., the mean and/or the median. The maximum QT/QTc increase from baseline provides an assessment of the worst potential for an adverse outcome when assessing the effect of a drug on QT/QTc intervals. However, "it may yield upwardly biased results and should only be used in placebo-controlled studies where the impact of diurnal patterns may be evaluated" (PhRMA, 2005, p. 253).

Hollister and Montague (2005) noted that the maximum difference approach may not be optimal if there are too few or two many sampling time points. In the first case the true maximal effect may be missed, and in the second case there is an increased chance of a false positive. As the QT, QTc, and the length of the cardiac cycle, represented by the time from one R-wave to the subsequent R-wave (the *RR* interval), are highly correlated, it is recommended that all three of these measures be summarized in the analysis. (While various point-to-point measurements could theoretically be used to represent the length of the cardiac cycle, the *RR* interval is typically used because the R-wave is typically the most readily identified landmark in the ECG.) Since the maximum QTc difference could correspond to different time points among participants, Hollister and Montague (2005) proposed that the QT and RR values obtained at the same time as the maximum QTc difference be summarized for these analyses.

At this point, it is worthwhile to expand on an important technical detail regarding the operational definition of Endpoint 4, the maximum QT/QTc increase from baseline, since it may be a source of confusion. The use and handling of replicate QT/QTc intervals around a nominal time point were discussed in Section 7.9. Typically, the value of QT/QTc for a given time point is the result of having averaged the values of the replicates, i.e., of having created a smoothed value. In defining Endpoint 4 on a per-participant basis, the largest increase from baseline to the on-treatment value (the resulting smoothed valued) is identified. However, Morganroth (2005) advocated a different use of the replicate values. By his method, the smoothed value corresponding to the time point with the largest change for an individual replicate value would be selected. Morganroth noted that this analysis "is done by looking at the largest positive change from baseline on-treatment at any time point (average the ECGs around that time point for better time point precision) in each subject and then calculating the mean 'maximum' change for all subjects in each treatment arm" (Morganroth, 2005, p. 220). While this analysis may initially seem identical to that described for Endpoint 4 it is not necessarily the same.

Endpoints 3, 5, and 6 may be helpful in some instances. However, all three have the disadvantage of potentially missing the time of maximal effect due either to limited sampling e.g., around the expected T_{max}, or to averaging over multiple time points. Readers are referred to PhRMA (2005) and Hollister and Montague (2005) for additional discussions.

Thus, the choice of endpoint upon which the primary analysis will be based is an important consideration in the design of a TQT study. The PhRMA QT working group commented as follows regarding the choice of the endpoint and its relationship with the effect of concern (PhRMA, 2005, p. 252):

> It is important to note that the commonly used threshold of 5–10 msec as the minimal difference of clinical significance is not applicable to all of the described QT/QTc summary measures. While 5 to 10 msec might be appropriate for AUC and time-averaged endpoints, analysis based on a maximum QT/QTc change from baseline may call for a larger threshold. Because of the dependency of threshold on the endpoint, it is important that the choice of threshold is linked to the specific endpoint being analyzed.

Since the current version of ICH E14 was released in 2005, there have been a number of published papers commenting on its implementation, including the work of the PhRMA QT working group and others. A representative view of more current thinking on this topic has been presented by Zhang (2008), who stated that the primary endpoint for the TQT study should be "the time-matched mean difference between the drug and placebo after baseline adjustment at each time point." This view is most consistent with Endpoint 1 in Table 7.1. In her description of the endpoint, however, Zhang (2008) referred explicitly to the participant-level summary measure as the baseline-adjusted QTc value for a particular subject at a particular time while on either the drug or placebo (participants in crossover trial will have both). Note that the endpoints described by the PhRMA QT working group also were to be subjected to a baseline covariate adjustment, as described earlier.

7.11   CONSIDERATIONS FOR STATISTICAL ANALYSIS OF TQT STUDY RESULTS

Data are numerical representations of information, and clinical data are numerical representations of clinically relevant data. Once the number crunching of data commences, it is often the case that the units of measurement are not included in visual displays of the data, but it is important to keep in mind at all times the real meaning of these numbers. For example, an investigational antihypertensive drug may lead to a decrease of 10 mmHg in a study participant, and the value "−10" may appear in data printouts. However, the real meaning of the number is a 10 mmHg decrease in blood pressure.

Different forms of clinical data have different characteristics that permit, or do not permit, certain analyses to be meaningfully conducted on them. Clinical data can fall into several categories, including numerical (continuous and discrete) and categorical (nominal and ordinal) data. Continuous variables are measured on a continuous, uninterrupted scale and can take any value on that scale. For example, blood pressure and heart rate are continuous variables. So too are QT/QTc values. In contrast, discrete variables can only take on certain values, which are usually whole numbers. The number of visits a patient made to his or her physician in a specified time period will be a whole number, or integer, and is therefore a discrete numerical variable.

Many variables fall into categories. Ethnicity is one example of categorical data often collected in clinical trials (e.g., Caucasian, Hispanic, African American, Native American, etc.). Ethnicity provides an example of nominal categorical variables: each category has a unique name but the possibilities are not ordered in any meaningful way. When a nominal categorical variable can only be placed into one of two categories the term dichotomous, or binary, is applicable. An example of a dichotomous variable would be survival data following surgery in a survey where the only two possible answers are alive or not 12 months following surgery. When the possibilities in a category can be ordered in a meaningful way, the variable is called an ordinal variable. Categorization of an adverse event as mild, moderate, or severe is one example. So too is categorizing participants in a TQT study by their QT/QTc interval prolongation while being administered the investigational drug in terms of those whose value is below, say, 480 msec and those whose value is 480 msec or greater.

The ICH E14 guidance states that an overall analytical strategy for QT/QTc intervals from a TQT study should include analyses of continuous outcomes as well as categorical measures. A typical continuous outcome is change from the baseline

QTc. An example of a categorical measure is classifying each participant as having or not having a response of interest (e.g., change from baseline of 10 msec or greater). Some authors refer to this categorical analysis as an outliers analysis. However, this term is somewhat of a misnomer since, in this binary categorization, subjects whose QTc interval increased by 10 msec are considered outliers just as much as those whose QTc interval increased by 30 msec or more. Readers who are familiar with statistical terminology in general drug development may recognize that this categorical analysis can also be considered a responders analysis. However, a responder in most clinical studies is a subject whose response is considered favorable.

A categorical response (e.g., yes or no) can be defined for each participant for any value of QT/QTc exceeding a particular threshold or any change from baseline in QT/QTc exceeding a particular threshold. As with many other issues in ICH E14, the definition of appropriate upper limits for categorical responses is not without controversy: As noted, "There is not consensus concerning the choice of upper limit values for absolute QT/QTc interval and changes from baseline" (ICH E14, 2005, p. 10). Historically, a QTc of greater than 500 msec has been a value of concern (for both the drug-induced prolongations of current interest and in cases of inherited LQT syndromes as discussed in Chapter 4). However, ICH E14 proposed multiple limits as a reasonable approach to the existing uncertainty. The limits for the categorical responses proposed in this guidance are as follows (p. 10):

> Absolute QTc interval:
  - QTc > 450 msec.
  - QTc > 480 msec.
  - QTc > 500 msec.

> Change from baseline QTc interval:
  - Change from baseline QTc > 30 msec.
  - Change from baseline QTc > 60 msec.

7.11.1   Descriptive Statistics: Methods

Descriptive summary statistics for endpoints of interest involving continuous data are typically presented for each treatment separately. These descriptive statistics include the sample size, the mean, and the standard error of the mean. As is the case for all statistical analyses, the statistical analysis employed for QT/QTc interval data from a TQT study needs to account for the study design used in that particular study. For example, whenever a crossover design was employed, the analysis should account for the statistical associations inherent in the design. Hollister and Montague (2005) recommend that crossover studies be analyzed using a mixed effects model with a random effect for subject, fixed effects for sequence, period, and treatment, and a covariate for the baseline value of the dependent variable. For parallel-group studies, they suggest the use of an analysis of covariance (ANCOVA) model with effects for treatment, any other fixed effects (e.g., sex), and a covariate for the baseline value.

Use of either the mixed effects model or the ANCOVA model provides estimates of the mean change from baseline QTc, adjusted for baseline (i.e., baseline-corrected) and a standard error for this estimate. As in all clinical studies, primary interest in the TQT study lies with the treatment effect, i.e., the QTc effect observed over and above that which would be expected through chance variation, which is estimated by the response to the placebo treatment. For continuous outcomes. the point estimate of the treatment effect is the difference in mean responses for the test and placebo treatments, adjusted for baseline.

For illustration, consider each individual time point separately, as proposed by Zhang (2008). In the case of a crossover study, the treatment effect is based on within-participant responses. That is, at a time point t, each participant will have a baseline-adjusted QTc value (or a baseline-adjusted change from baseline QTc value) while on the investigational drug and placebo. The treatment effect is then defined as the mean within-participant treatment difference in baseline-adjusted response at time t. In the case of a parallel-group study, the treatment effect is defined as the between-group difference in baseline-adjusted mean response at time t (e.g., QTc at time t or change from baseline QTc at time t). When using the baseline as a covariate in these analyses, the estimated treatment effect will be the same (for a particular time point t) whether the response is change from baseline QTc at time t or QTc at time t. In fact, the description of Zhang's endpoint of choice should result in the same treatment effect as Endpoint 1 in Table 7.1. The Greek symbol delta (δ) is often used in mathematical notation to indicate the calculation of a change. In this context, the term double delta is sometimes used since two aspects of change are involved. For the continuous outcomes discussed, the estimated treatment effect represents a best estimate of the magnitude of QTc prolongation attributed to the investigational drug. (Sponsors reading this chapter are reminded that the appropriate endpoint of interest should be discussed with regulators during the design stage of a TQT study.)

The point estimate of the treatment effect is liable to sampling variation, which needs to be accounted for since the objective of the TQT study is to rule out QTc effects that would potentially be of concern. Accordingly, CIs are constructed about the point estimate of the treatment effect, and these CIs form the basis of inferential statistical procedures employed, discussed in the following section.

Categorical responses for absolute QT/QTc or change from baseline QT/QTc are summarized descriptively using the number and percentage of participants with each response. The ICH E14 guidance suggests that categorical analyses be presented separately for participants with normal and with elevated QT/QTc intervals at baseline: Participants with an elevated QT/QTc at baseline may have less opportunity for further prolongation of the QT/QTc interval than participants whose starting state was normal. To enable meaningful comparisons, response rates should be presented separately for each baseline group (normal vs. elevated). The PhRMA QT working group (2005) suggested that a similar approach be taken with other important covariates of interest, e.g., age and sex.

7.11.2   Inferential Statistics: Methods, Results, and Interpretation

Inferential statistics play a central role in the analysis and interpretation of the TQT study since, as was noted earlier in Section 7.8, the primary objective is to rule out, with 95% statistical confidence, effects of an investigational new drug on the QTc interval that would be of regulatory concern, i.e., prolongation of the QTc interval by about 5 msec. As noted in ICH E14 (p. 5):

> It is difficult to determine whether there is an effect on the mean QT/QTc interval that is so small as to be of no consequence. However, drugs that prolong the mean QT/QTc interval by around 5 msec or less do not appear to cause TdP. On that basis, the positive control (whether pharmacological or non-pharmacological) should be well-characterized and consistently produce an effect on the QT/QTc interval that is around the threshold of regulatory concern (5 msec).

> Based on similar considerations, a negative 'thorough QT/QTc study' is one in which the upper bound of the 95% one-sided confidence interval for the largest time-matched mean effect of the drug on the QTc excludes 10 msec. This definition is chosen to provide reasonable assurance that the mean effect of the study drug on the QT/QTc interval is not greater than around 5 msec. When the largest time-matched difference exceeds the threshold, the study is termed 'positive'. A positive study influences the evaluations carried out during later stages of drug development, but does not imply that the drug is pro-arrhythmic.

For this reason, the guidance suggests that inferential statistics in the form of confidence intervals about the between-treatment mean QT/QTc effect be used to rule out changes of 10 msec or more with a high degree of confidence.

However, the rationale for the choice of 10 msec in ICH E14 is a rather curious one. A one-sided 95% CI with an upper limit less than 10 msec can only reasonably rule out an increase of 10 msec or greater: Such a CI reflects no explicit assurance about a change in QT/QTc of 5 msec. A one-sided upper confidence limit (discussed in Section 7.7.3) is constructed using a point estimate, such as the mean change from baseline QTc, plus a margin of error. The margin of error is the product of the standard error of the estimate, a parameter that reflects sampling error, and a precision coefficient corresponding to $100(1 - \alpha)\%$ confidence. That is, a one-sided $100(1 - \alpha)\%$ confidence limit is formulated as:

CI = Point estimate + [precision coefficient for 100(1 - α)% confidence][standard error]

The precision coefficient is larger for intervals with higher confidence than for intervals requiring less confidence (which is a more mathematical expression of the observation made in Section 7.7.2 that two-sided 99% CIs placed around a point estimate are always wider than 95% CIs). If the CI is based on a standard normal distribution—this will usually be the case, and discussion of this point is therefore not needed here—the precision coefficient associated with a one-sided 95% CI is 1.645. If the resulting upper limit is less than 10 msec, one can use algebra to calculate what the precision coefficient must be to ensure that the upper limit ruled out a prolongation of 5 msec. Since the point estimate and standard error would not change, the result is obtained by dividing 1.645 by 2 (which halves the acceptable upper limit of the interval). The resulting precision coefficient is 0.822, which corresponds to a one-sided 80% confidence limit. Provided that the point estimate is less than 5 msec, a statistical definition of reasonable assurance then equates to 80% confidence that the true mean QT/QTc effect does not exceed 5 msec.

Ruling out 5 msec with 95% confidence would require a larger study (assuming no real QTc effect). The criterion of 10 msec may be thought of as a worthwhile compromise, as it is not entirely clear that an effect on mean QTc as large as 10 msec conveys additional risk for TdP. Shah (2005a) characterized various changes in QTc from baseline in the following manner:

> ➢ 5 msec: No risk.
> ➢ 6–10 msec: Unlikely to be a risk.
> ➢ 11–15 msec: Possible risk.
> ➢ 16–20 msec: Probable risk.
> ➢ 21–25 msec: Almost definite risk.
> ➢ 26 msec: Definite risk.

In a similar manner, Hollister and Montague (2005, p. 251) used the following characterizations:

> ➢ Less than 5 msec: So far no TdP.
> ➢ Changes of 5–10 msec: No clear risk.
> ➢ Changes of 10–20 msec: Uncertainty.
> ➢ Greater than 20 msec: Substantially increased likelihood of being pro-arrhythmic.

As noted earlier, the most appropriate margin for the endpoint of interest may be less than 10 msec (depending on the potential benefit) and it should be defined with the endpoint of interest in mind. For the sake of illustration and simplicity, however, the margin of 10 msec is used in subsequent discussions in this chapter.

From the standpoint of a sponsor, the ideal outcomes from a TQT study would be as follows:

> ➤ A QTc prolongation effect for the supratherapeutic dose of the test drug as large as 10 msec can be ruled out with 95% confidence.
> ➤ A QTc prolongation effect for the therapeutic dose of the test drug as large as 10 msec can be ruled out with 95% confidence.
> ➤ A QTc prolongation effect for the positive control of zero could be ruled out with 95% confidence. That is, the study had assay sensitivity.

The following null and alternative statistical hypotheses, those used in hypothesis testing for noninferiority testing (e.g., see Durham and Turner, 2008), correspond to the first two of these ideal outcomes, i.e., to rule out a mean QTc effect as large as 10 msec for a given dose (here, m represents the mean):

$$H_0 : m_{Test} - m_{Placebo} \geq 10$$
$$H_A : m_{Test} - m_{Placebo} < 10$$

The null hypothesis is typically tested through the construction of an upper one-sided 95% CI about the between-treatment difference in mean baseline-adjusted change from baseline QT/QTc (calculated as the mean for the test drug treatment minus the mean for the placebo treatment). The upper bound of the 95% CI is used to make an interpretation about the trial (recall from Section 7.7.3 that the upper limit or bound of a 95% one-sided CI is equivalent to the upper limit of a two-sided 90% CI). If the upper limit of the interval excludes (i.e., lies to the left of) 10, the null hypothesis is rejected and it is possible to conclude with high (95%) confidence that prolongations longer than 10 msec are unlikely, provided that the study was designed such that prolongation could have been detected. If the upper limit of the interval encloses (i.e., lies precisely on or to the right of) 10, the null hypothesis may not be rejected, and therefore prolongations as great as 10 msec may not be ruled out. When such a result is obtained for the largest time-matched difference (the endpoint suggested by ICH E14), the study is considered positive, meaning positive for QT/QTc prolongation. In calculating the confidence interval, the point estimate (e.g., the difference in baseline-adjusted means) and its standard error will be obtained from an appropriate statistical model, which will depend on the study design (parallel vs. crossover) and the use of appropriate covariates (e.g., baseline QT/QTc).

If the test drug is found not to increase the QTc interval using the method described above, it is then important to establish assay sensitivity before declaring that the study was negative for QTc prolongation. The following null and alternative statistical hypotheses correspond to the third ideal outcome, i.e., to rule out a mean QTc effect for the positive control of zero or less:

$$H_0 : m_{Positive\,Control} - m_{Placebo} \leq 0$$
$$H_A : m_{Positive\,Control} - m_{Placebo} > 0$$

The null hypothesis is typically tested through the construction of a lower one-sided 95% CI about the between-treatment difference (calculated as positive control minus placebo) in the mean baseline-adjusted change from baseline QT/QTc. In this case, the lower limit of the CI is used to make an interpretation about the assay sensitivity. Note that the lower limit of a 95% one-sided CI is equivalent to the lower limit of a two-sided 90% CI. If the lower limit of the interval excludes (i.e., is greater than) zero, the null hypothesis is rejected and it is possible to conclude with high (95%) confidence that the positive control prolonged the QTc appropriately, and therefore to conclude that the study had appropriate assay sensitivity. If the study had such assay sensitivity and there was no evidence of QTc prolongation for the test drug, the study can be considered negative. On the other hand, if the lower limit of the interval encloses the value of zero, the null hypothesis may not be rejected and, therefore, assay sensitivity was not established.

There is room for debate regarding how the positive control should be treated in the TQT study. In the above description, assay sensitivity will be established if there is evidence that the positive control increased the mean QTc by any positive amount. However, if one considers that assay sensitivity can only be established if the positive control has an effect of 5 msec or more, the hypotheses of interest are:

$$H_0 : m_{Positive\,Control} - m_{Placebo} \leq 5$$
$$H_A : m_{Positive\,Control} - m_{Placebo} > 5$$

The PhRMA QT working group (PhRMA, 2005) noted that the assumption that the positive control will always yield a mean effect equivalent to its labeling is not appropriate when one considers measurement and sampling error. They continued as follows (PhRMA, 2005, p. 255):

> Positive control application in studies involving 20–30 subjects should *not* be expected to yield point estimates uniformly consistent with QTc-labeling for positive control agents. Mean effect sizes should be expected to vary between 2 to 3 msec above or below the true mean due to random variation and precision of measurement.

7.12   THE ISSUE OF MULTIPLICITY

A number of analyses are described in ICH E14, including the primary analysis of the largest time-matched difference in QT/QTc. As noted in Section 7.10, where the concept of multiple-hypothesis testing or multiplicity was introduced, the more of these responses that are tested, the more likely it becomes that a Type I error will be committed. In drug development there is often concern about committing a Type I error when testing a number of doses with respect to a single efficacy measure. In that context, committing a Type I error may mean that a less optimal dose is carried forward into further studies. In the context of the TQT study, a Type I error resulting from multiple tests of various changes in QT/QTc could have different but equally salient implications: The development program may be required to include intensive cardiac monitoring in future studies, or the development program could be halted altogether.

The ICH E14 guidance addresses this potential difficulty, at least partially, by identifying a single primary endpoint for consideration: "the effect of an investigational drug on the QT/QTc interval is most commonly analyzed using the largest time-matched mean difference between the drug and placebo (baseline-adjusted) over the collection period" (ICH E14, 2005, p. 9). However, as we have seen, the TQT study comprises more than just a single hypothesis comparing the mean effect between one dose of the test drug and the placebo: Other hypotheses tested (regardless of the endpoint considered as primary) include the comparison of a supratherapeutic dose to placebo and the comparison of a positive control to a placebo to evaluate assay sensitivity. The 2005 PhRMA report proposed a sequential testing, or serial gatekeeping, strategy to retain the experimentwise Type I error rate at the traditional $\alpha = 0.05$ level when evaluating a single endpoint, such as the one favored in the ICH E14 guidance (see Westfall et al., 1999, for more detailed discussions of serial gatekeeping strategies).

The serial gatekeeping strategy takes advantage of the notion that the three ideal conclusions from the study listed in Section 7.3.4 have a natural ordering by which they can be tested. First, it is assumed that the mean effect on QTc for the therapeutic dose of the test drug is only of interest if QTc prolongation with the supratherapeutic dose of the test drug has been ruled out first. Second, it is assumed that assay sensitivity only needs to be established if the results suggest no QTc prolongation for both the supratherapeutic dose and the therapeutic dose. Assuming that 10 msec is the effect to be ruled out in terms of QTc interval prolongation, the serial gatekeeping strategy proceeds as follows:

Step 1: Rule out a QTc effect for the supratherapeutic dose.
The null and alternative statistical hypotheses in this case are as follows:

$$H_0 : m_{High} - m_{Placebo} \geq 10$$
$$H_A : m_{High} - m_{Placebo} < 10$$

The null hypothesis is tested using an upper 95% one-sided CI about the difference in mean change from baseline QTc. If the upper limit includes 10, the null hypothesis is not rejected and the testing procedure stops. The study is then considered positive for QT/QTc prolongation. If the upper limit is less than 10, the null hypothesis is rejected in favor of the alternative and the testing strategy continues to Step 2.

Step 2: Rule out a QTc effect for the therapeutic dose.
The null and alternative statistical hypotheses are the same as in Step 1, i.e., they are as follows:

$$H_0 : m_{Test} - m_{Placebo} \geq 10$$
$$H_A : m_{Test} - m_{Placebo} < 10$$

The null hypothesis is again tested using an upper 95% one-sided CI about the difference in mean change from baseline QTc. If the upper limit includes 10, the null hypothesis is not rejected and the testing procedure stops. The study will be considered positive for QT/QTc prolongation. If the upper limit is less than 10, the null hypothesis is rejected in favor of the alternative and the testing strategy continues to Step 3.

Step 3: Test for a QTc effect for the positive control to establish assay sensitivity.
The null and alternative statistical hypotheses in this step are different and are as follows:

$$H_0 : m_{Positive} - m_{Placebo} \leq 0$$
$$H_A : m_{Positive} - m_{Placebo} > 0$$

At this stage, the null hypothesis is tested using a lower 95% one-sided CI about the baseline-adjusted difference in mean change from baseline QTc. If the lower limit is less than or equal to zero, the null hypothesis is not rejected and the study has failed to establish assay sensitivity. If the lower limit is greater than zero, the null hypothesis is rejected in favor of the alternative. In this case, the TQT study has established assay sensitivity.

In conclusion, rejection at each of the three steps in sequence provides compelling evidence that the test drug does not have an effect on QTc. This approach certainly has great appeal, but it requires the evaluation of the mean effect to be limited to a single endpoint. In the case of the ICH E14 guidance, this endpoint is the maximum change from baseline.

An alternative interpretation of the meaning of the endpoint favored in ICH E14 was presented by Zhang (2008), who noted that "in practice, we examine the largest upper bound of the 95% one-sided confidence interval instead of the upper bound of the largest mean difference." Use of this approach means that the specific endpoint (i.e., change at a specific time point) is not identified *a priori*, but involves interpretation of a 95% one-sided CI at every time point. Therefore, in this strategy, even the primary comparison of the test drug versus placebo results in multiple testing. One proposed strategy for this type of analysis is the Intersection-Union test (IUT), which has been studied by Hutmacher et al. (2008). For the IUT the null hypothesis is stated in the form of composite hypotheses considering all of k time points (again using 10 msec as an effect of interest):

$$H_0 = \cup H_{0,k}; \quad H_{0,k} : m_{Test,k} - m_{Placebo,k} \geq 10$$

The alternative is also in a composite form, considering all k time points:

$$H_A = \cap H_{A,k}; \quad H_{A,k} : m_{Test,k} - m_{Placebo,k} < 10$$

The test would consider k (one for each time point) one-sided 95% CIs, as before. If the upper limit of the CI for any one of the k intervals exceeded 10 msec, the null hypothesis could not be rejected and the study would be considered positive. All CIs would need to exclude 10 msec to reject the null hypothesis and claim a negative study, provided assay sensitivity could be established. In this case, rejection of the null hypothesis (H_0) is interpreted by concluding that there is no evidence at any time point of a mean QTc effect of 10 msec or more. Hutmacher et al. (2008) studied this particular design through simulations (parallel and crossover designs under various assumptions) and discovered that there were "large positive [study] rates for some of the parallel TQT study designs simulated, even when no QT prolongation existed" (Hutmacher et al., p. 223). The authors concluded as follows (p. 224):

> This report reveals significant limitations of the IUT in TQT studies. The limitations are revealed particularly for parallel designs when variability is large, potentially due to running the trial in patients. The sample sizes of these TQT studies could be extremely large to achieve acceptable power. Under these circumstances, alternative analytical approaches such as exposure-response modeling could provide more power to interpret the drug signal and evaluate the risks and benefits of a therapy.

This recently published research highlights the need to continue to research appropriate statistical methodologies which identify truly torsadogenic drugs (true positives) without leading to abandonment of potentially promising new drugs due to a spurious positive result from the TQT study (false positives).

7.13   SAMPLE SIZE CONSIDERATIONS

Strictly speaking, sample size estimation is a concern of study design and not of statistical analysis. However, the appropriate sample size is defined based upon the primary statistical objective of the study. The primary objective in the case of the TQT study was defined in Section 7.8. The sample size estimation for the TQT study should consider the following: estimates of variability for the endpoint of interest; the size of the effect to be detected or ruled out; and a desired level of power (e.g., 80% or 90%). The acceptable Type I error is usually 5% ($\alpha = 0.05$), consistent with a one-sided confidence limit. Care should be taken to utilize the variance estimate from the same endpoint intended for the study (e.g., maximum change from baseline QTc). A single method or formula for sample size estimation cannot be recommended, but two examples are provided below as a general guide for the sizes of the TQT study.

In the case of a single-dose crossover study of a mild QTc-prolonging drug reported by the PhRMA QT working group, estimates of the within-subject standard deviation ranged from 3.8 to 5.2 msec (depending on the endpoint evaluated). Using the largest of these estimated standard deviations, the authors stated (PhRMA, 2005, p. 255):

> A well-controlled crossover study should employ at least 22 subjects [per group] to detect a 5 or more msec baseline-corrected increase from placebo with at least 90% power at a 5% significance level.

Morganroth (2005, p. 219) cited an estimated standard deviation of less than 8 msec. In his experience, he noted this estimate typically results in 30–40 subjects per arm to provide 80% power to detect an effect of 5 msec.

7.14   ADVERSE EVENTS

The TQT study should include assessment and recording of adverse events. As described in the ICH E14 (p. 8), "ECG changes recorded as adverse events should be pooled from all studies for analysis" in an integrated analysis of safety. The guidance suggested that ECG interval data be pooled only among those studies with equally rigorous collection and analysis procedures. A detailed discussion of adverse events is provided in Chapter 8.

7.15   INTERPRETATIONS AND IMPLICATIONS OF TQT STUDY RESULTS FOR FUTURE STUDIES DURING THE PREAPPROVAL CLINICAL DEVELOPMENT PROGRAM

A negative TQT study would have few additional consequences for the development of the drug in future trials, as it "will almost always allow the collection of on-therapy ECGs in accordance with the current practices in each therapeutic area to constitute sufficient evaluation during subsequent stages of drug development" (ICH E14, 2005, p. 3). However, as the guidance noted, if the TQT study is negative but nonclinical data were strongly positive, additional intensive monitoring of ECG changes may still be required by a regulatory agency.

A positive TQT study would require additional ECG monitoring throughout the remainder of the drug's preapproval clinical development program. In particular, changes to the QT/QTc interval should be evaluated in the target population of interest, "with particular attention to dose- and concentration-related effects" (ICH E14, 2005, p. 6). This expanded study should include a range of doses and subjects who may have other risk factors for TdP. Extreme values from such a study would be examined more closely than mean changes. This additional investigation could be performed in the course of other studies, e.g., early therapeutic exploratory or therapeutic confirmatory trials, provided that the participants with ECGs were "in substantial numbers" and that the timing of the ECG collection coincided with the expected time of peak drug effects. Studies conducted after a positive TQT study should also aim to capture relevant cardiac adverse events as well as any marked QT/QTc prolongation, e.g., QTc intervals greater than 500 msec.

Positive results from the TQT study necessitate separate analyses of ECG and adverse event data for various subgroups of participants, including the following (ICH E14, 2005, p. 6):

> ➢ Participants with electrolyte abnormalities (e.g., hypokalemia, or low potassium electrolyte balance).
> ➢ Participants with congestive heart failure.
> ➢ Participants with impaired drug-metabolizing capacity or clearance (e.g., renal or hepatic impairment, drug interactions).
> ➢ Female participants.
> ➢ Participants less than 16 years of age and those over 65 years of age.

7.16   TORSADOGENIC LIABILITY EVALUATION WHEN A TRADITIONAL TQT STUDY CANNOT BE CONDUCTED

Under E14 guidance, the TQT study is typically to be carried out in healthy participants, as opposed to individuals at increased risk of arrhythmias, and is to be used to determine whether or not the effect of a drug on the QT/QTc interval in the target patient population should be studied intensively during later stages of drug development. However, the E14 guidance also commented as follows (Section 2.4, p. 7):

There are some drugs that cannot be studied in a "thorough QT/QTc study" in healthy volunteers due to safety or tolerability concerns (e.g., cytotoxic cancer drugs). In such cases, the "thorough QT/QTc study" can often be conducted in patient populations. When this is not possible, the importance of detecting and modifying this safety risk means that other ways of detecting effects on the QT/QTc interval need to be developed. These might include the collection of ECGs at multiple time points under tightly controlled settings that target a broad range of doses early in development.

This is essentially saying that when a TQT study cannot be done, the sponsor should be as thorough as possible. This is the approach taken with many oncology compounds, as discussed below and in Section 7.16.2.

This section of the guidance makes it clear that the development of oncology drugs may require alternative methods of QT liability assessment. The phrase "require alternative methods" in the previous sentence is important. In circumstances where a TQT study cannot be done in healthy participants, or cannot be done at all, this does not release sponsors from the need to evaluate QT liability to the best of their ability: rather, their assessments must (still) be as thorough as possible. The guidance actually provides two suggestions for potential alternative QT liability assessment:

> ➢ Conduct a TQT study using participants with the disease or condition of interest. Such a population may or may not be at increased risk of arrhythmias relative to healthy participants.
> ➢ Collect (even) more data relevant to the investigational drug's potential to impact cardiac functioning at the beginning of clinical testing. This intensive data collection will likely focus on extensive analysis of pharmacokinetic/pharmacodynamic data in relation to ECG measurements.

These two suggestions might be regarded as being at the two ends of a continuum of alternative strategies. Sponsors must employ careful planning and judgment here in determining the best approach for drug studies on a case-by-case basis. It is highly advisable to start a dialog with a regulatory agency as soon as possible so that the agency can provide feedback on an acceptable strategy rather that determining at a later stage that the strategy employed by the sponsor was not acceptable: that is, it is advisable for sponsors to gain mutual understanding and agreement on the most appropriate and acceptable approach (see the discussions in Section 7.16.1). Sponsors bear the responsibility of explaining why a standard TQT study cannot be done, and the related burden of explaining how they will provide sufficient alternative evidence of an acceptable level of QT liability. Once again, the concept of an acceptable level of risk arises at this point in our discussions: The smaller the likely therapeutic benefit of the investigational drug, or if other drugs already provide similar benefit, the greater the requirement to show minimal QT liability. Conversely, if a drug is the only candidate to date that promises to provide therapeutic benefit to a population with an extreme medical need, a certain degree of QT liability may be judged acceptable by a regulatory agency.

When deciding if it is possible to conduct a TQT study for a given investigational drug in a patient population, attention must be paid to the degree of risk tolerance in that population. Some patient populations may have immediately life-threatening conditions (e.g., blast crisis), while others may have conditions that are life-threatening at some point in the future (e.g., solid lung tumor). Also, others may already be on treatment with one (or more) drugs, and the goal is to investigate whether the new drug will provide additional therapeutic benefit if given as adjuvant therapy. Some populations may not be able to tolerate days without therapy in order to obtain baseline ECG data for time-matched comparisons. Data from some populations may be particularly confounded by factors such as the disease state itself, concomitant medications, and electrolyte balance (a state of hypokalemia means that there is less potassium available to the body for use in generating hERG current). It is more appropriate to conduct a TQT study in some of these populations than in others.

If a regulatory agency agrees that extensive and rigorous pharmacokinetic/ ECG data may be an acceptable alternative to conducting a TQT study, or part of such an alternative, the sponsor needs to take advantage of the best means of collecting such data. Human pharmacology studies provide the optimal, and likely the unique, opportunity to collect such data. As well as the thorough pharmacokinetic evaluations typically conducted in all human pharmacology studies, in this case rigorous ECG data are collected. Extensive statistical evaluation will be conducted, examining measures of central tendency and looking for outliers. The QT liability is then estimated from the technique of pharmacokinetic/pharmacodynamic (PK/PD) modeling. Such modeling is conducted for both low and high concentrations of the drug since this helps to determine the magnitude of any QT prolongation effect relative to the concentration. If an active control is being used, it is a good idea to consider PK/PD modeling for that compound too. The reason for this approach is that it helps to validate assay sensitivity. The logic here is similar to that for employing moxifloxacin in the regular TQT study: it is necessary to show that one's assay can detect a QT interval prolongation effect of around 5 msec, i.e., the effect that is well documented with moxifloxacin.

It is worth noting here that PK/PD or exposure-response modeling is becoming more and more a part of the regular TQT study too, and regulators can also ask for this modeling to validate the moxifloxacin arm. One aspect of incorporating such modeling is that it can be used to help assess for a false-positive QT liability signal. (See Garnett et al., 2008, discussed in Section 14.2.7.)

The results of PK/PD or exposure-response modeling techniques can be integrated with those from later preapproval studies: such an integrated approach is generally helpful but is particularly necessary when the regular TQT study is not (cannot be) conducted. This need for an integrated approach emphasizes the point that the sponsor is wise to start a dialog with the regulatory agency as early as possible, not when human pharmacology studies have been completed: they may have to be conducted again if inadequate data were collected. Future research will examine whether such integrated QT liability assessments can adequately characterize postmarketing arrhythmogenic risk.

7.16.1   The FDA's QT Interdisciplinary Review Team

We noted in the previous section that it is highly advisable for a sponsor to start a dialog with the regulatory agency as soon as possible when planning a TQT study, and perhaps even more so when the sponsor feels that it might not be appropriate to conduct a traditional TQT study to evaluate QT liability in the case of a particular investigational drug, so that the agency can provide feedback on the sponsor's proposed strategy. Such feedback from the FDA is facilitated by a relatively new body within the agency called the Interdisciplinary Review Team (IRT) that was founded in June 2006.

The IRT is responsible for reviewing study protocols and completed study reports related to QT liability assessment, including the traditional TQT study and alternative methods of assessment. It is made up of a statistician, clinical pharmacologist, medical officer, project manager, and data manager. When a sponsor submits a protocol or study report to the appropriate therapeutic review division within CDER, the division passes the document on to the IRT. The IRT then reviews the document and provides comments for the review division. The IRT's comments are considered nonbinding advice by the review division. The division takes the IRT's comments into consideration when forming its response to the sponsor, and communicates its response directly to the sponsor.

7.16.2   QT Assessments for Oncology Drugs

The oncology therapeutic area provides an instructive example of the considerations needed when it may not be possible to conduct a standard TQT study. The summary provided here is based on a presentation by Finkle (2008), who made it clear that, at that point in time, this approach had not been sanctioned by the FDA.

Some oncology compounds are too toxic to be given to healthy participants, so a modified approach is needed. (It should be noted, however, that others are not: therefore, the term oncology compound does not mean that a sponsor gets an automatic regulatory waiver from conducting a standard TQT study.) When a sponsor believes that a modified approach is warranted, a cogent scientific and clinical rationale must be provided to the regulatory agency. This rationale must to address each specific component of the standard approach that the sponsor believes should be different, and do this on a case-by-case basis for each investigational drug. As noted earlier, when preparing a plan for regulatory consideration a sponsor must be as thorough as possible in its evaluation of QT liability.

If conducting the TQT study in a patient population is proposed, two points to consider are as follows. First, the patients will differ from healthy participants in a standard TQT study in several ways that are relevant to assessment of QT liability. Their disease may have a direct influence, as may concomitant diseases. Also, they may be taking (many) concomitant medications, and their electrolyte levels may vary considerably from those of healthy participants, which can influence ionic currents. Second, the environment in which the TQT study will be conducted will likely differ considerably from the environment used for a standard TQT study. The standard TQT study is typically conducted in very tightly controlled settings in an inpatient medical center similar to those used for human pharmacology studies (recall the discussions in Section 7.1): A patient TQT study would be conducted in an environment typical of real-world patient care.

Given these difficulties in obtaining the ECG data obtained during a standard TQT study, one strategy is to collect even more relevant data than usual during the nonclinical development program and the early clinical program. With regard to early clinical trials, the collection of rigorous ECG data, using replicate data collection and manual adjudication (rather than the automated or semiautomated systems discussed in Section 7.9), may be appropriate, along with the collection of rigorous pharmacokinetic data. This strategy means that the need to implement it must be identified before these early clinical studies are done. This emphasizes the (even greater than usual) need to plan the developmental strategy carefully and to contact the regulatory agency as early as possible to get their acceptance of the proposed plan.

In later preapproval trials ECG analysis still needs to be done, and thorough statistical analysis, exposure response modeling, and interpretation, and presentation of the results are needed. One point of interest here is relevant to the ongoing discussions of benefit-risk balance assessments. Given that these drugs are being developed for serious, even life-threatening conditions, the benefit-risk balance is generally favorable. Therefore, regulatory acceptance of a greater degree of risk, as defined here by the extent of QT prolongation, may occur: that is, it may be the case that the upper bound of the one-sided 95% CI calculated should exclude increases greater than, say, 15 or 20 msec, rather than the prescribed value of 10 msec for a standard TQT study.

More extensive discussion of this topic is currently being prepared by the Cardiac Safety Research Consortium, discussed Section 7.20.

7.17   TORSADOGENIC LIABILITY EVALUATIONS FOR BIOLOGICALS

At the time of writing, this issue is one of considerable deliberation. As noted at the end of Section 7.20, which discusses the Cardiac Safety Research Consortium, this consortium is currently preparing a "Points to Consider" document on this topic, and we refer readers to that document when it becomes available.

7.18   LABELING IMPLICATIONS OF QT LIABILITY ASSESSMENTS

Sager et al. (2005) noted that the results of the TQT study will often be included in the drug's labeling (see also Malik and Camm, 2001). Sager et al. (2005, p. 392) further noted that "This will be particularly true when the results of the thorough QT study are positive, in which case there may also be specific warning information."

Readers who are familiar with drug labeling will be well aware that a considerable amount of information is presented in extremely small print (for those of you who are not familiar with drug labeling, it is an interesting exercise to read such a label for the first time). Kovacs (2008) commented that labeling information is generally vague and not always as helpful to a prescribing physician as one would like. Statements concerning changes in the QTc interval can be particularly challenging to a prescribing physician and his or her patient. The vast majority of physicians who prescribe noncardiac drugs are not cardiologists, and may not be well versed in the conduct, analysis, and interpretation of data from a TQT study.

This is also true for the typical patient. We noted in the preface that one of our intentions in this book is to explain and demystify proarrhythmic cardiac safety; so far, this has taken us approximately 200 pages of text! Kovacs (2008) also discussed the patient information literature provided with drugs. In one particular case, the information told patients to tell their doctor before taking the drug if they, or any members of their family, had a rare heart condition known as prolongation of the QTc interval. Before you started reading this book, did you know what a QT/QTc interval was? And, in either case, are you presently aware of the QTc status of yourself and your family members? It is true that family members of someone who has been identified as having inherited LQTS may be aware of this, but the vast majority of patients will likely have no idea what it means.

7.19   TRENDS IDENTIFIED FROM RECENT DRUG APPROVALS

This chapter has highlighted a number of aspects of the TQT study which are subject to interpretation, debate, and further research. Given these issues, we believe that a summary review of recently approved drugs may shed some light on current regulatory thinking. To that end, we accessed the FDA web site (www.fda.gov) on March 5, 2008, and reviewed the available labeling for the 17 new molecular entities (NME) that were approved during the calendar year 2007. Of these 17 drugs, labeling was available for 14 of them. Data on QT investigations were included in the label in eight cases. The QT study included in the label was conducted in healthy subjects in seven cases: the eighth, for an oncology drug, was conducted in patients. A positive control was used in four of the studies (three of these were moxifloxacin, and the other was an unspecified oral positive control). Of these eight TQT studies, the design employed could be identified in four: three were crossover designs and one was a parallel design, with the remainder being unspecified. As noted throughout this chapter, these data suggest that there is no single universally acceptable study design that may be advocated to characterize an investigational drug's effect on the QT/QTc interval.

7.20   THE CARDIAC SAFETY RESEARCH CONSORTIUM

The Cardiac Safety Research Consortium (CSRC) was established in September 2006 by a Memorandum of Understanding between the FDA and Duke University. A result of the FDA's 2006 Critical Path Initiative, the CSRC is a public-private partnership that focuses on the cardiac safety of drugs and medical devices. While several of the CSRC's initial projects have focused on drug proarrhythmic cardiac safety, this is certainly not their only long-term focus, which will be much broader. One example of this wider interest is investigating any relationship between drug-eluting stents and adverse clinical outcomes. The following information is a summary of a presentation given by Dr. Michael Krucoff (Duke Clinical Research Institute, and Co-Chair of the CSRC's Executive Committee) during a Webinar entitled *Cardiac Safety in Large Molecules: New Regulatory Expectations, New Strategies*, held on February 26, 2008, hosted by Pharmaceutical Executive and sponsored by Quintiles. During this Webinar, presentations concerning the cardiac safety of large-molecule drugs were also given by Drs. Chris Cabell, John Finkle, Norman Stockbridge, and Hugo Vargas, and we also acknowledge their contributions to our thinking and to the writing of several sections of this book. The mission of the CSRC is to advance scientific knowledge on cardiac safety for new and existing medical products by building a collaborative environment based upon the principles of the FDA's Critical Path Initiative and other public health priorities. This approach marks a new paradigm in approaching a wide range of critical cardiac safety issues. Representatives from industry, regulatory agency personnel, and academicians contribute to the collaborative activities of the consortium, bringing together a diverse set of perspectives, opinions, and potential options for addressing issues within cardiac safety. The key objectives of the consortium are to:

> ➢ Facilitate focused and pragmatic research that will inform regulatory processes.
> ➢ Create common nomenclature, standards, and draft documents related to cardiac safety evaluation. These documents include "Points to Consider" documents, addressed shortly.
> ➢ Develop knowledge and improve evaluative sciences in relation to cardiac safety and product development.
> ➢ Establish an infrastructure and operational processes that will support the accomplishment of all the other objectives.

The consortium funds research intended to provide knowledge in keeping with its mission. This research is proposed and conducted under the auspices of the consortium's Scientific Oversight Committee. Another committee, the Medical Products Development Strategy Committee (MPDSC), facilitates the preparation of strategy documents, including "Points to Consider" and "Best Practices" documents, based on the research funded by the consortium and other relevant available information.

The driving force behind the need for such strategy documents has been well exemplified by discussions in this chapter and the previous chapter focusing on nonclinical drug development programs. Despite the existence of official guidance documents from regulatory agencies and other influential and authoritative organizations, these documents do not always provide practical guidance for all foreseeable circumstances, and developers of medical products are not always sure of the optimal way to implement their content. Since the creation of new guidance documents typically takes several years, there is an immediate need for as much clarity as possible in many development scenarios for which guidance is absent or less than optimal.

The MPDSC's intention is therefore to facilitate the creation of strategy documents to provide such clarity. The MPDSC emphasizes that their documents are not proscriptive: they are in no way binding, nor should they be regarded as sanctioned by regulatory agencies. The documents' goals are to highlight areas where there is not presently a consensus of opinion on the optimal way to address an issue, provide ideas for research to provide knowledge currently lacking in certain areas, and to demonstrate the pragmatic implementation of data collection, analysis, and interpretation resulting from the collaborative research facilitated by the consortium.

Three examples of such documents are in progress at the time of writing. The first addresses QT assessment in oncology drug development, the second addresses QT assessment for biologicals, and the third discusses the evaluation of ventricular arrhythmias in early phase development. A fourth document focusing upon the use of troponins in clinical development will be underway shortly.

7.20.1 The Digital ECG Warehouse

The digital ECG warehouse is a repository of around 2 million (in May 2008) digital ECG waveforms that can be used for research purposes. These waveforms were submitted to the FDA during regulatory submissions and have been placed in the warehouse following the sponsors' permission and with full deidentification procedures conducted first. The FDA partnered with Mortara Instrument Inc. to provide this warehouse, in which ECGs from different source sponsors are all stored in a similar format. See Cabell et al. (2005, p. 175) for further discussion of this warehouse and the possibilities it affords "to improve the science surrounding important components of the drug approval process such as cardiac safety evaluation."

7.21   SHORT QT SYNDROME

Up to this point, our discussions in the domain of proarrhythmic cardiac safety have deliberately focused on QT interval prolongation, with the emphasis on the word prolongation. We have discussed both inherited LQTS and acquired (drug-induced) cases, and we have examined the underlying biological mechanisms leading to decreases in KCNH2/hERG current, related drug design activities, and the nonclinical and preapproval clinical evaluation of a drug's QT/torsadogenic liability. At this point, however, it is appropriate to take our discussions in the opposite direction (figuratively and literally) and consider QT interval shortening.

While medical and drug development attention has focused on the LQTS channelopathy and drug-induced QT prolongation for some time, more recently an inherited syndrome called short QT syndrome (SQTS) has been identified (see Gussak et al., 2000; Gaita et al., 2003; Bjerregaard and Gussak, 2008). Several forms of SQTS have now been named, including SQT1, SQT2, and SQT3 (e.g., see Bunch and Ackerman, 2007, Table 1, p. 337; Shah, 2007a). As the name suggests, a defining feature of these syndromes is a shorter than usual QT interval. Like LQTS, SQTS can also lead to syncope, and to arrhythmias and sudden death. Since both LQTS and SQTS confer a proarrhythmic liability, the nature of the relationship between the length of the QT interval and such liability therefore appears to be a nonlinear one that resembles the letter U. In this case, the lowest liability occurs when the QT interval is normal as indicated schematically by the bottom of the U curve. As one moves from this point in either direction, one moves toward a proarrhythmic liability.

In Section 4.3.5 we noted that there is an association between LQT2 and acquired (drug-induced) QT interval prolongation: As noted there, they are "partially phenocopies stemming from either pharmacologically or genetically mediated perturbations in the I_{Kr} potassium channel" (Bunch and Ackerman, 2007, p. 341). The mechanism of action in each case is a loss of function in the KCNH2/hERG channel, a loss of function in the hERG current, and a lengthening of repolarization. A question of interest, therefore, is: will an acquired (drug-induced) partial phenocopy of inherited SQTS be found? Shah (2007b, p. 1101) commented as follows:

> Although the significance of a short QT interval has hitherto remained elusive, recent description of congenital forms of short QT syndromes, and the arrhythmias associated with these syndromes, has begun to unravel an uncanny parallel with drug-induced prolongation of QT interval and its consequences.

As Shah (2007b, p. 1101) also noted, "The molecular basis of a parallel between congenital forms of long QT and short QT syndromes is immediately apparent." As in the case of LQTS, alterations in the ionic currents flowing through various ion channels (including sodium and calcium channels) play a role in the various forms of SQTS. However, as we did for LQTS, we will limit our attention to the KCNH2/hERG channel and current. Whereas LQT2 results from a loss of function in the repolarizing KCNH2/hERG current due to a mutation in the KCNH2/hERG protein, SQT1 results from a gain of function in the same current due a different mutation in the KCNH2/hERG protein. (Note: The numbering of these syndromes here is correct: while a loss of function in the KCNH2/hERG channel leads to the second numbered LQTS, i.e., LQT2, a gain of function in the same channel leads to the first numbered SQTS, i.e., SQT1).

Kang et al. (2005) reported results from nonclinical studies showing that the drug compound RPR260243 shortened the QT interval, commenting that "We believe RPR260243 represents the first known HERG channel activator" (Kang et al., 2005, p. 827). Zhou et al. (2005) described several other drugs that also shortened the QT interval. What might be the implications of SQTS and drug-induced QT shortening for future drug development? Shah (2007b, p. 1101) commented as follows:

> As new compounds that shorten QT interval progress further into clinical development and reach regulatory authorities for approval, questions will inevitably arise on the significance of drug-induced shortening. Therefore, it is not surprising that drug-induced shortening of the QT interval is emerging as another issue of potential clinical and regulatory concern.

It is interesting to speculate how exactly regulatory guidance may evolve. For example, might TQT studies be required to include assessment of an investigational drug's potential to induce QT interval shortening in addition to its potential to induce QT interval prolongation? If so, additional regulatory, methodological, and statistical issues will need to be addressed. First, the threshold of regulatory concern for a drug-induced decrease in QT interval will need to be established. While the threshold of regulatory concern for QT prolongation is stated in ICH E14 as around (positive) 5 msec, and an increase of 10 msec or less needs to be demonstrated, it is not immediately clear that the threshold for QT shortening would be analogously set at around (negative) 5 msec. Second, would an additional active control drug treatment be needed, i.e., a drug that is known to reduce the QT interval, in order to establish assay sensitivity in regard to QT shortening as well as QT interval prolongation? If so, the study design issues become more complex. Third, regardless of the magnitude of a new regulatory threshold(s) of concern, additional statistical testing would need to be conducted since, in this case, both a statistically significant increase and a statistically significant decrease in QT become of interest: currently, only a statistically significant increase is of interest. This further heightens the potential impact of multiplicity issues. The implications of these and other considerations for regulatory guidance on statistical analysis and interpretation of QT shortening may be seen in due course.

7.22   FURTHER READING

7.22.1   Clinical Practice regarding Long QT Syndrome

Roden, D.M., 2008, Long-QT syndrome, *New England Journal of Medicine*, 358: 169–176. [For readers who are interested in clinical treatment aspects, we recommend this paper by Dan Roden, MD, as an excellent starting point.]

7.22.2   Acquired QT Interval Prolongation and General QT Topics

Aerssens, J. and Paulussen, A.D., 2005, Pharmacogenomics and acquired long QT syndrome, *Pharmacogenomics*, 6:259–270.

Altin, T., Ozcan, O., Turhan, S., et al., 2007, Torsade de pointes associated with moxifloxacin: A rare but potentially fatally adverse event, *Canadian Journal of Cardiology*, 23:907–908.

Antonelli, D., Atar, S., Freedberg, N.A., and Rosenfeld, T., 2005, Torsade de pointes in patients on chronic amiodarone treatment: Contributing factors and drug interactions, *Israel Medical Association Journal*, 7:163–165.

Antzelevitch, C., 2007, Ionic, molecular, and cellular bases of QT-interval prolongation and torsade de pointes, *Europace*, 9(S4):4–15.

Antzelevitch, C., Sicouri, S., De Diego, J.M., et al., 2007, Does T_{peak}-T_{end} provide an index of transmural dispersion of repolarization? *Heart Rhythm*, 4:1114–1116.

Bass, A.S., Tomaselli, G., Bullingham, R., and Kinter, L.B., 2005, Drug effects on ventricular repolarization: A critical evaluation of the strengths and weaknesses of current methodologies and regulatory practices, *Journal of Pharmacological and Toxicological Methods*, 52:12–21.

Busti, A.J., Tsikouris, J.P., Peeters, M.J., et al., 2006, A prospective evaluation of the effect of atazanavir on the QTc interval and QTc dispersion in HIV-positive patients, *HIV Medicine*, 7:317–322.

Cabell, C.H., Noto, T.C., and Krucoff, M.W., 2005, Clinical utility of the Food and Drug Administration Electrocardiogram Warehouse: A paradigm for the critical pathway initiative, *Electrocardiology*, 38(S):175–179.

Camm, A.J., 2005, Clinical trial designed to evaluate the effects of drugs on cardiac repolarization: Current state of the art, *Heart Rhythm*, 2:S23–S29.

Couderc, J.P., Vaglio, M., Xia, X., et al., 2007, Impaired T-amplitude adaptation to heart rate characterizes $I_{(Kr)}$ inhibition in the congenital and acquired forms of the long QT syndrome, *Journal of Cardiovascular Electrophysiology*, 18: 1299–1305.

Dale, K.M., Lertsburapa, K., Kluger, J., and White, C.M., 2007, Moxifloxacin and torsade de pointes, *Annals of Pharmacotherapy*, 41:336–340.

Extramiana, F., Badilini, F., Sapara, N., Leenhardt, A., and Maison-Blanche, P., 2007, Contrasting time- and rate-based approaches for the assessment of drug-induced QT changes, *Journal of Clinical Pharmacology*, 47:1129–1137.

Extramiana, F., Haggui, A., Maison-Blanche, P., et al., 2007, T-wave morphology parameters based on principal component analysis reproducibility and dependence on T-offset position, *Annals of Noninvasive Electrocardiology*, 12: 354–363.

Extramiana, F., Maison-Blanche, P., Haggui, A., et al., 2006, Control of rapid heart rate changes for electrocardiographic analysis: Implications for thorough QT studies, *Clinical Cardiology*, 29:534–539.

Fitzgerald, P.T. and Ackerman, M.J., 2005, Drug-induced torsades de pointes: The evolving role of pharmacogenetics, *Heart Rhythm*, 2:S30–S37.

Gianotti, N., Guffanti, M., Galli, L., et al., 2007, Electrocardiographic changes in HIV-infected, drug-experienced patients being treated with atazanavir, *AIDS*, 21: 1648–1651.

Gupta, A., Lawrence, A.T., Krishnan, K., Kavinsky, C.J., and Trohman, R.G., 2007, Current concepts in the mechanisms and management of drug-induced QT prolongation and torsades de pointes, *American Heart Journal*, 153:891–899.

Gussak, I., Litwin, J., Kleiman, R., Grisanti, S., and Morganroth, J., 2004, Drug-induced cardiac toxicity: Emphasizing the role of electrocardiography in clinical research and drug development, *Journal of Electrocardiography*, 37:19–24.

Holzgrefe, H.H., Cavero, I., Buchanan, L.V., Gill, M.W., and Durham, S.K., 2007, Application of a probabilistic method for the determination of drug-induced QT prolongation in telemetered cynomolgus monkeys: Effects of moxifloxacin, *Journal of Pharmacological and Toxicological Methods*, 55:227–237. [This article also appeared in the Further Reading section in Chapter 6.]

Hondeghem, L.M., 2007, Relative contributions of TRIaD and QT to proarrhythmia, *Journal of Cardiovascular Electrophysiology*, 18:655–657.

Jalaie, M. and Holsworth, D.D., 2005, QT interval prolongation: And the beat goes on, *Mini Review of Medicinal Chemistry*, 5:1083–1091.

Jost, N., Papp, J.G., and Varro, A., 2007, Slow delayed rectifier potassium current (IKs) and the repolarization reserve, *Annals of Noninvasive Electrocardiology*, 12:64–78.

Judson, R.S., Salisbury, B.A., Reed, C.R., and Ackerman, M.J., 2006, Pharmacogenetic issues in thorough QT trials, *Molecular Diagnostics and Therapeutics*, 10:153–162.

Indik, J.H., Pearson, E.C., Freid, K., and Woolsey, R.L., 2006, Bazett and Fridericia QT correction formulas interfere with measurement of drug-induced changes in QT interval, *Heart Rhythm*, 3:1003–1007.

Kannankeril, P.J., and Roden, D.M., 2007, Drug-induced long QT and torsades de pointes: Recent advances, *Current Opinions in Cardiology*, 22:39–43.

Kligfield, P., Tyl, B., Maarek, M., and Maison-Blanche, P., 2007, Magnitude, mechanism, and reproducibility of QT interval differences between superimposed global and individual lead ECG complexes, *Annals of Noninvasive Cardiology*, 12:145–152.

Kounas, S.P., Letsas, K.P., Sideris, A., Efraimidis, M., and Kardaras, F., 2005, QT interval prolongation and torsades de pointes due to a coadministration of metronidazole and amiodarone, *Pacing Clinical Electrophysiology*, 28: 472–473.

Ly, T. and Ruiz, M.E., 2007, Prolonged QT interval and torsades de pointes associated with atazanavir therapy, *Clinical Infectious Diseases*, 44:e67–e68.

Malik, M., 2005, Detection of drug-induced proarrhythmia: Balancing preclinical and clinical studies, *Heart Rhythm*, 2:773–776.

Malik, M., Hnatkova, K., Batchvarov, V., et al., 2004, Sample size, power calculations, and their implications for the cost of thorough studies of drug induced QT interval prolongation, *Pacing and Clinical Electrophysiology*, 27:1659–1669.

Milic, M., Bao, X., Rizos, D., Liu, F., and Ziegler, M.G., 2006, Literature review and pilot studies of the effect of QT correction formulas on reported beta2-agonist-induced QTc prolongation, *Clinical Therapeutics*, 28:582–590.

Morganroth, J., 2007, Cardiac repolarization and the safety of new drugs defined by electrocardiography, *Clinical Pharmacology and Therapeutics*, 81:108–113.

Morganroth, J., Dimarco, J.P., Anzueto, A., et al., 2005, A randomized trial comparing the cardiac rhythm safety of moxifloxacin vs. levofloxacin in elderly patients hospitalized with community-acquired pneumonia, *Chest*, 138:3398–3406.

Patane, S., Marte, F., Di Bella, G., Curro, A., and Coglitore, S., 2008, QT interval prolongation, torsades de pointes and renal disease, *International Journal of Cardiology*, February 4 [E-publication ahead of print].

Remme, C.A. and Bezzina, C.R., 2007, Genetic modulation of cardiac repolarization reserve, *Heart Rhythm*, 4:608–610.

Roden, D.M., 2005, Proarrhythmia as a pharmacogenomic entity: A critical review and formulation of a unifying hypothesis, *Cardiovascular Research*, 67:419–425.

Roden, D.M., 2006, Long QT syndrome: Reduced repolarization reserve and the genetic link, *Journal of Internal Medicine*, 259:59–69.

Shah, R.R. and Hondeghem, L.M., 2005, Refining detection of drug-induced proarrhythmia: QT interval and TRIaD, *Heart Rhythm*, 2:758–772.

Sicouri, S. and Antzelevitch, C., 2008, Sudden cardiac death secondary to antidepressant and antipsychotic drugs, *Expert Opinion on Drug Safety*, 7: 181–194.

Somberg, J., 2007, Screening drugs for QT prolongation, *American Journal of Therapeutics*, 14:419–420.

Struijk, J.J., Kanters, J.K., Andersen, M.P., et al., 2006, Classification of the long-QT syndrome based on discriminant analysis of T-wave morphology, *Medicine, Biology, Engineering, and Computers*, 44:543–549.

Topilski, I, Rogowski, O., Rosso, R., et al., 2007, The morphology of the QT interval predicts torsade de pointes during acquired bradyarrhythmias, *Journal of the American College of Cardiology*, 49:320–328.

Vaglio, M., Couderc, J.P., McNitt, S., et al., 2008, A quantitative assessment of T-wave morphology in LQT1, LQT2, and healthy individuals based on Holter recording technology, *Heart Rhythm*, 5:11–18 van den Berg, M.P. and van Tintelen, J.P., 2006, Quantification of repolarization morphology in the long QT-syndrome in the genomic era, *Hearth Rhythm*, 3: 1467–1468.

Viskin, S. and Rosovski, U., 2005, The degree of potassium channel blockade and the risk of torsade de pointes: The truth, nothing but the truth, but not the whole truth, *European Heart Journal*, 26:536–537.

Wernicke, J.F., Faries, D., Breitung, R., and Girod, D., 2005, QT correction methods in children and adolescents, *Journal of Cardiovascular Electrophysiology*, 16: 76–81.

7.22.3   A Collection of Papers from Volume 39 of the *Drug Information Journal*

Agin, M.A., 2005, The importance of QT/QTc prolongation: A case study, *Drug Information Journal,* 39:385–386.

Dmitrienko, A.A., Sides, G.D., Winters, K.J., et al., 2005, Electrocardiogram reference ranges derived from a standardized clinical trial population, *Drug Information Journal,* 39:395–405.

Hosmane, B. and Locke, C., 2005, A simulation study of power in thorough QT/QTc studies and a normal approximation for planning purposes, *Drug Information Journal,* 39:447–455.

Johanson, P., Armstrong, P.W., Barbagelata, N.A., et al., 2005, An academic ECG core lab perspective of the FDA initiative for digital ECG capture and data management in large-scale clinical trials, *Drug Information Journal,* 39: 354–351.

Patterson, S., Agin, M., Anziano, R., et al., 2005, Investigating drug induced QT and QTc prolongation in the clinic: Statistical design and analysis considerations: Report from the Pharmaceutical Research and Manufacturers of America QT Statistics Expert Team, *Drug Information Journal,* 39:243–266.

Patterson, S.D., Jones, B., and Zariffa, N., 2005, Modeling and interpreting QTc prolongation in clinical pharmacology studies, *Drug Information Journal,* 39: 437–445.

Sager, P.T., Nebout, T., and Darpo, B., 2005, ICH E14: A new regulatory guidance on the clinical evaluation of QT/QTc interval prolongation and proarrhythmic potential for non-antiarrhythmic drugs, *Drug Information Journal,* 39:387–394.

Strnadova, C., 2005, The assessment of QT/QTc interval prolongation in clinical trials: A regulatory perspective, *Drug Information Journal,* 39:407–433.

Wei, G.C.G., 2005, Model-based correction to the QT interval for heart rate for assessing mean QT interval change due to drug effect, *Drug Information Journal,* 39:139–148.

7.22.4   QT Interval Shortening

Bjerregaard, P. and Gussak, I., 2005, Short QT syndrome: Mechanisms, diagnosis and treatment, *Nature Clinical Practice: Cardiovascular Medicine*, 2:84–87.

Cerrone, M., Noujaim, S., and Jalife, J., 2006, The short QT syndrome as a paradigm to understand the role of potassium channels in ventricular fibrillation, *Journal of Internal Medicine*, 259:24–38.

Cordeiro, J.M., Brugada, R., Wu, Y.S., Hong, K., and Dumaine, R., 2005, Modulation of $I_{(Kr)}$ inactivation by mutation N588K in KCNH2: A link to arrhythmogenesis in short QT syndrome, *Cardiovascular Research*, 67:498–509.

Gussak, I. and Bjerregaard, P., 2005, Short QT syndrome: 5 years of progress, *Journal of Electrocardiography*, 38:375–377.

Hong, K., Bjerregaard, P., Gussak, I., and Brugada, R., 2005, Short QT syndrome and atrial fibrillation caused by mutation in KCNH2, *Journal of Cardiovascular Electrophysiology*, 16:394–396.

Itoh, H., Horie, M., Ito, M., and Imoto, K., 2006, Arrhythmogenesis in the short-QT syndrome associated with combined HERG channel gating defects: A simulation study, *Circulation Journal*, 70:502–508.

McPate, M.J., Duncan, R.S., Milnes, J.T., Witchel, H.J., and Hancox, J.C., 2005, The N588K-HERG K+ channel mutation in the "short QT syndrome:" Mechanism of gain-in-function determined at 37 degrees C, *Biochemical and Biophysical Research Communications*, 334:441–449.

Perez Riera, A.R., Ferreira, C., Dubner, S.J., et al., 2005, Brief review of the recently described short QT syndrome and other cardiac channelopathies, *Annals of Noninvasive Electrocardiology*, 10:371–377.

8

GENERAL SAFETY ASSESSMENTS

8.1 INTRODUCTION

Following the previous chapter's focus on the TQT study, a central component of preapproval proarrhythmic cardiac safety evaluations, this chapter reviews other safety assessments made in preapproval clinical development programs. Some of these may prove helpful in identifying drug effects that might contribute to some of the cardiac events included in our generalized cardiac safety category.

From a regulatory perspective, all pertinent data collected during nonclinical studies and preapproval clinical trials—human pharmacology, therapeutic exploratory, and therapeutic confirmatory trials—contribute to an investigational drug's safety profile, and they will all be considered by a regulatory agency when marketing approval has been requested by a sponsor. In general, the evaluation of safety of an investigational therapy is rather open-ended, with the general philosophy being to "cast a wide net." For this reason, unlike the specific objectives that are listed for efficacy evaluation in a study protocol, specific details about safety analyses are not necessarily identified in advance of the study being conducted. However, if the evaluation of safety is the primary objective of the study, e.g., a TQT study, prespecification of a particular safety analysis is especially important. When that is the case, specific evaluations, e.g., collection of ECGs, will be well thought out in advance, as will the statistical approach used to evaluate the effect of concern.

The data discussed in this chapter are representative of the wide array of safety data typically collected during therapeutic exploratory and therapeutic confirmatory trials. As noted in the first paragraph, some of these data can be of particular relevance in generalized cardiac safety assessments. As noted in Section 4.10, major independent risk factors for the development of atherosclerosis include elevated blood pressure, elevated plasma total cholesterol and LDLc, and low plasma HDLc: these parameters can be readily assessed as safety data in preclinical trials. (In trials of investigational antihypertensive drugs and drugs intended to improve cholesterol profiles, such measures would be considered efficacy data.) While the actual development of atherosclerotic plaques takes a considerable length of time, and preclinical trial treatment periods are relatively short, data collected during the treatment periods may be particularly noteworthy in the case of drugs that, if approved, would typically be used on a long-term basis. As well as being evaluated by regulatory agencies at the time a marketing application is made, these data may be revisited at a later time if the investigational drug is approved and a

Integrated Cardiac Safety: Assessment Methodologies for Noncardiac Drugs in Discovery, Development, and Postmarketing Surveillance. By J. Rick Turner and Todd A. Durham
Copyright © 2009 John Wiley & Sons, Inc.

possible link is suspected between the drug and generalized cardiac events seen once it is on the market.

It should be noted here that the word revisited in the previous sentence does not imply that the regulatory agency did not consider these data appropriately when deciding to give marketing approval. This eventuality does not represent a second guessing of the agency's original decision, nor does it imply that the decision was wrong. Regulatory agencies can only use the totality of data available at a specific point in time when making a marketing approval decision, and such decisions involve a judgment call regarding the investigational drug's overall benefit-risk balance. At some point later in time a regulatory agency may use these data in conjunction with additional (postmarketing) data and reach a different decision about the drug's overall benefit-risk balance.

8.2   STATISTICAL ANALYSIS AND INTERPRETATION IN DRUG DEVELOPMENT

Turner (2007, pp. 4–5) provided an operational definition of the discipline of Statistics in the context of drug development, one that encapsulates all of the considerations of study design, research methodology, and analysis and interpretation of the results obtained. Statistics can be thought of as an integrated discipline that is important in all of the following activities:

> ➢ Identifying a research question that needs to be answered.
> ➢ Deciding upon the design of the study, the methodology that will be employed, and the numerical representations of biologically important information (data) that will be collected.
> ➢ Presenting the design, methodology, and data to be collected in a study protocol. This study protocol specifies the manner of data collection and addresses all methodological considerations necessary to ensure the collection of optimum-quality data for subsequent statistical analysis.
> ➢ Identifying the statistical techniques that will be used to describe and analyze the data in an associated statistical analysis plan, which should be written in conjunction with the study protocol.
> ➢ Describing and analyzing the data. This includes analyzing the variation in the data to see if there is compelling evidence that the drug is safe and effective. This process includes evaluation of the statistical significance of the results obtained and, very importantly, their clinical significance.
> ➢ Presenting the results of an individual clinical study to a regulatory agency in a clinical study report and presenting the results to the clinical community in journal publications and presentations. From the regulatory perspective, this activity can be extended to presenting the results of an entire nonclinical and clinical development program to a regulatory agency in a marketing application.

These activities can be directly translated into the following central tenets in the analysis of efficacy data (the focus of Turner, 2007) and the analysis of safety data, our present focus:

> Study design and statistical analysis are intimately and inextricably linked: the design of a study determines the analysis that will be used once the data have been collected during the study.
> Research methodology is intimately related to both design and analysis. If the data acquired during the study are not of optimum quality, the subsequent statistical analysis simply cannot produce the optimum-uality information that leads to optimum-quality decision making.
> Quantitative numerical representations of biologically important information provide the rational basis for evidence-based decision making.

8.2.1   The Central Role of Biology in Clinical Research

The last bullet in the previous section contained the phrase "biologically important information." Clinical trials investigate topics of clinical relevance, and clinical relevance is intimately related to biological relevance. The goal of drug development is to produce a biologically active drug whose benefit-risk balance is positive. This sentiment can be expanded to mean producing a biologically active drug whose benefit-risk balance is favorable from a public health perspective (i.e., will be approved by regulators) and will likely be found by prescribing physicians to be favorable for the vast majority of their individual patients on a case-by-case basis: when it is found not to be favorable for an individual patient, the physician will look for other treatment modalities that do have such a balance for that patient.

Biological and clinical considerations therefore pervade all of our discussions, even when terms such as methodological assessments, study design, and statistical analysis are used. These are fundamental tools used in this context with the sole purpose of providing biologically and clinically relevant information to prescribing physicians so that these physicians can make informed decisions on a patient-by-patient basis. Piantadosi (2005, pp. 9--0) made the following observation about clinical trials and the need for study design, methodology, and analysis:

> Experimental design and analysis have become essential because of the greater detail in modern biological theories and the complexities in treatments of disease. The clinician is usually interested in small, but biologically important, treatment effects that can be obscured by uncontrolled natural variation and bias in non-rigorous studies. This places well-performed clinical trials at the very center of clinical research today.

8.2.2   A Simpler Definition of Clinical Research.

Various authoritative but often complex definitions of the field of clinical research can be found (e.g., see http://www.nichd.nih.gov/health/clinicalresearch/index.cfm, accessed March 10, 2008; Gallin, 2002, p. 1; Schuster, 2005, p. xvii). A simpler definition might be that clinical research comprises any research undertaken with the intent of improving the care provided to patients. While initially appearing paradoxical, given the usual association of the word clinical with humans, this definition readily embraces the nonclinical research discussed in this book: the reason for conducting these nonclinical research studies is the intent to improve the care provided to human patients (therapies for use in veterinary medicine can also benefit from such research). As discussed in Chapter 6, *in vitro* and *in vivo* animal studies are necessary and logical forerunners of preapproval clinical trials. Another clear application of information from animal studies is that this information sometimes appears in an approved drug's labeling. If there are no human data available to answer a question that prescribing physicians may ask when considering the use of the drug for an individual patient, provision of animal data can provide the physician with (at least) some information to aid in deciding whether or not to prescribe the drug for that particular patient.

Therefore, while we agree with Piantadosi (2005) that clinical trials are indeed at the very center of clinical research today, the definition of clinical research provided here also embraces the research performed in drug discovery and design and research conducted in postmarketing settings. It therefore has an inherent lifecycle drug development perspective, a perspective in keeping with our discussions throughout this book.

8.2.3   Statistical Analysis and Interpretation of Safety Data in Drug Development

Chow and Liu (2004, p. 3) noted the following concerning a drug-related tragedy in the United States:

> The concept of testing marketed drugs in human subjects did not become a public issue until the Elixir Suflanilamide disaster occurred in the late 1930s. The disaster was a safety concern of a liquid formulation of a sulfa drug that caused more than 100 deaths. This drug had never been tested in humans before its marketing.

This tragedy had a major impact on legislation in the United States, leading to the Federal Food, Drug and Cosmetic Act in 1938. The Kefauver-Harris Drug Amendment to this act was passed in 1962. This amendment strengthened the safety requirements for new drugs and added an efficacy requirement for the first time.

In Europe, tragedies such as that involving the drug thalidomide in the 1960s (recall the discussions in Section 1.7) also led to legislation regarding the safety of pharmaceuticals. Given that the strengthening of legislation regarding drug safety was, and still is, extremely important, Senn (2007, p. 383) observed a paradoxical trend in the development of statistical theory relating to clinical trials:

> It is a curious fact that whereas the original inspiration for much legislation covering drug development has its origin in concerns about the safety of pharmaceuticals…much of the statistical theory of planning clinical trials has to do with investigating efficacy rather than safety.

There are several reasons for this that are, in themselves, very reasonable:

> ➢ Drug development programs are designed with therapeutic needs in mind.
> ➢ While some adverse events may be expected based on the mechanism of action of the therapeutic benefit, others that are unexpected may also occur,
> ➢ Unexpected adverse events are typically rare and thus hard to detect.

Nevertheless, as Senn (2007, p. 384) continued with regard to safety, "The subject is extremely important. Safety issues can cause drugs to be abandoned and companies to fail. If there are problems with a drug, then the sooner they are discovered the better." With some notable exceptions (e.g., O'Neill, 1995, 1998), it has traditionally been considered that simple descriptive analysis of safety data from preapproval clinical trials is acceptable, while more formal analyses are needed for efficacy data. Senn (2007, pp. 388–389) argued that, despite the undeniable difficulties associated with safety issues—including the rationale that formal analyses of safety data are often inappropriate because prespecified hypotheses are not available—formal analysis of safety data should not automatically be ruled out:

> In the end some sort of decision may be required and it would be difficult to maintain that the problems which a formal analysis would have to face have gone away by virtue of their being ignored…Whereas for many well-designed trials a description of the results may be adequate for making a judgment of efficacy; when it comes to analysing safety data it is often the case that only an extremely complex investigation can make any sense of them at all.

We do not present "extremely complex" approaches in this chapter: as stated in the book's preface, our approach is introductory, and our discussions of statistical analysis are conceptual rather than computational. However, following considerations of the traditional descriptive approach to safety data, we do discuss some formal methods of analyzing safety data to illustrate the contribution of inferential (hypothesis testing) statistical approaches in the assessment of the risk for adverse events.

Readers who are interested in the computational details of these approaches can find relevant discussions in Durham and Turner (2008).

8.3   PHYSICAL EXAMINATIONS

Physical examinations are typically conducted at the start of a clinical trial. They may also be conducted at later points, such as the end of the treatment phase and/or the end of a follow-up phase. Data collected from physical examinations include a subjective assessment by the physician investigator as to whether the participant has normal or abnormal function for each body system examined, including the cardiovascular system that is of particular interest in this book. Data are recorded as categorical data: the value for each participant is either normal or abnormal. These data are typically summarized by tabulating the number and the percentage of participants with each result. Additionally, if one (or more) of a participant's body systems is considered abnormal, additional descriptions of each abnormality are recorded.

8.4   CLINICAL LABORATORY TESTS

Participants in many clinical trials provide blood and/or urine samples at every clinic visit. A wide range of clinical chemistry tests can be conducted, including liver (hepatic) and kidney (renal) tests. Typically, the analyses conducted for clinical laboratory data are not based solely on measures of central tendency (means and medians) but also on individual observations, since it is quite possible that the average value for all participants in a treatment group could be normal—formal definitions of normal ranges for a given study must be presented in the study's protocol—while the values for certain participants could be clearly abnormal. A table of summary descriptive statistics that includes the minimum and maximum along with the mean and/or median values is therefore informative. Since treatment group minimums and maximums, by definition, each come from only one participant, minimums and/or maximums for a particular parameter(s) that are extreme can lead to additional scrutiny of values of that parameter for all other participants. This is typically accomplished with the use of a comprehensive listings that provide all values of all laboratory tests for all participants in the trial along with the dates and times of each sample's collection.

Clinicians on a clinical trial's study team review clinical laboratory data collected during the trial, and if a clinically significant observation, i.e., an observation of clinical concern, is noted for an individual participant, the clinician would look closely at all of that participant's values throughout the trial. The clinician would be interested to see whether the participant's values returned to normal levels at some later point in the trial or remained abnormal. The reviewer would also determine whether there were any accompanying adverse events (adverse events are discussed in Section 8.6).

8.4.1 Analyses of Clinical Laboratory Data

Clinical laboratory samples collected during a multicenter trial could theoretically be analyzed by laboratories associated with and geographically close to each site (sometimes called local labs), but this is not an optimal strategy since each local lab has its own handling procedures, assays, and reporting conventions. The use of a site's local lab poses no difficulties when the emphasis is on medical care and the values obtained are for an individual patient under the care of a physician. However, in clinical research, the focus of interest lies with using data from a group of participants to make optimally informed conclusions and decisions that are generalizable to large populations of potential patients, and differences between local labs may preclude meaningful combination of data from all participants across a number of investigative sites that may be spread across the country or, increasingly, spread across several countries and continents.

A statistical approach to standardizing laboratory values from a number of different local labs (each potentially with its own reference ranges) has been described by Chuang-Stein (1992). However, standardization is time-consuming, and the use of a number of local labs can introduce unwanted sources of variability that are neither easily quantified nor accounted for. To overcome these difficulties, the use of a single core, or central, lab is desirable. In this strategy, samples from all investigative sites in a given trial are sent for analysis at the core lab. The advantages of using a core lab include:

> ➢ All samples are handled in a similar fashion.
> ➢ The assays used are consistent over time and across participants.
> ➢ The reporting conventions, e.g., the units of measurement used, are uniform (cholesterol, for example, is measured in different units in different countries).

Techniques for proper sample collection, storage, and handling—including shipment of the samples to the core lab, a nontrivial consideration in multicenter trials involving investigative sites spread across multiple countries—should be included in the study protocol. Once the samples reach the core lab, they are analyzed and data are recorded in a database that includes participant identifiers, study visit, date and time of sample collection, test name, result, reporting units, and the value of the reference or normal range. (With regard to the ECGs discussed in Chapter 7, the "shipping" of these to a core lab is less cumbersome since digital ECGs can be transmitted electronically.)

The determination of reference range values is based on the distribution of test values in large samples. Reference ranges are determined using large databases from a general population. The (reasonable) assumption is made that the values in such a population are normally distributed (see Turner, 2007, pp. 93–96, for a straightforward discussion of the normal distribution, a particularly noteworthy distribution in the discipline of Statistics). The lower limit (often written as LL) of the reference range is typically the value below which the lowest 2.5% of values from individuals in the general population fall. Similarly, the upper limit (UL) of the reference range is the value above which the highest 2.5% of values fall. Reference ranges for certain clinical chemistry parameters may be defined differentially by characteristics such as age and sex.

Several analytical strategies for clinical laboratory data are recommended in the 1996 ICH Guidance E3, *Structure and Content of Clinical Study Reports*. The approaches to describing clinical laboratory data include:

> ➤ Measures of central tendency (means, medians) for all groups at all time points examined.
> ➤ Identification of individual values that are so extreme that they would be considered clinically significant.
> ➤ Shift analysis (discussed in the following section).
> ➤ Responders analysis (discussed in Section 8.4.3).

It is also possible to conduct similar analyses using change from baseline values at given time points. These change scores are typically calculated as the value at the time point of interest minus the baseline value. This form of analysis can highlight consistent and systematic changes from the start of the study.

It is perhaps helpful to note here that for parameters that increase during the treatment period, this calculation, i.e., mean treatment value minus mean baseline value for a given group of participants, leads to a positive value: in contrast, for parameters that decrease, it leads to a negative value. Care needs to be taken when reporting and discussing all results, especially the results for a parameter that decreases. Imagine the scenario where the mean treatment group baseline value for a particular clinical laboratory value is 100 units and the group's mean value during the treatment period is 90 units. The calculation leads to a mean change value of -10 units, with the minus sign being very important since it indicates a decrease. However, another way of expressing this change is to use the phrase "a mean decrease of 10 units." In this latter case the minus sign is not used, since the word decrease indicates the direction of the change. Both expressions of the change are correct, but care is needed to ensure that the chosen representation of the change is expressed unambiguously.

8.4.2   Shift Analysis

The objective of a shift analysis is to identify any systematic pattern in how participants' values change from one category—low, normal, or high relative to the reference range—to another over time. Shift analyses can be conducted for parameters that are a central focus of a clinical trial for which a change during the treatment period is of interest, and also for parameters for which no appreciable change is indicative of the drug's safety. With regard to the first of these scenarios, consider a trial of an antihypertensive investigational drug. Since participants enrolled in this trial would likely have relatively high blood pressure at the time of their recruitment for the trial, their baseline blood pressure measurements would likely be high relative to the normal range as defined in the study protocol. The sponsor would be interested to see whether blood pressures for participants in the drug treatment group would come down over the treatment period and fall inro the normal range at the end.

As an example of the second scenario, one in which no appreciable change in a parameter of interest is indicative of the drug's safety, consider a trial of an investigational drug for a psychiatric condition. The sponsor would hope, for example, not to see a trend for blood pressure or LDLc to increase, or for HDLc to decrease, across the treatment phase: that is, the sponsor would hope not to see a pattern of change from baseline to the end of the treatment phase that would indicate a safety concern.

8.4.3   Responders Analysis

A responders analysis examines how many participants show a change of a certain magnitude in a parameter of interest. Change scores can be calculated for various times during the treatment phase, but for simplicity here the scenario of calculating only one change score, from baseline to the end of the treatment phase, is considered.

The rationale for wanting to know how many participants have a change score of a certain magnitude is that a consistent but relatively minor change in a parameter may not be of clinical concern. As an example of this scenario, treatment with hydrochlorothiazide, a diuretic used for the treatment of hypertension, is often associated with increases in blood glucose that are not of clinical concern. Expressed in a different manner, one that fits with our ongoing discussions of benefit-risk balance assessments throughout the book, individual physicians may well decide that the therapeutic benefit from hydrochlorothiazide therapy outweighs concern about the increased blood sugar, that the drug therefore has a favorable benefit-risk balance, and hence prescribe the drug to their patients.

In a responders analysis a change score is calculated for each participant, and, in the simplest case in which only two categories of response are employed, each participant is categorized either as a responder or as a nonresponder. Such categorization requires the *a priori* designation of what constitutes a responder, and this information must be provided in the study protocol or the associated statistical analysis plan. Note that the change in the parameter that categorizes a participant as a responder can be an increase of a certain magnitude or a decrease of a certain magnitude: Whether or not an increase or a decrease in the laboratory value is indicative of potential harm depends on the laboratory test itself. For example, an increase in blood pressure may be indicative of potential harm, as might a decrease in HDLc.

Consider a hypothetical example in which an increase of 10 units of measurement or more in a particular parameter of interest categorizes a participant as a responder, and an increase of less than 10 units of measurement categorizes a participant as a nonresponder. The number and percentage of responders and nonresponders in both the drug treatment group and the placebo group are typically presented. A possible extension of this two-category approach would be to categorize a participant with an increase of 10 units of measurement or less as a nonresponder, a participant with an increase of greater than 10 units but less than 20 units of measurement as a responder, and a participant with an increase of 20 units of measurement or greater as a hyperresponder (or some similar term). Theoretically, any number of levels of response is possible, but the use of three to five categories is most common. A responders analysis is most useful for clinical interpretation when the categories at either extreme represent clear benefit or harm. The intermediate categories may then represent responses for which the clinical relevance is less obvious. As noted in Section 7.11, the use of various threshold effects in the TQT study is an example of a responders analysis.

8.5   VITAL SIGNS

Vital signs typically measured in clinical trials include blood pressure (both SBP and DBP) and heart rate, often measured at the wrist as pulse rate. Weight will likely also be of interest. Blood pressure and heart rate may be measured at baseline and at each of several clinical visits, while weight may be measured simply at baseline and at the end of the treatment phase. While blood pressure and heart rate are typically measured in the same units internationally (mmHg and bpm, respectively) weight can be measured in different units (e.g., pounds and kilograms). Therefore, for international multicenter trials a measurement convention needs to be established in the study protocol, or a conversion factor needs to be carefully applied where necessary in a method stated in the statistical analysis plan.

As for clinical laboratory data, several analytical methods can be employed for vital signs data. Measures of central tendency and of dispersion are appropriate for continuous data. Categorical data can also be of interest. Imagine a trial in which the treatment phase is 12 weeks long and participants visit their investigational site every two weeks. In this scenario a baseline value, taken before treatment commences, is followed by six values measured during the treatment phase. It may be of interest to the study team to know how many participants show clinically significant changes in blood pressure and heart rate during the treatment period. As for laboratory data, such categorization requires a precise *a priori* definition of a clinically significant change. The following are hypothetical definitions of clinically significant changes that are used here for illustrative purposes only:

> An increase from baseline in SBP ≥ 20 mmHg.
> An increase from baseline in DBP ≥ 12 mmHg.
> An increase from baseline in SBP ≥ 15 mmHg and an increase in DBP ≥ 10 mmHg.
> A pulse rate ≥120 bpm and an associated increase from baseline of at least 15 bpm.

The clinicians on the study team might also be interested in sustained changes in vital signs. Hypothetical examples of definitions of sustained changes might be:

> An increase from baseline in SBP ≥ 15 mmHg at each of three consecutive visits.
> An increase from baseline in DBP ≥ 10 mmHg at each of three consecutive visits.
> An increase from baseline in pulse rate ≥ 10 bpm at each of three consecutive visits.

Appropriate categorical analyses could then be conducted with data generated in this manner.

8.6   ADVERSE EVENT DATA

Adverse event data, unlike some safety parameters, are collected in all clinical trials of investigational drugs: these types of data are therefore the focus of the remainder of this chapter. Before commencing our discussions, as is the case in several places in this book, some nomenclature considerations are appropriate.

8.6.1   Nomenclature

The term adverse drug reaction is used in this book to refer to an unwanted occurrence seen in a patient who has been prescribed a certain drug (or drugs in cases where the adverse reaction results from a drug-drug interaction). Prescribing clinicians are concerned with adverse drug reactions, as are researchers conducting the postmarketing surveillance studies discussed in Chapters 10–12. However, during double-blind preapproval clinical trials, unwanted occurrences can be seen in drug treatment groups and placebo treatment groups, and, at the time that the adverse event occurs, neither the participant nor the investigator knows which treatment the participant is receiving. These unwanted occurrences are called adverse events. If an investigator thinks, based on prior available information such as that provided in the investigational drug's Investigator's Brochure that is supplied to all investigators before the trial commences, that a particular adverse event reported by a participant is likely to be related to the treatment the participant is receiving, the adverse event is recorded as possibly or probably drug related. This nomenclature is used for adverse events reported by all participants in the trial. It is therefore quite possible that a drug-related adverse event may be recorded for participants in the placebo treatment group. This seemingly paradoxical nomenclature is appropriate at that point in time since, as noted, neither the participant nor the investigator in a double-blind trial knows at that time which treatment group the participant is in.

Once the trial is completed and the treatment status of each participant is made known to the statisticians analyzing the data from the trial, the drug-related adverse event determinations that were made during the trial for participants in the placebo treatment group are shown not to be possible. However, such clarity is not provided for drug-related adverse event judgments that were made and recorded during the trial for participants in the drug treatment group. While it is certainly possible (highly likely in some cases) that the investigational drug led to the adverse event, this cannot be known with certainty in all cases.

8.6.2   The Use of Adverse Event Data in Clinical Practice

Adverse event data from preapproval clinical trials are used by both of the following:

> ➢ By regulatory agencies when judging whether an investigational drug's benefit-risk balance is positive, and therefore whether the drug should be approved for marketing.
> ➢ By a physician when deciding whether to prescribe an approved drug to an individual patient.

At this point in the book our interest lies with the second of these circumstances.

When a physician prescribes an approved drug for a patient, both of them will likely have questions concerning the drug's safety. These questions may include the following:

> ➢ How likely is it that the patient will experience an adverse drug reaction?
> ➢ Are the typical adverse drug reactions temporary or permanent?
> ➢ Will the risk of experiencing an adverse drug reaction likely change with the length of time the drug is taken?
> ➢ Are there specific clinical parameters that should be monitored particularly closely while the patient is taking the drug?
> ➢ How likely is it that the patient will experience an adverse drug reaction that is so serious that it may be life-threatening?

Shortly after the drug has received marketing approval, the best available data upon which answers to these questions can be based are the adverse event data gathered during the preapproval clinical trials, and this information is provided to physicians and patients in the drug's package insert, also called the labeling. This situation changes in due course as additional and more detailed safety evaluation takes place during postapproval clinical trials and postmarketing surveillance of the drug's use in clinical practice, but it may take several years to acquire, collate, and present such data to regulatory agencies and thus to potentially modify the labeling. Therefore, this chapter discusses how adverse event data included in the drug's labeling when it is first approved might be used by a prescribing physician.

8.6.3 Regulatory Definitions of Different Categories of Adverse Events

The 1996 ICH Guidance E6(R1), *Guideline for Good Clinical Practice*, provides the following definition of the term adverse event (p. 2):

> Any untoward medical occurrence in a patient or clinical investigation subject administered a pharmaceutical product and which does not necessarily have a causal relationship with the treatment. An adverse event (AE) can therefore be any unfavourable and unintended sign (including an abnormal laboratory finding), symptom, or disease temporally associated with the use of a medicinal (investigational) product, whether or not associated with the medicinal (investigational) product.

Similarly, the 1994 ICH Guidance E2A, *Clinical Safety Data Management: Definitions and Standards for Expedited Reporting*, provides the following definition of a serious event (p. 3):

> A serious adverse event (experience) or reaction is any untoward medical occurrence that at any dose:

➤ Results in death,
➤ Is life threatening,
  (NOTE: The term "life threatening" in the definition of "serious" refers to an event in which the patient was at risk of death at the time of the event; it does not refer to an event which hypothetically might have caused death if it were more severe.)
➤ Requires inpatient hospitalization or prolongation of existing hospitalization,
➤ Results in persistent or significant disability/incapacity, or
➤ Is a congenital anomaly/birth defect.

8.6.4   Collection of Adverse Event Data

The collection of adverse events data can be based on observation by the investigator (e.g., abnormalities found during physical examinations, from

ECG recordings, or from clinical lab values) or by participant self-report. It is advisable to elicit adverse events from study participants using a standardized script to ensure that adverse events are collected as accurately as possible. For example, a question such as "Have you noticed anything different or had any health problems since you were last here?" is a way of asking a participant about potential adverse events without leading him or her to answer in a certain way. Study personnel who interact with subjects are trained to capture the essence of any self-reported adverse events on a case report form, one of the most important documents in clinical trials. To standardize adverse event descriptions, they are coded using medical dictionaries such as the *Medical Dictionary for Drug Regulatory Affairs* (MedDRA) coding dictionary. Information typically collected includes:

> The adverse event description itself, e.g., rash on the left forearm, shortness of breath, dry mouth, vomiting.
> The severity or intensity of the adverse event, e.g., mild, moderate, severe.
> The date and time of onset.
> The outcome of the adverse event (resolved without sequelae, resolved with sequelae, or ongoing).
> Any treatments administered for the adverse event.
> Any action taken with the study drug (e.g., temporarily discontinued, stopped, none).
> Whether or not the adverse event was considered serious according to a regulatory definition.

8.6.5   Describing the Risks of Adverse Events

Descriptive reports of adverse event data provide simple summary statistics such as the number and the proportion of participants in each treatment group experiencing these adverse events. Proportions are numbers between 0 and 1. The proportion of participants in the drug treatment group reporting an adverse event during the trial is calculated as expressed in Formula 8.1 (AE, a common abbreviation for adverse event, is used):

Proportion = Number of participants in the drug group reporting an AE   (8.1)
                      Total number of participants in the drug group

Similarly, the proportion of participants in the placebo treatment group reporting an adverse event during the trial is calculated as expressed in Formula 8.2:

Proportion = Number of participants in the placebo group reporting an AE (8.2)
                      Total number of participants in the placebo group

Proportions can be multiplied by 100 and expressed in percentage terms (e.g., the proportion 0.5 is equivalent to 50%), an approach typically taken when presenting adverse event information in drug labeling. It is important to note that, if a participant reports more than one adverse event, the participant is counted only once for purposes of this analysis.

Table 8.1 represents a typical presentation of adverse event data from a clinical trial, in this case the hypothetical trial ABC001. For each treatment group, the absolute numbers and percentages of participants experiencing various adverse events are presented. It should be noted that the low number of participants in each group has been deliberately chosen to make the few calculations presented here simple. Also, the number of participants in each group is not the same: In real trials these numbers will often be close but not identical. This difference in the number of participants highlights the unique information provided by the percentage values (in this example, rounded up to the nearest whole number) over and above that provided by the absolute numbers. For example, 50 participants in the drug treatment group ($N = 250$) would be 20% of that group, whereas the same absolute number of participants, i.e., 50, would be 25% of the placebo treatment group ($N = 200$).

TABLE 8.1. Overall Adverse Event Data (Numbers and Percentages) by Treatment Group, Clinical Trial ABC001

Adverse Events (AEs)	Placebo Treatment Group ($N = 200$)	Drug Treatment Group ($N = 250$)
Pretreatment AEs, n (%)	8 (4%)	10 (4%)
On-treatment AEs, n (%)	54 (27%)	74 (30%)
Drug-related AEs, n (%)	21 (11%)	34 (14%)
AEs leading to withdrawal, n (%)	5 (3%)	8 (3%)
Serious AEs (SAEs), n (%)	7 (4%)	12 (5%)

Table 8.2 presents additional data on individual adverse events, with the first row presenting data for "Any event." Note that, for both treatment groups, the individual events are presented in descending order of frequency as they occurred in the drug treatment group.

TABLE 8.2. Adverse Events (Numbers and Percentages) by Treatment Group, Clinical Trial ABC001

Adverse Events (AEs)	Placebo Treatment Group (N = 200)	Drug Treatment Group (N = 250)
Any event, n (%)	54 (27%)	74 (30%)
Headache, n (%)	24 (12%)	45 (18%)
Dizziness, n (%)	10 (5%)	38 (15%)
Upper respiratory infection, n (%)	24 (12%)	19 (8%)
Nausea, n (%)	23 (12%)	18 (7%)
Specified AE of special interest, n (%)	2 (1%)	12 (5%)

8.6.6 Comparing the Risk of Adverse Events between Groups: Risk Difference

Data such as those presented in Table 8.2 may appear in a drug's labeling (see Section 8.8.1 for more details). These data—as noted earlier, the only data available at this time—provide a way for prescribing physicians and their potential patients to begin to answer the first question posed in Section 8.6.2: how likely is a patient to experience an adverse drug reaction if prescribed this drug? Based on the data for the drug treatment group, the best guess of the likelihood of a patient treated with this drug experiencing any adverse drug reaction is 30%.

However, Table 8.2 also provides "any event" data for the placebo treatment group, i.e., it provides an additional piece of information over and above that provided by the drug treatment group's data. Since the placebo treatment group in the clinical trial did not receive the investigational drug, the occurrence of any event in that group can be conceptualized as providing best-guess information concerning what adverse events may be seen in an individual patient not treated with the drug: that is, it provides best-guess information concerning the background occurrence of adverse events. Therefore, it is possible to obtain best-guess information concerning how much more likely it is that a patient would experience any adverse event if treated with the drug as compared with not being treated with it. By subtracting the proportion of participants in the placebo treatment group experiencing any event (27%) from the proportion of participants in the drug treatment group experiencing any event (30%) the increased likelihood of experiencing any event if treated with the drug can be estimated. This quantity is called the estimated risk difference.

In general, the estimated risk difference is calculated as the proportion of participants in the drug group with the event of interest minus the proportion of participants in the placebo group with the event. When calculated in this manner, an estimated risk difference of zero indicates that the risk of an adverse event is the same in the drug treatment and placebo treatment groups, an estimated risk difference greater than zero indicates a greater risk for participants in the drug treatment group compared with participants in the placebo treatment group, and an estimated risk difference less than zero indicates that the risk of an adverse event is greater in the placebo treatment group than in the drug treatment group.

In this example, it can be seen that the estimated risk difference for any event is rather small (3%). If the physician and the patient believe that the patient will likely experience considerable benefit from the drug, the physician may decide to prescribe the drug for the patient. In other words, the physician performs a benefit-risk assessment for the specific individual patient and judges the benefit-risk balance to be positive.

A similar approach can be used to describe the occurrence of specific adverse events, including adverse events of special interest, defined on a case-by-case basis for investigational drugs. These adverse events of special interest may be related to a particular adverse event of clinical concern that has already been noted in nonclinical studies and/or earlier trials in the clinical development program, and/or an adverse event that has been noted for an approved drug that is in a similar chemical class as the investigational drug. By comparing the occurrence of the adverse event of interest in the drug treatment group with the occurrence of the adverse event in the placebo treatment group, it is possible to form an initial opinion concerning the increased likelihood of a patient experiencing the specific adverse event if treated with the drug compared with not being treated with the drug. Therefore, while an overall analysis of participants experiencing any event provides useful overall data, information from analyses of individual adverse events is potentially much more useful to prescribing physicians, who are likely to be more interested in the occurrence of some adverse events than others.

While this initial comparative strategy can be helpful, it has its limitations. First, the two estimates of risk (the percentages of participants in each group with the event) can be meaningfully compared only if participants in both groups were at risk for the adverse event for the same amount of time. Imagine a (deliberately extreme) scenario in which half of the participants in the drug treatment group in a preapproval clinical trial discontinued treatment after one day, while all of the participants in the placebo group completed the full study, which lasted one year. In this scenario, a comparison of such percentages is likely to be inaccurate and misleading. An alternate analysis strategy to deal with varying times at risk is described in Section 8.6.11.

Second, excess risk associated with the drug treatment can be expressed in a number of ways, each of which may affect one's perception of the drug's usefulness. The physician and patient are required to make subjective judgments concerning the difference between values that may be relatively similar. For example, is the difference between a 12% occurrence of an adverse event of interest in the drug treatment group and a 10% occurrence in the placebo treatment group, i.e., an estimated risk difference of 2%, enough to cause concern? Consider a second scenario of occurrences, one that involves 3% of participants in the drug treatment group experiencing an event and 1% in the placebo treatment group experiencing the event. Comparison of these values with the values of 12% and 10% used in the former example reveals several points, each of which leads to a potential conclusion:

> The estimated risk difference, 2%, is the same in both cases (12% minus 10% is 2%, and 3% minus 1% is also 2%). Consideration of this observation may lead to the conclusion that the potential consequences of the patient being treated with the drug versus not being treated with the drug are about the same in each scenario.

> The occurrence of the adverse event of interest in the second scenario (3%) is only one-quarter the occurrence of the adverse event in the first scenario (12%). Consideration of this observation may lead to the conclusion that the patient is considerably less likely to experience the adverse event if treated with the drug in the second scenario compared with the first.

> The occurrence of the adverse event in the drug treatment group is three times as great as in the placebo drug treatment group (3% versus 1%) in the second scenario. In the first scenario the difference was much less striking: An occurrence of 12% is only 1.2 times as great as an occurrence of 10%. Consideration of this observation may lead to the conclusion that the patient is considerably more likely to experience the adverse event if treated with the drug in the second scenario compared with the first.

Would you agree or disagree with these potential conclusions? And, if you were the prescribing physician or the patient, what would your feelings be concerning possible treatment with the drug and the likelihood of experiencing the adverse event of interest? (See also discussions in Sections 12.2.5 and 12.6.2.)

8.6.7   Comparing the Risk of Adverse Events between Groups: Relative Risk

The questions posed in the previous section are not easy to answer definitively on the basis of the data analysis conducted to this point: when considered in this manner, the available data cannot provide sufficient information to reach such an answer. In the second scenario discussed above, the estimated risk difference was 2%, which may not have seemed extreme. However, when these rates are considered in relative terms, participants treated with the investigational drug were three times as likely to experience the event as those who received placebo. This measure of risk is called a relative risk, and it is discussed in this section. First, however, it is appropriate to briefly discuss probabilities in order to fully understand relative risks.

Probabilities are an important and central component of inferential statistics, and are relevant to the calculation and interpretation of relative risks. Probabilities exhibit the following characteristics:

> They refer only to future events. Of relevance here is that the physician and patient would like to estimate the likelihood, i.e., the probability, that the patient will experience a particular adverse drug reaction at some point in the future after first taking a drug.
> Like proportions, they can range from 0 to 1. A probability of 0 indicates that a possible future event will certainly not occur, and a probability of 1 indicates that a possible future event will certainly occur. In most circumstances of interest in this book, probabilities fall somewhere in between these limiting values.
> Also like proportions, probabilities are often multiplied by 100 and expressed in percentage terms. Thus, the probability of a heads occurring if a fair coin is tossed in the air, i.e., 0.5, can also be represented as 50% (exactly the same as for the only other option, the probability of a tails).

A relative risk is a ratio of two probabilities. In its general form, the formula for the calculation of a relative risk can be written as:

$$\text{Relative risk} = \frac{\text{Probability of the event in group A}}{\text{Probability of the event in group B}} \qquad (8.3)$$

In the present context, this formula can be rewritten as:

$$\text{Relative risk} = \frac{\text{Probability of the adverse event in the drug treatment group}}{\text{Probability of the adverse event in the placebo treatment group}} \qquad (8.4)$$

As can be seen in Formula 8.4, we need to know two probabilities to calculate the relative risk. Since we do not have this knowledge *per se,* i.e., we do not know the true probabilities in the general population of which the patient is a member, we need to determine our best estimate of these probabilities. That is, we need to estimate the probability of experiencing an adverse event in the drug treatment group and the probability of experiencing an adverse event in the placebo treatment group. Our best estimates of these probabilities at this point in time are given by the observed proportions of adverse events reported in the drug's labeling.

The calculation of a relative risk point estimate, a computation that involves the division of one number by another number, results in a value that can range from zero to infinity. It is normally the case that the probability of an adverse event in the drug treatment group is regarded as the numerator, and is divided by the probability of an adverse event in the placebo treatment group, which is therefore used as the denominator. It is certainly possible to calculate the relative risk the other way, i.e., by using the value for the placebo treatment group as the numerator and the value for the drug treatment group as the denominator. However, from the point of view of ease of interpretation, that approach tends to be more tortuous (recall the discussions in Section 1.5.1 about the importance of the choice of numerator and denominator in such cases). In our discussions, we will follow the typical method of using the probability for the drug treatment group as the numerator and the probability for the placebo treatment group as the denominator.

If the probability of an adverse event in the drug treatment group is exactly the same as the probability of an adverse event in the placebo treatment group, the relative risk calculation will result in a point estimate of exactly 1, which we will write to two decimal places as 1.00. It is actually unlikely—and in larger samples extremely unlikely—that the two probabilities will be identical, which means that the relative risk point estimate will most likely be either greater or smaller than 1.00. If the probability of an adverse event in the drug treatment group is greater than the probability of an adverse event in the placebo treatment group, the relative risk point estimate will be greater than 1.00. If the probability of an adverse event in the drug treatment group is less than the probability of an adverse event in the placebo treatment group, the relative risk point estimate will be less than 1.00.

It was noted a short while ago that a relative risk point estimate can range from zero to infinity, and the reasons for these two extreme values are considered here. If there are zero occurrences of the adverse event in the drug treatment group and any occurrences in the placebo treatment group, the relative risk point estimate will be zero. If there are no occurrences of an adverse event of interest in the placebo treatment group and there are any occurrences in the drug treatment group, the relative risk point estimate will be infinity, since any positive nonzero number divided by zero is defined mathematically as infinity. Meaningful interpretation of this relative risk is not possible. (If there are zero occurrences of the adverse event in the drug treatment group and zero occurrences in the placebo treatment group, the relative risk estimate will be 1.00, since zero divided by zero is defined mathematically as unity. This value of 1.00 falls in between the two extreme values of 0.0 and 1.0.)

The adverse event data presented in Table 8.2 can be used to illustrate the concept of relative risk. Consider the adverse event of dizziness. As shown in Formula 8.4, this relative risk of experiencing the adverse drug reaction of dizziness can be best estimated as:

Relative risk = Probability of dizziness in the drug treatment group
                 Probability of dizziness in the placebo treatment group

Our best estimates of these two probabilities come from the proportions captured in Formulae 8.1.and 8.2, respectively. That is, relative risk is estimated as:

Estimated relative risk = Proportion of participants in the drug group experiencing dizziness
                          Proportion of participants in the placebo group experiencing dizziness

$$= \frac{\frac{38}{250}}{\frac{10}{200}} = \frac{(38)(200)}{(10)(250)}$$

$$= 3.04$$

It should be noted here that this answer, while certainly informative, is not the complete answer of interest to us. This answer is regarded as a point estimate, an estimate of relative risk calculated on the basis of precise results from a single set of data. In the situation of present interest, i.e., estimating whether a patient is more likely to suffer an adverse event if treated with a drug than if not treated with the drug, only relative risk point estimates greater than 1.00 are of interest. If the relative risk point estimate is precisely equal to zero (a very unlikely occurrence), the drug and placebo are equally safe, and if the relative risk point estimate is less than 1.00 the drug is safer than placebo, and therefore we do not need to be concerned. However, these statements require some qualification, qualification that is provided by the calculation of CIs around the point estimate. We encountered this procedure in the previous chapter when placing confidence intervals around a point estimate of the effect of an investigational drug on the QTc interval. The next section describes how CIs are placed around a relative risk point estimate.

8.6.8   The Use of Confidence Intervals to Compare the Risk of Adverse Events between Groups

In the calculation performed in the previous section, we used two observed proportions to estimate two probabilities in order to calculate a relative risk. This three-step process can be represented as follows:

➢ The proportion of participants experiencing dizziness in the drug treatment group was used to estimate the probability of a participant in that group experiencing the event.
➢ The proportion of participants experiencing dizziness in the placebo treatment group was used to estimate the probability of a participant in that group experiencing the event.
➢ The probability of a participant in the drug treatment group experiencing dizziness was then divided by the probability of a participant in the placebo treatment group experiencing dizziness to yield the relative risk point estimate.

This computational process yielded a precise answer, an answer resulting from the use of the actual data from the single trial. However, the calculated answer must itself be regarded as an estimate since it was obtained from two estimates. While the point estimate has been derived from actual data collected from a specific sample of participants, this sample is only one of many potential samples drawn from the population of individuals who could have participated (recall the discussions in Section 7.7). Importantly, had a different sample taken part in the trial, the precise value of the proportions calculated would almost certainly differ to a certain extent. Therefore, the calculated relative risk would almost certainly differ to a certain extent. It is therefore of interest to estimate to what extent different samples would likely provide different proportions, different probabilities derived from these actual proportions, and hence a different estimate of relative risk.

Interest here therefore lies in determining our best estimate of the respective probabilities, and hence of the relative risk, no matter what sample might have been selected. As was illustrated in the previous chapter, using the (known) data from an individual sample in a single study to estimate the unknown but true population value of any parameter is a hallmark of inferential statistics: we infer from the known data what the true but unknown value is for the population of interest from which the sample was drawn. The analytical strategy discussed here illustrates a methodology for making statistical statements concerning the relative frequency of adverse events of particular interest in different treatment groups.

A question of interest here is:

> Is there any statistically significant evidence that a participant in the drug treatment group was more likely to experience an adverse event than a participant in the placebo treatment group?

This question can be answered by placing CIs around the point estimate. Population parameters of interest regarding adverse events are the population risk difference (difference in proportions of participants experiencing an adverse event) and the population relative risk.

The exact calculation of the CI depends on the population parameter of interest since the method of calculation differs according to mathematical characteristics of the sample estimator used in the estimation. In some cases, e.g., the risk difference—and also the drug treatment effect on QT/QTc interval discussed in the previous chapter—the point estimate will lie at the center of a two-sided CI, equidistant from the lower limit and the upper limit. This is not the case with CIs placed around a relative risk point estimate. The point estimate will be somewhat closer to the lower limit. This occurs because the calculation of the lower and upper limits of the CI about the relative risk involves a scale that is not linear. We need not go into the mathematics of these calculations (it involves logarithmic scales, and hence nonlinearity), but it is useful to be aware when reading clinical communications presenting such data that the point estimate will not necessarily be equidistant from the lower limit and the upper limit.

CIs and hypothesis tests are closely related inferential procedures. Our discussions here are couched in terms of "100(1 minus α)%" or "100(1 – α)%" CIs, with this term representing the general case. As we saw in the previous chapter, two commonly used CIs are the 95% and 99% CIs. These intervals are calculated from the general case when the selected values for α are 0.05 and 0.01, respectively. Using the first case as an example, (1 – 0.05) results in 0.95, which becomes 95 when multiplied by 100.

In the case of a two-sided 100(1 – α)% CI the lower and upper limits represent the range of plausible values of the unknown population parameter. A hypothesis test may be carried out by positing a number of values of the population parameter in the null hypothesis. All values outside of the limits of the two-sided 100(1 – α)% CI would be rejected by a two-sided hypothesis test of size α. Conversely, values within the two-sided 100(1 – α)% CI would not be rejected. Thus, a CI can be used to test a number of values of the population parameter.

A graphical representation of the relationship between a two-sided 100(1 – α)% CI about a population parameter, q , and a two-sided hypothesis test of the null hypothesis, $H_0 : q = q_0$, is presented in Figure 8.1.

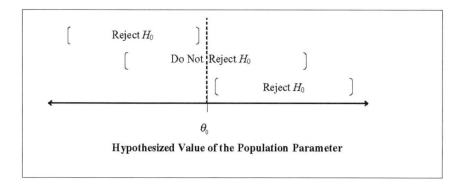

Figure 8.1. Relationship between confidence intervals and hypothesis tests.

In Figure 8.1 three hypothetical CIs (with lower and upper limits indicated by the brackets) are displayed with the corresponding statistical conclusion regarding the null hypothesis. The first interval lies entirely to the left of the hypothesized value of the population parameter, indicating that all of the plausible values of q

are less than q_0. Therefore, the null hypothesis is rejected. The second interval encloses the hypothesized value of the population parameter, indicating that q_0 is among the plausible values of q. Therefore, the null hypothesis is not rejected. The third interval lies entirely to the right of the hypothesized value of the population parameter, indicating that all of the plausible values of q are greater than q_0. Hence, the third CI is also consistent with rejection of the null hypothesis. It is important to note here that the quantification of plausibility corresponds to the desired level of confidence. If more confidence is required for the estimate of q, the result will be a wider interval estimate and, thus, a wider range of plausible values than would result from requiring less confidence. This statement is simply a different form of expressing the notion stated in Section 7.7.2 that two-sided 99% CIs placed around a point estimate are always wider than 95% CIs.

Once a CI has been placed around a point estimate, it is possible to make a statement as to whether or not there is a statistically significantly greater occurrence of events in the drug treatment group than in the placebo drug treatment group. Consider a scenario in which the relative risk point estimate is 1.50, and we have calculated a two-sided 95% CI around this point estimate. By definition, the upper limit of the CI will be greater than 1.50, and this interval is not of immediate concern when determining whether or not a statement of a statistically significant difference in risk can be made. The key determining point here is the location of the lower limit of the CI. If the lower limit is greater than 1.00, i.e., the range of values within the CI excludes unity, it is possible to state that the risk of the event is statistically significantly more likely to occur in the drug treatment group than in the placebo treatment group. The reason for this is that the lowest plausible value of the population relative risk, represented by the lower limit of the CI, is greater than the value (unity) that represents equally likely probabilities in the two groups.

Interpreting the two-sided 95% CI as a hypothesis test, one would conclude that there is a 5% chance that the population relative risk is really equal to 1.00. Therefore, one can conclude that the difference in the two proportions, expressed as a ratio (relative risk), is statistically significantly different from 1.00 at the $\alpha = 0.05$ level. In addition, there is a 2.5% chance that the population relative risk is less than the value represented by the lower limit and a 2.5% chance that the population relative risk is greater than the value of the upper limit of the CI.

The same logic holds true when a 99% CI is calculated around a relative risk point estimate. In this case, if the lower limit is greater than 1.00, it is possible to state at the $\alpha = 0.01$ level that the risk of the event is statistically significantly different from 1.00. Further, there is only a 0.5% chance that the true relative risk is less than the lower limit of the interval and only a 0.5% chance that the true relative risk is more than the upper limit of the interval. Since a 99% CI will be wider than a 95% CI it is possible that the difference in two proportions may be considered statistically significant at the $\alpha = 0.05$ level but not at the more conservative (i.e., more certain) $\alpha = 0.01$ level.

8.6.9 Interpretation and Use of Confidence Intervals by Prescribing Physicians

There are five possible scenarios when calculating CIs around a relative risk point estimate of interest, as listed shortly. It is reasonable to presume that the number of certain adverse events used to calculate the estimated relative risk is likely to be greater in the drug treatment group than in the placebo treatment group, which means that it is likely that the relative risk point estimate will lie above 1.00. Therefore, scenarios 4 and 5 are arguably the most likely of the five scenarios to occur. Nonetheless, we will consider the implications and reasonable interpretations of each of them. The scenarios are:

1. The point estimate lies below 1.00, and so do the lower limit of the CI and the upper limit of the CI.
2. The point estimate and the lower limit of the CI lie below 1.00, while the upper limit of the CI lies above 1.00.
3. The point estimate is precisely 1.00. As already noted, this scenario is not likely. The placement of the confidence intervals is not of importance here, although any variation in the data that led to identical proportions in the two treatment groups will ensure that the lower limit will lie below 1.00 and the upper limit above 1.00.
4. The lower limit of the CI lies below 1.00, while the point estimate and the upper limit of the CI lie above 1.00.
5. The point estimate lies above 1.00, and so do the lower limit of the CI and the upper limit of the CI.

Scenario 1 leads to the interpretation that there is statistically significant evidence that treatment with the drug will likely lead to less adverse drug reactions than not using it, i.e., the drug is not only safe, it is super-safe. This relative risk may not be likely, but if it should occur, it presents no cause for concern on the part of the prescribing physician and his or her patient. Scenarios 2, 3, and 4 all represent outcomes that lead to the statement that there is no statistically significant evidence that treatment with the drug will lead to more adverse drug reactions than not using it. The interpretation of these relative risks would likely be that the drug was acceptably safe to be prescribed.

The outcome in scenario 5, however, leads to a different interpretation. In this case, there is statistically significant evidence that treatment with the drug will likely lead to more adverse drug reactions than not using it. Put another way, there is statistically significant evidence that treatment with the drug will likely increase a patient's risk of experiencing the event. This outcome does indeed represent a cause for concern for the physician and patient.

We can now use the data in Table 8.2 to place CIs around the relative risk point estimate of 3.04 calculated in Section 8.6.7 for the adverse event of dizziness. The lower and upper limits of the two-sided 95% CI are 1.55 and 5.95 (as mentioned, the actual method of calculation need not be presented here). These CIs would typically be presented along with the point estimate as follows:

$$\text{Relative risk of dizziness (95\% CI)} = 3.04 \ (1.55, 5.95)$$

The interpretation of this expression is as follows: We are 95% confident that the interval (1.55, 5.95) encloses the true but unknown population relative risk of experiencing dizziness. Our best estimate is 3.04, i.e., the point estimate.

This example has illustrated how data that were collected during a preapproval clinical trial and subsequently presented in the drug's labeling can be used to estimate the (true but unknown) relative risk for a patient experiencing a particular adverse drug reaction if prescribed the drug. In many instances, communicating the risk of a patient experiencing an event ("AE of special interest" in Table 8.2) to a patient and his or her prescribing physician is done most clearly with an absolute measure, e.g., 5% of participants in the clinical trial's drug treatment group experienced the event, in conjunction with a relative measure, e.g., the relative risk of experiencing the event was 4.80, with a 95% CI of (1.09, 21.20). (The distance between the point estimate and upper bound is a result of using the logarithmic scale in the calculation of the CI, as noted in Section 8.6.8.)

8.6.10   The Odds Ratio

Another measure of association encountered in medical research and clinical communications is the odds ratio. The odds of an event is defined as the probability of the event occurring divided by the probability of the event not occurring, as shown in Formula 8.5:

$$\text{Odds} = \frac{\text{Probability of event A}}{1\text{- Probability of event A}} \tag{8.5}$$

The odds for a particular adverse event occurring in the drug treatment group can be defined as shown in formula 8.6:

$$\text{Odds of AE in the drug treatment group} =$$

$$\frac{\text{Probability of adverse event in drug treatment group}}{1\text{- Probability of adverse event in drug treatment group}} \tag{8.6}$$

Similarly, the odds for a particular adverse event occurring in the placebo treatment group can be defined as shown in Formula 8.7:

$$\text{Odds of AE in the placebo treatment group} = \qquad (8.7)$$

Probability of adverse event in placebo treatment group
1 – Probability of adverse event in placebo treatment group

The ratio of the two quantities shown in Formulae 8.6 and 8.7 is called the odds ratio (OR), calculated as shown in Formula 8.8:

$$\text{Odds ratio of AE} = \qquad (8.8)$$

(Prob. of adverse event in drug treatment group)(1 - prob. of adverse event in placebo group)
(1 – prob. of adverse event in drug treatment group)(prob. of adverse event in placebo group)

The odds ratio is an estimate of the relative risk defined in Formula 8.4. When the odds ratio is calculated in this manner, there are three possible interpretations of interest:

➢ An odds ratio of less than 1.00 indicates greater odds of the adverse event in the placebo group than in the drug treatment group.
➢ An odds ratio of 1.00 (unity) indicates that the odds of the adverse event are equal between the two groups.
➢ An odds ratio of greater than 1.00 indicates greater odds of the adverse event in the drug treatment group than in the placebo group.

Three other points to note about the odds ratio are as follows:

➢ As with the relative risk, an estimate of the odds ratio can be obtained by using the sample proportions of participants with the adverse event of interest.
➢ A $100(1 - \alpha)\%$ CI can be constructed about the odds ratio point estimate.
➢ The odds ratio and relative risk can be in close agreement, but only when the probability in one or both groups is low (e.g., less than 0.10).

Odds ratios are encountered in many areas of medical research because they can be estimated from logistic regression models which are intended to describe how the probability of a dichotomous outcome is related to one or more explanatory variables (e.g., age, sex, and treatment). Odds ratios are often used in meta-analyses, which are discussed in the following chapter.

8.6.11   Describing the Risk of Adverse Events Using Time-to-Event Analysis

Calculation of the relative risk of experiencing an adverse event, as expressed by a point estimate and its associated CIs, is one example of how inferential statistics can be used in the analysis of safety data. This section discusses an additional example, time-to-event analysis. The fundamental premise of time-to-event analysis is that it is informative to know when events happened as well as simply knowing that they did happen.

Consider a trial involving a 12-week treatment period in which the numbers of headaches (adverse events) were very similar in the drug treatment group and the placebo treatment group. Consider also a physician's interpretation of these data as presented in the drug's labeling. Based on the type of analysis considered so far in this chapter, if the data presented in the labeling indicated that the number and percentage of participants in the drug treatment group and the placebo group were relatively similar, the physician might reasonably conclude that a patient would not experience more headaches if prescribed the drug than if not prescribed the drug. However, how might that interpretation change if the physician also had access to the temporal patterning of headaches in the drug and placebo treatment groups? One scenario is that temporal patterning might be similar in both groups, with the headaches occurring relatively evenly throughout the trial. Another scenario is that the headaches reported by participants in the placebo treatment group occurred relatively evenly throughout the trial, but a large proportion of the headaches reported by participants in the drug treatment group occurred in the first three weeks of the trial, with the remaining headaches being relatively evenly distributed across the remaining nine weeks. It is possible that the physician's interpretation of the data in these two hypothetical scenarios may differ: in the second case, the physician might reasonably conclude that a patient prescribed the drug might experience more headaches than usual in the first few weeks of treatment. If the physician did come to this conclusion, he or she would share this information with the patient.

The number of events (adverse events or serious adverse events) occurring in a trial can be termed the rate of events: sometimes the term crude rate or incidence is used. As we have just seen, simply comparing the rates of events across two treatment groups does not tell the whole story, since this strategy does not address the potential temporal relationship between exposure to the study treatment and the adverse event of interest. Additionally, there are other relevant considerations here. First, a participant may withdraw from the trial before completion of the treatment period. Using our previous example of a 12-week trial, imagine that one participant withdrew at the end of Week 4 and that he or she had not reported a particular adverse event by the time of withdrawal. This participant was at risk of experiencing the adverse event only during the time of his or her participation: it is possible that, if withdrawal had not occurred, this participant would have reported the adverse event at some point during the subsequent eight weeks of the treatment period. Second, a sponsor may (legitimately) combine adverse event data from several clinical trials into one dataset in order to use all available data to provide as much information as possible from all trials conducted during the clinical development program. In this scenario, it is possible that different trials may have incorporated treatment periods of different lengths, and simply analyzing rates would not take this into account.

A more informative approach is to take into account the time of the event relative to the start of treatment, use the data from all participants, and account for varying lengths of time at risk for experiencing the event. O'Neill (1987) advocated such an approach, especially for serious adverse events, due to the shortcomings of simply describing the crude rate, or incidence, of the event. He commented as follows (p. 20):

> For drugs used for chronic exposure, one number or rate such as the crude rate is not likely to be informative without reference to time. To be useful as a summary measure of combined safety data from several studies and which would estimate an overall rate that describes experiences of all participants exposed for varying time periods, there is a need to stratify for time as well as other factors.

At the time of this writing, the results from this type of analysis are not typically provided in drug labeling. Therefore, they cannot help a prescribing physician reach informed treatment decisions unless the physician can access such information from additional sources. There are two possible sources of such information. First, sponsors may provide the information to regulatory agencies in support of their assertion that the investigational drug is acceptably safe. If the drug is approved, the regulatory agency may make this information public on its web site (this is current FDA practice). Second, sponsors may publish such information in clinical communications.

Accessing information from either of these sources raises another issue of relevance in clinical practice. The information provided in these sources may be presented in a more complex and idiosyncratic format than the fairly standardized format currently used in drug labeling. This places the onus for appropriate interpretation squarely on the physician. Therefore, a working knowledge and understanding of Statistics is vital for the physician, certainly at a conceptual level. As Campbell et al. (1999) noted:

> Statistics is not only a discipline in its own right but it is also a fundamental tool for investigation in all biological and medical science. As such, any serious investigator in these fields must have a grasp of the basic principles. With modern computers there is little need for familiarity with the technical details of statistical calculations. However, a physician should understand when such calculations are valid, when they are not, and how they should be interpreted.

The analysis method attributed to Kaplan and Meier (1958) enables us to analyze the time to the first reported adverse event while accounting for different lengths of time at risk for participants. (Note the phrase first reported in the previous sentence: it is possible that a participant may report several occurrences of an event, but interest here lies with the first occurrence. Analyzing multiple occurrences is another interesting challenge but is beyond the scope of the present discussions.) Readers are referred to Durham and Turner (2008) for an introductory discussion of the Kaplan-Meier analysis in the context of adverse event data.

It should be noted here that the Kaplan-Meier analytical strategy can also be used for analyzing efficacy data. Consider the example of a new drug used in the care of terminal cancer patients. The primary efficacy objective in such a clinical trial might be the median length of time following the commencement of treatment before patients died. While death is typically considered as a serious adverse event (recall the definition in Section 8.6.3), in this form of trial it is unfortunately the case that all patients will die: the question of interest is whether the new drug increases survival time compared with the active control treatment, i.e., the gold standard of treatment at that time. Given the knowledge that patients in both the drug treatment group and the active control group will die during this trial, the question of interest is the survival time while on therapy. If the investigational drug is associated with a statistically significant prolongation of life, i.e., a greater survival time, it may be approved by a regulatory agency.

8.7   ISSUES OF MULTIPLICITY

Given the large number of adverse events and other safety parameters evaluated in therapeutic exploratory and confirmatory trials, analysis of all of them (e.g., by calculating a two-sided 95% CI about the relative risk of every adverse event) would involve issues of multiplicity (recall the discussions of multiplicity in Section 7.10). The danger in this scenario is that far too much importance may be given to a result that is simply not representative of the truth.

There are several sophisticated statistical approaches that can be used to address the problem of multiplicity in this context. However, a more simple and useful strategy is to follow the lead of the main analytical strategies used for efficacy parameters in therapeutic exploratory and confirmatory trials. By the time that therapeutic exploratory and confirmatory trials are conducted, researchers ideally should have developed just one or two specific research questions and therefore have just one or two efficacy endpoints of interest. Conducting only one or two analyses reduces the chances of finding a statistically significant result that is not really there by chance alone. That is, adoption of an inferential statistical approach works well for analyzing efficacy data since one or two primary objectives have been declared *a priori*. Therefore, only one or two inferential analyses are conducted, and issues of multiplicity are minimized.

This observation suggests an inferential approach to the analysis of adverse event data in which researchers declare *a priori* one or two potential adverse events for investigation and present the appropriate prespecified hypothesis of interest in the study protocol. Such a hypothesis may be the result of knowledge gained in an earlier trial(s) in the clinical development program or it may relate to an adverse event of special interest.

8.8   REGULATORY CONSIDERATIONS FOR SAFETY DATA

When a manufacturer submits a marketing application to a regulatory agency, the written results of each study are submitted in the form of clinical study reports that describe and summarize the results. In addition, summaries of findings across studies are created, as discussed in the following section. However, the original raw data are also submitted in an electronic format that enables the regulatory body to perform its own statistical analyses of the data collected: the regulators can duplicate analyses that have been reported, and they can also conduct new analyses.

8.8.1   Pooling Adverse Event Data Across Studies for Purposes of Labeling

Estimates of the incidence of adverse events from all clinical studies are provided in licensing applications for a new drug. In the United States a licensing application for a drug is called a New Drug Application (NDA). An NDA will include complete study reports for all clinical studies of the new drug. In addition, all of the relevant safety information will be synthesized in an overview document called an Integrated Summary of Safety (ISS). In the ISS, adverse events are typically presented in a pooled fashion by combining the numerators (participants with a particular adverse event) and denominators (all participants exposed to a particular dose or concentration of the new drug) across a number of studies. Pooled analyses of adverse events require that all adverse events are coded using a common dictionary. The 2005 ICH E14 guidance discussed in the previous chapter stated that ECG changes reported as adverse events should be pooled from all studies. The guidance therefore suggested that the following specific adverse events be compared in participants receiving the investigational drug and the control treatments, since these events can be indicative of potential proarrhythmic effects: TdP, sudden death, ventricular tachycardia, ventricular fibrillation and flutter, syncope, and seizures.

Data from clinical studies can be pooled in a number of ways:

➢ Data from all studies, without regard for duration of exposure (i.e., time at risk), geographic region, population studied, or phase of development (e.g., human pharmacology, therapeutic exploratory, therapeutic confirmatory).

➢ Data from studies with a common duration of exposure. For example, data from all studies with treatment periods of three months or less may be pooled as short-term studies, and data from all studies with treatment periods of more than three months may be pooled as long-term studies. Pooling data in this manner is one way to account for the fact that the probability of experiencing an adverse event (as estimated by the percentage) is a function of the time at risk.

➢ Data from studies according to the phase of development. For example, data from all therapeutic confirmatory studies may be pooled separately from all others. Adverse event data from the therapeutic confirmatory trials may be more representative of the kinds of events that would be expected once a new drug is marketed. Participants are more similar within phases of development than among phases, the most obvious example being healthy participants in early pharmacology studies compared with participants with the disease or condition of interest in therapeutic confirmatory trials.

➢ Data from studies according to geographic region. Medical care can vary significantly from country to country (and also from region to region within countries). This diversity in care can translate into varying background rates of adverse events. These regional differences can be accounted for by pooling data from similar geographic regions.

➢ Data pooled according to some combination of the above factors. It may be most meaningful to pool data only from those studies that are thought to be most homogeneous. The strategy for pooling data for a licensing application is typically discussed with the regulatory agency reviewing the application.

Analyses based on pooled adverse events offer two advantages: increased precision for the treatment effect and the ability to examine specific subgroups of interest (e.g., sex, baseline disease severity). Both of these objectives are of interest to regulatory agencies and, ultimately, to prescribing physicians.

Importantly, an analysis of data pooled using individual observations in this manner is one form of meta-analysis: meta-analysis is discussed further in Chapter 9.

8.8.2   Regulatory Review Approaches to Safety Data

The FDA's view concerning safety reviews is presented in their guidance document on the safety review of new drug applications, *Conducting a Clinical Safety Review of a New Product Application and Preparing a Report on the Review*, which can be accessed at the FDA's web site, www.fda.gov. As this guidance states, most therapeutic exploratory and therapeutic confirmatory trials are carefully designed to establish that a new drug is efficacious while controlling the probability of committing a Type I or a Type II error. In the context of efficacy evaluations, a Type I error occurs when a statistical conclusion is made that the drug had an effect when, in truth, the drug is not efficacious. A Type II error occurs when the statistical conclusion is made that there is insufficient evidence to claim an effect of the drug when, in truth, the drug is efficacious. Unless safety concerns have arisen in earlier stages of the clinical development program, these trials typically do not involve assessments of safety that are as sensitive as those designed for establishing the efficacy of the investigational drug. Quoting from this FDA guidance:

> In the usual case, however, any apparent finding emerges from an assessment of dozens of potential endpoints (adverse events) of interest, making description of the statistical uncertainty of the finding using conventional significance levels very difficult. The approach taken is therefore best described as one of exploration and estimation of event rates, with particular attention to comparing results of individual studies and pooled data. It should be appreciated that exploratory analyses (e.g., subset analyses, to which a great caution is applied in a hypothesis testing setting) are a critical and essential part of a safety evaluation. These analyses can, of course, lead to false conclusions, but need to be carried out nonetheless, with attention to consistency across studies and prior knowledge. The approach typically followed is to screen broadly for adverse events and to expect that this will reveal the common adverse reaction profile of a new drug and will detect some of the less common and more serious adverse reactions associated with drug use.

Safety evaluations of investigational drugs focus primarily on estimating the risk of unwanted events associated with the drug and, more specifically, on the risk of those events relative to what would be expected in the patient population as a whole if the drug were to be approved.

8.8.3 Limitations of Preapproval Safety Data

Summarizing safety data in marketing applications is useful and necessary. However, the safety data collected during preapproval clinical trials have limitations regarding their usefulness once the new drug is marketed:

➤ Study populations involved in preapproval clinical trials are not necessarily similar to the target population of patients who will use the drug once it is available. Compared to patients, participants in clinical trials (even therapeutic confirmatory studies) are monitored more closely, are likely to be more compliant with study drug administration, and tend to have fewer concurrent illnesses and use fewer concomitant medications. (These issues are discussed in more detail in Chapter 9.)

➤ The number of participants exposed to a new drug in the entire safety database created from all preapproval clinical trials is too small to detect a potentially important increased risk in rare adverse drug reactions. The 1994 ICH Guidance E1, *The Extent of Population Exposure to Assess Clinical Safety for Drugs Intended for Long-term Treatment of Non-life-threatening Conditions*, recommends 1,500 individuals as the minimum number of individuals who should be exposed to a new investigational drug. However, consideration of the sample size needed to detect a significant difference at the $\alpha = 0.05$ level in adverse event rates with power of 80% (widely regarded as the lowest reasonable power for a clinical trial) reveals that this minimal sample size is clearly inadequate to detect rare but important safety risks that truly exist. If greater power (sometimes 90%) is desired, even larger sample sizes would be required.

Some illustrative data are provided in Table 8.3. This table displays various background rates of an event, ranging from the relatively low rate of 0.0001, i.e., 1 in 10,000, to a much higher rate of 0.30, i.e., 30 in 100. These background rates can be thought of as the proportion of placebo participants experiencing an adverse event. These rates can also be considered as the rates of adverse reactions in patients with the disease who do not take the new drug (assuming that the clinical trial participants come from populations similar to those of the patients likely to be treated with the approved drug: as discussed further in Chapter 9, this assumption is tenuous). The sample sizes per group required to detect (with power = 80%) a difference in rates (drug treatment group vs. placebo or active control) consistent with relative risks of 1.25, 2.00, and 3.00 are displayed for each background rate.

TABLE 8.3. Sample Size Required to Detect a Difference in Rates of Adverse Events

Background Rate	Sample Size per Group Required (80% Power) to Detect Effect for Each Relative Risk (RR)		
	RR = 1.25	RR = 2.00	RR=3.00
0.0001	2,825,271	235,430	78,472
0.0010	282,240	23,511	7,832
0.0100	27,937	2,319	769
0.0500	5,333	435	141
0.1000	2,507	199	62
0.2000	1,094	82	23
0.3000	623	42	10

Consider a serious adverse event that occurs with a probability of 0.001 (0.1%) among clinical trials participants with the disease or condition of interest. Based on the magnitude of the rate, this event could well reflect TdP: Shah (2005a, p. 260) reported that "the frequency of TdP with noncardiac drugs is largely unknown but it is typically well below 0.1% of the patients receiving such a drug." If the true relative risk of the adverse event is 2.00, i.e., the adverse event is twice as likely to occur in participants taking the new drug compared with placebo, a sample size of 23,511 per group would be required to detect a statistically significant difference in the two rates. This sample size is clearly much larger than the minimum number of exposures cited in ICH E1. The inadequacy of the preapproval sample size is magnified when considering rarer events or relative risks less than 2.00 that nonetheless may be of great concern.

The importance of these results can best be illustrated with a simple example. Imagine that the new drug is approved for marketing and the true background rate remains 0.001 (0.1%) in the target population of patients with the disease or condition of interest. If 100,000 patients take the new drug in the first five years following marketing approval (with the relative risk of 2.00 applying to the target population), introduction of the new drug would be expected to result in 100 more serious adverse reactions than would have been reported without the new drug. The reason for this is that the background rate among those not taking the new drug (0.001, or 0.1%) applied to 100,000 patients is 100 serious adverse drug reactions. Since the true relative risk is 2.00, we would expect 200 serious adverse drug reactions from 100,000 patients taking the new drug, which would result in an excess of 100 cases.

In reality, we will never know the true relative risk, but this example illustrates the limitations of the amount of data acquired in preapproval clinical trials. If the study population differs in important ways from the target patient population, especially ways that increase the risk of an adverse event (e.g., comorbid disease, use of concomitant drugs), it is likely that preapproval trials would poorly estimate the risk that applies to patients who will use the new drug.

8.9 THE CONTRAST WITH REGULATORY GUIDANCE CONCERNING PROARRHYTHMIC CARDIAC SAFETY

While this chapter has adopted a relatively broad strategy in discussing adverse events, it is appropriate to return to the specific topic of generalized cardiac safety in this section, and to highlight a difference in regulatory guidance as it applies to preapproval proarrhythmic cardiac safety investigations and to preapproval generalized cardiac safety investigations. As we saw in Chapters 6 and 7, there is internationally accepted regulatory guidance in the domain of proarrhythmic cardiac safety at both the nonclinical and preapproval clinical levels (ICH S7B and ICH E14, respectively). This is not the case for generalized cardiac safety. While very reasonable assumptions concerning safety risks can probably be made for noncardiac investigational drugs that have sizable impacts on cardiac and cardiovascular parameters in preapproval clinical trials, both sponsor and regulatory judgments and decisions regarding these occurrences must be made in a more subjective manner that changes in the QT/QTc interval, as discussed in the previous chapter: Whatever the degree of help provided by ICH E14, it does at least provide a "line in the sand" to assist decision making. To our knowledge, there are no analogous thresholds of regulatory concern for individual members of the overall lipid profile, blood pressure, or other parameters that are known to be (or may be reasonably suspected to be) associated with the long-term development of cardiovascular and cardiac disease, and there is no direct equivalent of the TQT study for such parameters.

This situation may contribute to the observation that generalized cardiac safety concerns arise more frequently in the postmarketing than the premarketing domain. The use of the biomarker QT/QTc prolongation has received specific regulatory attention, the current consequences of which are that drugs are either denied marketing approval or are tagged upon approval as having torsadogenic liability, thus (ideally) alerting physicians and potential patients to take this information into account when making benefit-risk balance assessments in clinical settings. In apparent contrast, it seems that generalized cardiac safety concerns currently arise more from observations and analyses of clinical endpoints, such as fatal and nonfatal myocardial infarctions: examples of such postmarketing investigations are discussed in Chapter 12.

8.10   AUTHORS' PERSPECTIVES

Consider a scenario in which an investigational drug is associated with a statistically significant prolongation of survival, but it is also associated with a fairly brutal side effect profile. A regulatory agency may approve the drug for marketing despite its side effect profile (its risk profile) since its therapeutic benefit (its benefit profile) is clear in statistical terms. This is a very reasonable decision on the part of the regulatory agency, since many patients may be willing to endure considerable side effects in order to extend their life and this drug is therefore a good option for them. However, other patients may decide that, in spite of the statistically significant evidence of the likelihood of extending their life for a certain amount of time, they would rather share a shorter period of time with their loved ones in relative comfort than a somewhat longer period of time in considerable discomfort.

As noted in the preface, while we have kept the vast majority of the text factual, we feel that it is appropriate to share our perspectives on occasion as long as we make it clear that we are doing so. This is one of those occasions. First, since no drug is immune from the possibility of side effects, regulatory agencies can legitimately approve drugs that have such side effects if there are also therapeutic benefits. The fundamental question a regulatory agency must address is one of benefit-risk estimation at the level of public health. That is, if the benefits to the entire population of patients likely to be prescribed the drug outweigh the risk to the entire population, approval of the drug is reasonable on one condition, i.e., full disclosure of information concerning both potential benefits and potential risks to prescribing physicians and potential patients. It is not the job of the regulatory agency to make therapeutic treatment decisions at the level of the individual patient: that is the job of the physician in consultation with his or her patient.

Second, physicians must take responsibility for remaining well informed about the benefits and risks of all drugs that they may potentially prescribe (given that this information has been made available to them by regulatory agencies). While regulatory agencies have the responsibility for full disclosure of this information (either directly from the agency or by telling the sponsor to make this information available and checking that they do so), physicians have the responsibility of becoming familiar with this information.

Third, physicians should engage in discussions about the benefits and risks of any therapeutic option with patients on an individual level (unless the patient clearly and rationally does not want to know, preferring the physician to do as he or she considers best). A benefit-risk assessment must be made each time a physician prescribes a drug to a patient, and any risks must be acceptable in relation to the likely benefits. While the phrase acceptable risk elicits a strong emotional response, deciding to take acceptable risks is actually part of our everyday lives. Everyone who travels in a motor car is exposed to the risk of an injury or worse on the journey and, consciously or unconsciously, deems the benefit of getting to the desired destination worth taking the risks involved in traveling there. Taking prescription medication also exposes us to risks and benefits, and it is preferable if these are considered explicitly and judiciously in conversation with a physician before beginning a treatment regimen. The acceptability of the risk of a particular side effect or adverse drug reaction depends on the benefit of that drug to an individual patient. The level of acceptable risk (i.e., an acceptably low probability) of experiencing a particular adverse drug reaction generally increases as the probability of benefit and/or the degree of benefit to the patient increases.

Fourth, patients have the final say in whether or not they would like to start a particular treatment regimen. Regulatory agencies should make all reasonable treatment options available along with all available information concerning benefits and risks, and physicians should recommend and discuss appropriate treatment options with their patients on an individual basis, but the sanctity of the patient's informed decision must be respected.

Lastly, sponsors should make every attempt to work with regulators to update information regarding the benefits and risks of drugs in a timely manner throughout a drug's lifecycle. Timely reporting of data obtained from clinical trials involves scientific, regulatory, and ethical considerations. Participants take part in clinical trials for the greater good. In return, sponsors have an obligation to allow individuals access to the most up-to-date information regarding a drug. When discussing the publication of the results from clinical trials in medical journals, Piantadosi (2005, p. 479) commented as follows:

> Reporting the results of a clinical trial is one of the most important aspects of clinical research. Investigators have an obligation to each other, the study participants, and the scientific community to disseminate results in a competent and timely manner.

While Piantadosi's comments are still absolutely true, there are additional means of communicating information about clinical trials to the general public, including government-sponsored web sites such as www.clinicaltrials.gov. When accessed on March 10, 2008, the site contained information on 52,510 trials with locations in 154 countries. There are also web sites maintained by individual sponsors. For example, GlaxoSmithKline's Clinical Trial Register can be accessed at http://ctr.gsk.co.uk/welcome.asp. Other means of communicating information to both physicians and the general public (i.e., potential patients) can also play important roles (see the discussion of the FDA's new Risk Communication Advisory Committee in Section 14.10.7). Hopefully, regulators and sponsors will continue to work diligently to create more and more such venues.

8.11   FURTHER READING

Dieterie, F., Marrer, E., Suzuki, E., et al., 2008, Monitoring kidney safety in drug development: Emerging technologies and their implications, *Current Opinion in Drug Discovery and Development*, 11:60–71.

Durham, T.A. and Turner, J.R., 2008, *Introduction to statistics in pharmaceutical clinical trials*, London: Pharmaceutical Press. See Chapter 7, *Early-phase clinical trials*, Chapter 8, *Confirmatory clinical trials: Safety data I*; and Chapter 9, *Confirmatory clinical trials: Safety data II*.

Lagakos, S.W., 2006, Time-to-event analyses for long-term treatments: The APPROVe trial, *New England Journal of Medicine*, 355:113–117.

Senn, S., 2007, *Statistical issues in drug development*, 2nd edition, Chichester, UK: John Wiley & Sons. See Chapter 23, *Safety data, harms, drug monitoring, and pharmaco-epidemiology*.

van der Laan, J.W., 2006, Safety assessment of pharmaceuticals: Regulatory aspects. In Mulder, G.J. and Dencker, L. (Eds.), *Pharmaceutical toxicology*. London: Pharmaceutical Press.

9

THERAPEUTIC USE TRIALS AND META-ANALYSES

9.1 INTRODUCTION

We have now discussed cardiac safety considerations during drug design, nonclinical development, and preapproval clinical development, the first three of four phases of lifecycle drug development introduced at the beginning of the book. At the start of our discussions of nonclinical safety assessments in Chapter 6 we acknowledged that, while the *in silico* strategies used in drug design are informative, they do have limitations. In a similar manner, at the start of our discussions of preapproval studies in Chapter 7 we acknowledged the limitations of nonclinical data. Following the same pattern, the limitations of preapproval clinical trials are discussed at the beginning of this chapter before we focus on postapproval investigations of a drug's safety.

This practice of acknowledging the limitations of respective phases in lifecycle drug development methodology before commencing discussions of the next phase is done in a positive rather than a negative spirit. Acknowledging the limitations of the respective investigational strategies does not negate their usefulness: it simply lays the groundwork for the discussion of how additional and complementary knowledge will be useful. Preapproval clinical trials are essential to the process of new drug development, providing the information concerning an investigational drug's safety and efficacy that forms the rational basis for regulatory decisions concerning marketing approval. It is simply important to realize their limitations as well as appreciating the very important information that they do provide: as Katz (2001, p. xi) noted, "to work skillfully with evidence is to acknowledge its limits." It is important not to completely discount the results from preapproval clinical trials at this point: postmarketing data add to and complement the information gained in preapproval trials (see Faich and Stemhagen, 2005).

Once a drug has been approved, the evaluation of its safety should continue throughout the entire time that the drug is on the market. Just because a drug has been found to be safe for several years does not mean that a safety issue(s) will not be identified in the future, perhaps when the drug is prescribed to other populations or when more precise assays become available: the observation that "it's been around forever without causing any problems" must not be allowed to be a cause for complacency. Additionally, as we noted earlier in the content of preapproval clinical trials, a drug's efficacy must also be assessed since its safety can only be meaningfully assessed in relation to its therapeutic benefit in the form of a benefit-risk balance assessment. In the postmarketing arena, the term effectiveness is used in relation to a drug's therapeutic benefit.

Integrated Cardiac Safety: Assessment Methodologies for Noncardiac Drugs in Discovery, Development, and Postmarketing Surveillance. By J. Rick Turner and Todd A. Durham
Copyright © 2009 John Wiley & Sons, Inc.

This chapter discusses two strategies for assessing postmarketing safety (additional strategies are addressed in the following chapter). One strategy involves conducting therapeutic use trials. One form of such postapproval clinical trials involves relatively small numbers of participants who represent populations that were not represented in the drug's preapproval clinical trials. A second form of therapeutic use trials involves many more participants than took part in preapproval clinical trials: the greater number of participants in these trials permits more safety information to be collected and also more information regarding the drug's therapeutic benefit.

The second strategy addressed in this chapter is the statistical technique of meta-analysis, an approach that combines data from several trials to provide a larger participant sample than took part in any one of the individual trials incorporated in the analysis. Meta-analysis has assumed a high-profile status in assessments of drug safety, and this strategy is therefore discussed in some detail.

9.2   NOMENCLATURE CONSIDERATIONS

As in the preapproval arena, an attempt to reconcile different terminologies that appear in the literature in the postapproval domain may be useful. Additionally, in this section we clarify what we mean by the use of certain terms.

9.2.1   Adverse Events and Adverse Drug Reactions

In preapproval clinical trials, which are typically double-blinded (neither the participant nor the investigator knows which treatment the participant is receiving in the trial), events of concern from a safety perspective are recorded as adverse events, the nomenclature used in Chapter 8. At the time that they are recorded, the investigator cannot know that an adverse event is actually due to the investigational drug since, by definition in a double-blinded trial, neither the investigator nor the participant knows which drug treatment, i.e., the investigational drug or the control treatment, a participant is receiving. In contrast, in the postmarketing arena, it is known that a patient reporting an adverse outcome is taking the drug of interest. Therefore, the term adverse drug reaction is typically used here.

9.2.2   Therapeutic Use Trials, Surveillance Studies, Phase IV Studies: What's in a Name?

Table 1.1 (see Section 1.2.3) provided the nomenclature used in the ICH classification of clinical trials, a classification system that we have adopted throughout the book. In this system the term therapeutic use trial is used, for example, for comparative effectiveness studies, studies of mortality/morbidity outcomes, studies of additional endpoints, and large simple trials. If one were using the more traditional phase terminology, these investigations would be regarded as Phase IV studies. However, as Glasser et al. (2007) observed, defining exactly what studies can be referred to as a Phase IV study is complex. These authors commented as follows (Glasser et al., 2007, p. 1074):

> In the past, postmarketing research, postmarketing surveillance, and pharmacovigilance were synonymous with phase IV studies because the main activities of the regulatory agency (e.g., FDA) were focused on the monitoring of adverse drug events and inspections of drug manufacturing facilities and products. However, not all FDA-mandated (classical phase IV trials) research consists of randomized controlled trials (RCTs), and not all postmarketing activities are limited to safety issues (pharmacovigilance), so these terms required clarification.

Glasser et al. (2007) proceeded to discuss various nomenclatures for postmarketing study designs, including:

> - FDA-mandated or negotiated studies. Examples given included studies of drug-drug interactions and drug responses in special populations (e.g., pediatric and elderly populations).
> - Non-FDA-mandated or negotiated studies. There are two categories of study designs:
>   - Randomized controlled trials. Examples given included equivalence and noninferiority trials (e.g., see Durham and Turner, 2008, pp. 187–189) and large simple trials, discussed in Section 9.4.1.
>   - Surveillance studies. Examples given included pharmacovigilance, effectiveness, drug utilization, and observational epidemiology studies.

As will be seen in the following chapter, however, the terminology described in Glasser et al.'s paper is not universally adopted. Accordingly, the precise terminology used when describing a postmarketing study design and presenting its results is likely less important than an accompanying unambiguous statement of the intent of the study and the methodology used. Such studies can be experimental or nonexperimental in nature (these terms are discussed in Section 10.2), and both types of study provide valuable information about the safety and effectiveness of drugs that are approved and used by patients.

9.3   LIMITATIONS OF PREAPPROVAL CLINICAL TRIALS

Olsson and Meyboom (2006, p. 229) made the following observation about preapproval clinical trials:

The randomized controlled clinical trial is the method of choice for the objective and quantitative demonstration of the efficacy and tolerability of a new medicine. None the less, such studies have limitations in discovering possible adverse events that may occur, in particular those that are rare or develop after prolonged use, in combination with other drugs, or perhaps due to unidentified risk factors. Clinical trials are inherently limited in duration and number of patients, and, significantly, patients are selected prior to inclusion. In other words, the conditions of a trial are artificial compared with the real-life use after the introduction of a medicine.

Even the best-designed and best-conducted preapproval clinical trials are limited in their ability to provide information that truly represents the safety and effectiveness of the drug once it has been widely prescribed and is being taken by many more individuals than participated in the preapproval clinical trials. There are various reasons for this, including:

➤ The inclusion and exclusion criteria that are used in preapproval clinical trials can be extensive, meaning that these clinical trials typically employ relatively homogeneous participant samples. For example, potential participants who have other illnesses or medical conditions, including renal and hepatic impairment, are typically excluded. The age range of participants can be fairly limited, and potential participants who are taking certain concomitant medications are likely to be excluded from the trial.

➤ Participants in preapproval trials are relatively more compliant than patients who may use the drug: they are included in the trial because they are thought to be able to comply with all study procedures, including taking the study drug and attending all scheduled clinic visits.

➤ Preapproval trials typically contain relatively small numbers of participants. While the 3,000–5,000 subjects employed in a therapeutic confirmatory trial may seem large relative to the couple of hundred participants who were employed in earlier human pharmacology studies, this is still a small number compared with the number of patients who may take the drug if and when it is approved. Also, if participants were randomized in the typical 1:1 manner to the drug treatment group and the control treatment group, only half of the participants in therapeutic confirmatory trials would have received the investigational drug.

➤ In real-life situations, drugs are typically not taken by patients in the (relatively) tightly controlled manner in which the investigational drug is administered in preapproval clinical trials.

➤ Preapproval clinical trials often use surrogate endpoints. Examples include measurements of blood pressure when the ultimate goal of a new antihypertensive is reduction of stroke and myocardial infarction and the use of T4 lymphocyte counts in lieu of survival in AIDS. During the relatively short duration of many preapproval trials, it is typically easier to collect data on these parameters since the actual clinical endpoints of interest (e.g., myocardial infarction and death) may not be seen. The use of surrogate endpoints may be acceptable when there are few if any treatment options for potentially serious conditions or when not much is understood about a disease process. The use of surrogate endpoints, however, raises its own issues.

➢ Patients may take a new drug for much longer periods of time than the treatment periods in preapproval clinical trials, especially in the case of chronic diseases. The long-term safety of a drug that is suitable for chronic administration is therefore not known at the time that the drug is approved.

Despite appearing in this list of limitations, the first one actually has a sound scientific basis. Participant homogeneity provides a relatively good opportunity to evaluate the true biological efficacy of the drug since the results are insulated to some degree from extraneous influences. However, at the same time, this scientific strength of preapproval trials is also one of their major limitations from both efficacy and safety perspectives: the lack of heterogeneity makes it difficult to generalize (extrapolate) the trial's results to patients who may be prescribed the approved drug: As Katz (2001, p. xi) noted, "If our patient is older than, younger than, sicker than, healthier than, ethnically different from, taller, shorter, simply different from the subjects of a study, do the results pertain?" This is one of the main reasons that therapeutic use trials involving more heterogeneous participants are conducted.

The third reason listed has particular implications from a safety perspective. The limited sample size of even the largest preapproval clinical trials means that there is a (very) low probability of observing rare adverse events. The rule of threes (e.g., see Strom, 2005a, p. 35) is instructive here. In these preapproval trials the sample size that would be needed to be 95% confident that a single case of an identified adverse event of interest would be seen is roughly three times the reciprocal of the frequency of the event in the general population. That is, for an event that occurs in 1/1,000 individuals, a sample size of around 3,000 subjects would be needed to be 95% confident of observing at least one adverse event. Based on this rule, the sample sizes that would be needed to observe at least one adverse event in a preapproval clinical trial when the frequency of the event is 1/10,000 or less (i.e., sample sizes on the order of 30,000 or greater) would be much larger than is feasible. Expressed the other way, it is very unlikely that adverse events with low frequencies of occurrence will be observed during these trials. As described in Chapter 8, the ability to detect an important safety signal (i.e., a treatment effect consistent with a relative risk of as great as 2.00) for a fairly common adverse effect is even greater than the sample sizes needed to detect a rare event. Rare side effects are probabilistically much more likely to surface once the drug is widely used by hundreds of thousands of patients. Unfortunately, some of these rare side effects may be extremely serious and can be fatal.

The fourth reason listed highlights another paradox in the clinical development arena. The desirable nature of tightly controlled preapproval clinical trials, while necessary and informative in indicating the true biological efficacy of the drug, limits the generalizability of any therapeutic benefit seen. Participants in preapproval trials are expected (actually recruited) to be compliant, i.e., to receive the study treatments as scheduled in the study protocol: potential participants who do not have the physical or mental faculties to comply with the protocol procedures are not typically enrolled. However, patients taking drugs prescribed by their physicians typically do not take their medications in as controlled a manner as was evident in the preapproval trials (the topic of adherence to prescribed drug regimens is discussed in Chapter 13). Therefore, a clinically important biological effect that was observed in well-controlled preapproval clinical trials may not be reflected in the drug's widespread therapeutic profile. Faich and Stemhagen (2005, p. 231) expressed this notion as follows: preapproval clinical trials study a drug under ideal circumstances and are concerned with answering the question "Can it work?" while postmarketing investigations are interested in answering the question "Does it work?" Effectiveness trials—sometimes called large-scale trials, mega trials, large simple trials, or public health trials—typically employ simple methods of assessment and data capture while collecting data from a large number of patients from heterogeneous populations.

The fifth reason in our list addresses the issue of the employment of surrogate endpoints. During relatively short-term preapproval trials, the biological activity (therapeutic benefit) of the investigational drug is often evaluated via surrogate endpoints rather than clinical endpoints. Machin and Campbell (2005) defined a surrogate endpoint as a biomarker, or any indicator, that is intended to substitute for clinical endpoints and to predict their behavior. While the use of surrogate endpoints can be valuable in this context, certain considerations are important. First, an appropriate surrogate must be chosen. Biological plausibility is an important aspect of a surrogate endpoint's appropriateness: there should be evidence that the surrogate endpoint is on the causal pathway to the clinical endpoint of interest. Detailed knowledge and understanding of the pathophysiology of the disease or condition of interest and of the drug's mechanism of action are beneficial in this context. Additionally, it is important that the surrogate endpoint predicts the clinical endpoint consistently and independently (Oliver and Webb, 2003). Some surrogate endpoints are well established, e.g., high blood pressure is a well-established cardiovascular surrogate endpoint (e.g., see Kannel and Sorlie, 1975, for discussion of results from the Framingham Heart Study), but this degree of confidence is not always evident for other biomarkers of potential interest. Biomarkers are discussed further in Section 14.17.

The sixth reason listed, i.e., that patients may take a new drug for a chronic condition for much longer periods of time than the treatment periods in preapproval clinical trials, is simply a consequence of the relatively short length of time for which a preapproval trial is (can be) conducted. The ICH E1 guidance provided recommendations for the minimum number of participants to be exposed in preapproval trials of investigational drugs intended for chronic use: at least 1,500 participants should be exposed to the drug for some period of time, 300–600 participants should be exposed for at least six months, and at least 100 participants should be exposed for at least one year. If all 1,500 participants (the minimum number that should receive any exposure) were all exposed to the investigational drug for one year, the treatment experience would still only be 1,500 patient-years (1,500 participants multiplied by one year of exposure) prior to marketing authorization.

In postmarketing surveillance the concept of patient-years is used to estimate the incidence of an adverse drug reaction, which is defined as the number of new adverse drug reactions divided by the number of patient-years of exposure. Recall that the crude rate or incidence defined in our discussions in Chapter 8 treated the element of time as equal among all participants in a given trial (a tenuous assumption that could be addressed by employing time-to-event analyses). As noted, the ICH E1 guidance provides some idea of the minimal number of participants who are required to be exposed to an investigational drug during a preapproval clinical development program: however, this minimum number of exposures is inadequate to detect rare events or clinically important relative risks for rate events. This limitation of the recommendations in ICH E1 is explicitly identified in the guidance document. As a given drug is on the market for longer and longer periods, more data can be collected concerning its long-term use safety profile.

It is appropriate here to consider the importance of 1,500 patient-years in the context of the preapproval and postmarketing settings. The drug development process is complex and lengthy. As a result, 1,500 participant-years of exposure may take many participants and many calendar years to acquire. However, if just 1,500 patients use a newly marketed drug during the first year of its introduction, the same amount of safety data will be acquired in one year. It is not hard to imagine that a successful new treatment will be prescribed to many more than 1,500 patients in the first year. If so, an amount of safety experience can be acquired in just a few months equal to that acquired over many years during the preapproval clinical program. Extending this line of thinking, it does not take much time for the amount of safety data on a newly marketed drug to comprise the large majority of the total known safety information.

The previous comment addressed the amount of safety data. It is also of relevance to consider the extent to which the quality of safety data may differ from preapproval to postmarketing settings. This issue is discussed later in the chapter.

9.4   THERAPEUTIC USE TRIALS

Therapeutic use trials may be required studies or optional studies. As examples of required studies, a regulatory agency may demand that certain therapeutic use trials be conducted (commenced) immediately after marketing as a requirement of the drug's approval. This may be done to clarify safety and efficacy issues that remained after the therapeutic confirmatory trials reported in the marketing application but that the regulatory agency believed were not sufficient to prevent or delay marketing of the drug. The sponsor may also wish to conduct studies to gain additional information in patient groups not represented in preapproval trials, e.g., elderly patients, patients with compromised liver function, and patients taking additional drugs concurrently. Optional therapeutic trials may be done for specific safety reasons to investigate an adverse drug reaction (or signal, a term that is discussed in the following chapter) that has unexpectedly arisen · during postmarketing surveillance after marketing. Therapeutic use trials differ considerably in design and size and include small open-label trials, classical clinical trials, and massive multicenter comparator trials. Our discussions focus on large simple therapeutic trials.

9.4.1   Large Simple Therapeutic Trials

Piantadosi (2005, p. 124) addressed the rationale for large simple (large-scale) trials, comparing and contrasting their rationale with that for therapeutic confirmatory trials:

> The expense and complexities of clinical trials limit their wide applicability. However, there is a broad need for reliable and unbiased inferences like those that usually result from well-performed randomized comparisons. This tension has led to large-scale trials which test the worth of interventions in large populations without the extensive data collection and other infrastructure needed for many trials.

Large-scale clinical trials conducted following a drug's marketing approval are also referred to as simplified clinical trials, mega trials, practical trials, public health trials, and low-tech trials (see Faich and Stemhagen, 2005). Like preapproval trials, large-scale trials are experimental studies: participants receive random treatment allocation, and observations are made under conditions in which the influence of interest is controlled by the research scientists. However, large-scale trials have several characteristics that distinguish them from preapproval trials. Probably the most immediately noticeable difference when reading publications presenting the results from these trials is the number of participants in them. Large-scale trials employ sample sizes that are much bigger than those employed in preapproval trials (examples of trials employing between 33,000 and almost 60,000 participants are provided in this chapter's Further Reading section). This characteristic can allow the statistically significant identification of relatively small but clinically meaningful effect sizes and thereby provide important information concerning a drug's effectiveness. These trials are also very important in initial postmarketing safety monitoring since many more subjects are exposed to the drug than was the case in preapproval trials, thereby making detection of rare adverse drug reactions more likely.

In order to conduct and complete trials including so many participants, the study protocols are often much simpler than those used in preapproval trials, a characteristic that can lead to one of the terms used to describe these trials, i.e., simplified clinical trials. These trials employ simplified and less restrictive eligibility criteria, which leads to a more heterogeneous participant sample and results that are more representative of the population as a whole. These studies can be regarded as evaluation tools to see whether a drug treatment that is biologically sound (one that can work) will be effective when used outside the realm of preapproval developmental trials (i.e., it will work). These studies have increased external validity due to their large and diverse study samples (Piantadosi, 2005).

The message conveyed by the word simplified in the term simplified trials should be clarified here. The term refers to the fact that the time and procedural demands on both participants and investigators are less than in confirmatory trials: it does not imply that they are simple to design and implement. For example, instead of visiting an investigational site every week throughout a 12-week treatment period in a preapproval trial and having many measurements made at each visit, participants in large-scale trials may visit the site only at the beginning and the end of their participation in the trial and have far fewer measurements taken at each of these two visits. In addition, participants receive treatments in a much more naturalistic setting, one that is much more representative of how patients in general will be treated than the measurement- and attention-intensive environment of preapproval therapeutic exploratory or confirmatory trials.

The design of large-scale trials has its own challenges and complexities. For example, deciding to what extent to relax the tight eligibility criteria and the tight control of drug administration that are hallmarks of preapproval trials is not a simple process, and it can be quite problematic (Piantadosi, 2005). Friedman et al. (1998) noted that the feasibility of large simple trials is contingent upon a relatively easily administered intervention and an outcome that is easily ascertained and commented as follows (Friedman et al., 1998, p. 56):

> If the intervention is complex, requiring either special expertise or effort, particularly where adherence to protocol must be maintained over a long time, this kind of study is less likely to be successful. Similarly, if the response variable is a measure of morbidity that requires careful measurement by highly trained investigators, a large simple trial is not feasible.

The authors noted further that for a large simple trial to be useful, appropriate attention must be paid to data collection and documentation, just as in preapproval clinical trials (Friedman et al., 1998, p. 57):

The investigator also needs to consider that the results of the trial must be persuasive to others. If other researchers or clinicians seriously question the validity of the trial because of inadequate information about participants or inadequate documentation of quality control, then the study has not achieved its purpose....Undoubtedly, many clinical trials are too expensive and cumbersome, especially multicenter ones. The advent of the large, simple trial is an important step in enabling many meaningful medical questions to be addressed in an efficient manner. In other instances, however, the use of large numbers of participants may not compensate for reduced data collection and quality control. As always, the primary question being asked dictates the optimal design of the trial.

Large simple therapeutic trials can be quite useful, then, but like other investigations of a drug throughout its lifecycle, they should have a clear objective and careful planning.

9.5   Introduction to Meta-analysis

Piantadosi (2005, p. 530) observed that "The number of randomized clinical trials probably approaches 10,000 per year." Given the enormous amount of information published in medical journals, it has become very difficult (and arguably impossible) for practicing clinicians to keep fully abreast of the information published by reading every paper of relevance to their particular specialty. Systematic reviews provide a useful complement to individual articles that publish original empirical data by reviewing a collection of articles related to a specific question. Systematic reviews are typically descriptive in nature. As Matthews (2006, p. 212) observed, these reviews "collate, compare, discuss, and summarize the current results in that field." A considerable problem in the creation of such reviews is retrieval of all relevant articles published in the medical literature, although the advent of computerized databases has made this task much less arduous. However, obtaining data that were not included in a publication (a point addressed shortly) and obtaining unpublished manuscripts addressing the question of interest remains challenging.

While narrative reviews can be very useful in their own right, they can also form the first step in a two-step process. The second step involves conducting a meta-analysis. Meta-analysis is a statistical technique that can be used to combine data from many publications (studies) and use these data to conduct a new analysis that was not possible on the basis of any of the individual datasets. The EMEA has published a "Points to Consider" document that addresses the use of meta-analyses (EMEA CPMP, 2001). This guidance document addresses the use of meta-analyses in a preapproval setting (for efficacy or safety), but its general descriptions of meta-analyses serve as a useful reference for this chapter.

A meta-analysis is "a formal evaluation of the quantitative evidence from two or more trials bearing on the same question. This most commonly involves the statistical combination of summary statistics from various trials but the term sometimes is also used to refer to the combination of raw data" (EMEA CPMP, 2001, p. 2). The EMEA identified the following regulatory purposes of meta-analyses (EMEA CPMP, 2001, p. 1):

> ➢ To provide a more precise estimate of the overall treatment effects.
> ➢ To evaluate whether overall positive results are also seen in prespecified subgroups of participants.
> ➢ To evaluate an additional efficacy outcome that requires more power than the individual trials can provide.
> ➢ To evaluate safety in a subgroup of participants or a rare adverse event in all participants.
> ➢ To improve the estimation of the dose-response relationship.
> ➢ To evaluate apparently conflicting study results.

Our discussions focus on just one of these purposes: the evaluation of safety.

9.6   THE BASIC STEPS IN META-ANALYSIS

The appropriate implementation of meta-analysis and the appropriate interpretation of the results obtained are not straightforward. The technique has both strengths and weaknesses, and both advocates and detractors. If all of the components involved in conducting a meta-analysis are performed appropriately, and the extent to which the results are helpful is not overstated (that is, any limitations are appropriately acknowledged and shared whenever and wherever communicating the results), the results can be informative and instructive. Unfortunately, however, it is easier than one might suspect to conduct a meta-analysis inappropriately and then to overstate the results in a variety of circumstances.

Piantadosi (2005, pp. 529–538) has written eloquently and authoritatively on the topic of meta-analysis. As noted in the previous section, a large number of clinical trials are now conducted, and synthesizing the results from many studies can be difficult and confusing. Inconsistency between published studies addressing the same research question is not uncommon for several reasons. First, somewhat different study designs may be employed. Second, the treatment effect of interest (the desirable biological change due to the drug) may be relatively small numerically even though it is of considerable clinical importance: such treatment effects can have considerable public health benefits if they are seen in a very large number of patients with a common disease. While the methodological advantages of randomized trials provide a very good means of evaluating treatment effects, small treatment effects can sometimes be obscured if the variability among participants' responses during the trial is of sufficient magnitude.

One way to combat inconsistencies seen between studies is to combine the data from all of the studies and conduct a new analysis on these data (the pooled data analysis approach). The size of the new dataset will be (much) larger than the size of any of the individual datasets, and the analysis of larger datasets lends itself more readily to the identification of relatively small but clinically meaningful treatment effects. That is the good news about meta-analysis. The bad news, as noted earlier, is that a certain degree of methodological sophistication is necessary to conduct a good meta-analysis, and it is (all too) easy to conduct a poor meta-analysis. Even though a meta-analysis does not require a new trial to be conducted, it is still a research method in its own right. Therefore, like all formal research methods, it "needs to proceed from a foundation of planning and design" (Piantadosi, 2005, p. 531). Kay (2007, p. 237) similarly noted that "to ensure that a meta-analysis is scientifically valid it is necessary to plan and conduct the analysis in an appropriate way. It is not sufficient to retrospectively go to a bunch of studies that you like the look of and stick them together!"

The basic steps required for the conduct of a meta-analysis are listed here. Weakness in any one of them can undermine the validity and strength of the analysis:

➤ Formulation of the purpose of the meta-analysis and specification of an outcome for the analysis. This outcome is used in data analysis, which is one of the subsequent steps in this list.
➤ Identification of all relevant studies.
➤ Establishing inclusion and exclusion criteria for studies to be included in the analysis. This includes determining and detailing approaches to ensure consistent quality of the studies and how to handle poor-quality studies.
➤ Data abstraction and acquisition.
➤ Data analysis.
➤ Evaluating homogeneity.
➤ Evaluating robustness.
➤ Dissemination of results and conclusions.

The first step, formulating a prespecified objective or purpose for the meta-analysis, is necessary to ensure that the results of the meta-analysis are credible. All other steps of the meta-analysis are governed by a clearly stated objective. These other steps are discussed in turn.

9.7 IDENTIFYING ALL RELEVANT STUDIES: PUBLICATION BIAS I

Identification of relevant studies can be a complex task, especially since the results of clinical trials are published in so many journals. Computerized searches can locate published articles, but there is a (strong) possibility that not all relevant studies may have been published and are therefore not readily accessible to the investigators performing the meta-analysis. The issue of publication bias is a particularly important one in this context.

Piantadosi (2005, pp. 582–583) defined publication bias as a "tendency for studies with positive results, namely those finding significant differences, to be published in journals in preference to those with negative findings." Stewart et al. (2005, p. 262) commented as follows:

> It is clear that the publication process can distort the underlying findings of research. Overt or subconscious pressures such as the wish to bolster research ratings, the need to sell journals or simply the desire to deliver good news can lead to results being presented in an over-favourable light, or to publishing only those papers that will deliver a message of progress or improvement. This is of course potentially very damaging, and in the context of systematic review it is important that we do all we can to minimize sources of potential bias, including those associated with publication and reporting.

Bowers et al. (2006) noted that publication bias can result from various other sources in addition to the simple observation that journals tend to favor positive studies. These include:

➤ Studies with positive results are more likely to be published in English language journals (and hence located more readily by various computer search engines).
➤ Studies with positive results are more likely to be cited in other publications.
➤ Some studies are never submitted for publication. These may include studies that fail to show a positive result and that have unfavorable results (as judged by those conducting the study).

If the typical $p < 0.05$ level of statistical significance is adopted by many studies examining the same treatment effect, a statistical argument can be made that 1 in every 40 trials would be expected to result in a statistically significant positive effect by chance alone, even if there is no true treatment effect. As Durham and Turner (2008) noted, studies with low power are more likely to have misleading results (e.g., positive results from truly ineffective drugs) than studies with high power. This can be a problem for meta-analyses since small, early clinical studies tend to be underpowered to detect effect sizes of clinical importance. Further, Ioannidis (2005) identified a number of reasons why published results may be misleading, including low power, small effect sizes, and flexibility in designs, analysis, and outcomes. Given that trials demonstrating positive results are more likely to be published, there is an immediate problem of distortion in the cumulative clinical literature (Matthews, 2006). This observation makes it very important that researchers conducting a meta-analysis (meta-analysts) try very hard to locate any unpublished study reports.

9.8   ESTABLISHING INCLUSION AND EXCLUSION CRITERIA: PUBLICATION BIAS II

In addition to making every effort to locate and obtain reports (published or unpublished) of all relevant studies, formalized *a priori* inclusion and exclusion criteria are needed to determine which studies will be included in the meta-analysis. There is an illuminating parallel here with the methodology used in conducting a clinical trial. For a given trial, unambiguous inclusion and exclusion criteria used to determine which potential participants enter the trial and which do not must be stated *a priori* in the study's protocol. The same is true for the conduct of a meta-analysis: there has to be a clearly defined set of rules for choosing, from among all the study reports that could be located and obtained, those studies whose results will be included in the meta-analysis. This is one of many parallels between the conduct of experimental studies that collect original data and the conduct of a meta-analysis: both are investigative studies that need to follow carefully circumscribed rules.

The establishment of these formalized inclusion and exclusion criteria requires a judgment call to be made, and this need for (subjective) judgment opens the door to a second form of publication bias, an omission bias. Citing Garattini and Liberati (2000) as an original source, Halpern and Berlin (2005, p. 311) commented as follows:

> Most of the discourse regarding bias in meta-analysis has focused
> on factors causing the selective publication of certain results.
> However, it is also possible that bias may stem from the selective
> conduct of evaluations likely to yield specified results.

One arguably straightforward approach to circumvent this omission bias is to use every study identified in the original search for all relevant studies. The ease of this strategy, however, can be countered by the genuine (and well-meaning) realization that some studies are clearly better (which needs to be operationalized in a precise manner by the meta-analysts) than others, and that some poorer studies probably should not be included if the best information is to be provided to the clinicians who will read the meta-analysis and therefore may base treatment decisions (at least in part) on its results. A related argument could be made for a scenario in which meta-analysts who would like to find a particular result select "appropriate" studies for inclusion in their meta-analysis. Both publication bias and omission bias highlight the need for appropriate circumspection when presenting the results and interpretations of one's meta-analysis. Whitehead (2002) described a number of analytic approaches intended to identify selection bias among the studies included in the meta-analysis and methods to modify the analysis if bias is suspected.

9.9   DATA ABSTRACTION AND ACQUISITION: INDIVIDUAL PARTICIPANT DATA

Data extraction and acquisition also has its challenges when planning and conducting a meta-analysis. Many published studies present summary statistics as opposed to presenting the underlying data, i.e., the participant-level data. This is a relatively common publishing practice, especially in the case of trials employing thousands of participants. However, as Piantadosi (2005, p. 530) noted, "it is now clear that more than the published information is usually necessary to perform rigorous overviews." A meta-analysis conducted using participant-level data has the advantages of standardizing the way in which the treatment effect is reported (e.g., use of the same outcome and the measure of the treatment effect) and the ability to examine subgroups. This requires the meta-analysts to obtain and analyze participant-level data (not simply aggregate data across treatment groups) from each study to produce a credible result (see also Stewart and Clarke, 1995).

Stewart et al. (2005) provided a comprehensive introduction to the use of individual participant data (in their terminology, individual patient data or IPD). When conducting an IPD meta-analysis, the original raw data are collected directly from the investigators conducting the original research studies, combined by the meta-analysts according to the protocol for the meta-analysis, and reanalyzed. When conducted in a rigorous manner, "IPD meta-analyses of randomized controlled trials are likely to offer a 'gold standard' of research synthesis" (Stewart et al., 2005, p. 261).

One meta-analysis method for combining data from a number of studies involves pooling participant-level data to produce an overall estimate of a treatment effect. An example of this type of meta-analysis was noted in Section 8.6.8. When sponsors submit a marketing application (e.g., an NDA) to regulatory agencies, an ISS often includes an analysis of pooled adverse event data. This is accomplished by pooling the coded adverse events from a number of studies and generating a statistical table from the pooled dataset. A simple example would be to generate a table that included the crude rates, or incidences, of all adverse events reported in all studies of an investigational drug. The incidence could be compared among the dose groups of the investigational drug and the control groups (e.g., placebo or active controls). In essence, the numerator (the number of participants reporting each adverse event) and the denominator (the number of participants at risk) are pooled across all studies. To account for the element of time, a similar pooled data analysis may be produced separately for short-term studies or long-term studies. Alternatives to this approach include a time-to-event analysis, such as the Kaplan-Meier estimation of the survival distribution. A pooled data analysis provides the ability to describe subgroup effects (e.g., age or sex) since these participant-level data would be available in a pooled dataset.

However, unless a sponsor is implementing a meta-analysis of several of its own studies, it can be quite difficult for meta-analysts to gain access to IPD for every study of interest. Since such detailed data are not routinely published, a considerable effort is likely to be needed to acquire them. For this reason, meta-analyses based on summary measures of the treatment effect gathered from published studies are currently more commonly reported. Accordingly, our discussions from this point forward pertain to such meta-analyses.

9.10   DATA ANALYSIS

There are a number of analytical elements that contribute to an appropriate and credible meta-analysis. In keeping with this book's general approach, we do not address these elements in detail (readers interested in a thorough statistical exposition of meta-analyses of randomized clinical trials are referred to Whitehead, 2002). However, we believe that it is appropriate for us to provide some statistical background on meta-analyses for two reasons. First, as noted in Section 9.1, meta-analysis has assumed a high-profile status in assessments of drug safety, and you are therefore likely to encounter such analyses when reading the drug safety literature. Second, our discussions in Chapter 12 include drug safety case studies in which meta-analyses play a considerable role, and some degree of familiarity with the technique will enable you to fully appreciate those discussions. As in other places in this book when some statistical description is beneficial, we have kept the mathematical notation to the bare minimum. Five formulae are presented for illustrative purposes, but no calculations are performed.

9.10.1   Choice of the Summary Statistic Representing the Treatment Effect of Interest

When designing and planning a meta-analysis, meta-analysts must choose the summary measure, or statistic, that will represent the treatment effect of interest. It is this summary statistic that is abstracted from each study included in the analysis, along with some estimate of its variability. In the following discussions, we will use the example of a treatment effect involving a comparison of participants' response to a drug (i.e., the test treatment) and their response to a control treatment (placebo).

This methodology can be used in assessments of therapeutic benefit. When evaluating a drug's effectiveness using continuous data, such as the change in SBP in response to an antihypertensive investigational drug, a useful summary statistic is the difference between the mean response of the treatment group and the mean response of the placebo group, i.e., the between-group difference in means. When evaluating a drug's effectiveness using survival data, i.e., the length of time that patients receiving the drug live following a particular diagnosis or a particular surgical intervention, a useful summary statistic is the log hazard ratio. This value is the logarithm (to base e) of the actual hazard ratio. The advantage of using log scores is that nonlinear relationships become more linear when the logarithms of the initial (raw) data are used (for example, a true exponential curve plotted on a graph becomes a perfect straight line when the logarithms of the raw data are plotted). Put another way, some asymmetrical relationships become symmetrical when logarithms are used.

In this book our interest lies with safety data. For adverse events, i.e., dichotomous data where the event is either experienced or is not experienced, useful summary statistics include the risk difference, the log relative risk, and the log odds ratio. Whitehead (2002) identified a number of reasons that make the log odds ratio preferable for meta-analysis of dichotomous outcomes. Two of the reasons cited are:

> Test statistics based on the log odds ratio best fit the approximate statistical distributions, which permit the calculation of confidence intervals. We have already noted the contribution of confidence intervals to the meaningful interpretation of point estimates in Chapters 7 and 8.
> The log odds ratio is symmetrical about 0.0. In contrast, the odds ratio is finite from 0.0 to 1.00, with values less that 1.00 indicating less risk for the test treatment group, and infinite from 1.00 to infinity, with values greater than 1.00 indicating greater risk for the test treatment group. (Recall the discussions in Section 8.6.8 regarding the asymmetry of odds ratios and relative risks.)

When the summary statistic used in a meta-analysis is on the log scale of measurement it is also useful to report results on the original scale of measurement (e.g., relative risk or odds ratio) to aid in the interpretation of the results.

9.10.2   The Data Used in a Meta-analysis

Two items of data are obtained from each study incorporated into a meta-analysis:

> A measure of the treatment effect in that specific study.
> An estimate of the variance associated with the treatment effect.

If we designate the total number of studies incorporated into the analysis as s, there will be s study-specific estimates of the treatment effect of interest, which we will denote as $\hat{q}$ and the same number of study-specific estimates of the variances associated with the treatment effects, which we will denote as $\text{var}(\hat{q})$. These data are the inputs of the meta-analysis. Any given treatment effect and its associated variance can be denoted by adding the letter i to $\hat{q}$, and $\text{var}(\hat{q})$, i.e., $\hat{q}_i$, and $\text{var}(\hat{q}_i)$. The possible values of i start at 1, and proceed to the total number of studies in the analysis, i.e., s. That is, $i = 1, 2, 3, \ldots .s$. The ultimate goal of the meta-analysis is to estimate the value of the treatment effect over all of the studies, i.e., q.

To obtain a single estimate of the treatment effect (e.g., the log odds ratio) over all of the studies included in a meta-analysis, we need to make a decision concerning whether to regard "study" as a fixed effect or a random effect in our analysis: This decision dictates how the study-specific estimates of the treatment effect will be weighted in the overall estimate. Before explaining the consequences of this decision, it may be helpful to clarify some terms introduced in the previous sentence.

Fixed Effects and Random Effects. As just noted in the previous section, the ultimate goal of a meta-analysis is to estimate the value of the treatment effect over all of the studies. This involves using the treatment effect found in each of the studies included in the meta-analysis. The individual values of treatment effect will likely (almost certainly) be somewhat different across the group of studies included, and it is of interest to know exactly how they differ. In statistical terms, this is the source of variation of primary interest in the meta-analysis: the result of the meta-analysis is influenced by the degree of variation here.

However, in addition to these values being different, the studies themselves are different, and we can therefore call 'study' a factor in our meta-analysis. Each study included in the meta-analysis will have many unique characteristics, such as the precise number of participants in each treatment group within the study, the precise length of the treatment periods, the investigational site(s) where the study was conducted, and even perhaps the precise way in which the treatment effect of interest was calculated. That there may be differences among studies comes as no surprise to us: even before looking at this information for each study, we fully expect that they will differ in some ways. Importantly, we are not ultimately interested in quantifying the extent to which they vary: that is, the result of the meta-analysis will not, for example, be a statement of how much the treatment periods in the trials differed. However, even though the factor study is therefore not ultimately of interest to us, this source of variation does need to be taken into account in the mathematics of calculating the result that is of interest, i.e., the estimated value of the treatment effect over all of the studies. The question then becomes: How are we going to take this source of variation into account? We can choose to do this in one of two ways: by regarding the factor study as either a fixed effect or a random effect in our analysis.

The specification of how the study-specific estimates will be combined across the studies is called a meta-analysis model. Choosing whether study will be treated as a fixed effect or as a random effect is one part of the model, and each choice has implications:

> ➤ If study is treated as a fixed effect, the study-specific estimates, $\hat{q}_i$ for $i = 1$, $2, ..., s$, are considered a sample of estimates arising from a population with a single fixed parameter, q, representing the true, but unknown treatment effect.
> ➤ If study is treated as a random effect, the underlying population parameter, q, is allowed to vary from one study to the next.

Kay (2007, p. 234) addressed how the choice between a fixed effects model and a random effects model impacts the result of interest generated by the meta-analysis:

> The fixed effects model considers the studies that have been combined as the totality of all the studies conducted. An alternative approach considers the collection of studies included in the meta-analysis as a random selection of the studies that have been conducted or a random selection of those that could have been conducted. This results in a slightly changed methodology, termed the random effects model. The mathematics for the two models is a little different…The net effect, however, of using a random effects model is to produce a slightly more conservative analysis with wider confidence intervals.

Whitehead (2002, pp. 153–154) addressed the advantages and disadvantages of the fixed effects model and the random effects model as follows:

> The overall estimate from the fixed effects model provides a summary of the results obtained from the particular sample of patients contributing data. Extrapolation of the results from the fixed effects model to the total population of patients makes the assumption that the characteristics of patients contributing data to the meta-analysis are the same as those in the total patient population. A common argument in favour of the random effects model is that it produces results which can be considered more generalizable. However, the underlying assumption of the random effects model is that the results from studies in the meta-analysis are representative of the results which would be obtained from the total population of treatment centres, and study centres are usually not chosen at random… One advantage of the random effects model is that it allows the between-study variability in the treatment difference estimates to influence the overall estimate and, more particularly, its precision. Therefore, if there is substantial variability, this will be reflected in a wide confidence interval.

Weighting Individual Studies According to the Analysis Model Chosen. Each study included in a meta-analysis contributes the same input to the analysis, i.e., the treatment effect found in that study. Therefore, if we have 50 studies, there will be 50 treatment effects included in the analysis. However, each item of information does not necessarily carry the same weight when determining the result of the meta-analysis: some items are accorded more influence than others. Studies that are weighted more heavily will exert a greater influence on the final result of the analysis than those that are weighted less heavily. The weighting accorded to each individual study, i.e., to each study-specific treatment effect, is determined mathematically according to the rules of the meta-analysis model adopted. As seen in the previous section, two meta-analysis models are of interest: the fixed effects model and the random effects model.

In the fixed effects model, the weight (w) assigned to each study is the inverse of the variance of the estimate, calculated as follows:

$$w_i = \frac{1}{\mathrm{var}(\hat{q}_i)} \tag{9.1}$$

This expression indicates that the more precise the treatment effect estimate (i.e., the smaller the variance), the greater the study's contribution will be to the overall estimate of the treatment effect. Larger studies tend to yield more precise estimates so this weighting implies that the overall estimate will be more consistent with the largest data sources.

In the random effects model, the calculation of the weight (w) assigned to each study involves an additional component, namely, an estimate of the between-study variance in underlying parameters, represented by $\hat{t}^2$. The weight assigned to each study in this model is calculated as follows:

$$w_i = \frac{1}{\mathrm{var}(\hat{q}_i) + \hat{t}^2} \tag{9.2}$$

In this case, therefore, the weight assigned to each study is a function of the inverse of the variance of the estimate (the sole item used in the fixed effects model) and an estimate of the between-study variance in the underlying parameters, which represent the true but unknown treatment effects (recall that the random effects model presumes that these can vary). The methods of estimating $\hat{t}^2$ are beyond the scope of this chapter, but it is appropriate to note that if this quantity is zero, the weight assigned to each study is identical to the weight assigned under the fixed effects model.

9.10.3 Obtaining the Overall Estimate of the Treatment Effect of Interest

Whichever model is chosen, i.e., whichever method of calculating the weights assigned to each individual study's results is employed, the overall estimate of the treatment effect based on all of the studies can then be obtained as a weighted average of the study-specific estimates of the treatment effect. This value is the point estimate in the final answer, an answer that will also incorporate confidence intervals, as seen shortly.

The point estimate is calculated from Formula 9.3:

$$\hat{q} = \frac{\sum_{i=1}^{s} \hat{q}_i w_i}{\sum_{i=1}^{s} w_i}$$

(9.3)

All of the symbols used in this formula have been introduced in the text with the exception of Σ. This symbol is an enhanced version of the Greek letter sigma, and it is used in mathematical notation as a summation instruction. The information placed directly below and above the symbol indicates which values should be summed. Consider first the numerator. The information below and above the Σ symbol, i.e., $i=1$, and s, respectively, indicates that the letter i should take every (whole) value between 1 and s, where s represents the total number of studies. Therefore, if there are 50 studies included in the analysis, i will take the values 1, 2, 3, ...48, 49, 50. This means that, for each of the 50 studies, the study-specific value of $\hat{q}_i w_i$ will be calculated, and all of these values will be added together. Now consider the denominator. The information placed directly below and above the Σ symbol is the same as that used with the symbol in the numerator, so i will again take the values 1, 2, 3, ...48, 49, 50. Hence, for each of the 50 studies, the study-specific value of w_i will be calculated, and all of these values will be added together. The value obtained for the numerator is then divided by the value obtained for the denominator to yield the value of $\hat{q}$, the point estimate of the treatment effect of interest.

Having calculated the point estimate, it is now appropriate to place confidence intervals around this point estimate. This calculation involves two steps. The first step is the calculation of the standard error of the point estimate, represented as $se(\hat{q})$, as shown in Formula 9.4:

$$se(\hat{q}) = \sqrt{\frac{1}{\sum_{i=1}^{s} w_i}}$$

(9.4)

The second step involves multiplying $se(\hat{q})$ by a precision coefficient, *PC*. The resultant value is then added to, and subtracted from, the point estimate $\hat{q}$. This yields the upper and lower limits of a CI around $\hat{q}$:

$$CI = \hat{q} \pm PCse(\hat{q})$$

(9.5)

The product of the precision coefficient and the standard error is called the margin of error. The margin of error is determined by two items: the degree of confidence that we wish to employ and a measure of the extent to which the study-specific values of the treatment effect estimate the true but unknown population value. With regard to the first item, the typical CIs used in such analyses are 95% and/or 99%, which means that 95% CIs and/or 99% CIs are calculated using the actual value of the precision coefficient obtained from the standard normal distribution. For illustration, we provide two values that are representative of the precision coefficients seen for these confidence levels in meta-analyses: the precision coefficient used in the calculation of 95% CIs is typically around 1.96, and it is typically around 2.58 for 99% CIs.

With regard to the second item, the standard error of the estimate of the combined treatment effect is a function of the variances of the study-specific estimates. The more precise the study-specific estimates are, the smaller the standard error of the estimated combined treatment effect will be. Equivalently, uncertainty with regard to the study-specific estimates will translate into uncertainty about the combined estimated treatment effect.

This information permits the calculation of a two-sided CI for the chosen level of confidence to be placed around the overall treatment effect point estimate. In conjunction with the point estimate, the positive value and the negative value of the margin of error lead to the upper limit and the lower limit of the CI, respectively. The upper limit results from using the positive value of the margin of error, i.e., adding a certain value to the point estimate, and the lower limit from using the negative value of the margin of error, i.e., subtracting the same value from the point estimate.

Two points about these calculations are noteworthy. First, whichever level of confidence is chosen, the respective calculations result in confidence interval limits that are symmetrically placed around the point estimate. Second, given that the precision coefficient for a 99% CI is greater than the precision coefficient for a 95% CI, the upper and lower limits of a 99% CI placed around the point estimate will be further away from the point estimate than the upper and lower limits of a 95% CI. That is, a two-sided 99% CI placed around a point estimate is always wider than a two-sided 95% CI, a statement originally made in Section 7.7.2 and reiterated in Section 8.6.8.

Finally here, it is important to remind ourselves that if the CI is calculated in this manner for a summary statistic measured on the log scale (e.g., the log odds ratio), it will not be symmetric when transformed into the original scale of measurement (e.g., the odds ratio). In the case of the log odds ratio, exponentiation of the point estimate and the confidence limits results in corresponding estimates on the odds ratio scale.

9.10.4   Evaluating Homogeneity

In the statistical theory underpinning meta-analysis, an assumption is made that the study-specific estimates of the treatment effect are (relatively) homogeneous. Homogeneity exists when the study-specific estimates of the treatment effect are similar in magnitude (and sign) to the estimate of the treatment effect obtained by combining the estimates from all studies. Heterogeneity can arise from differences in studies, such as study populations, the quality of measurement, and reporting conventions. Since the objective of a meta-analysis is to calculate a well-justified combined estimate of the treatment effect of interest, it is typical to conduct a test for homogeneity as part of a meta-analysis.

Once a combined estimate of the treatment effect has been calculated, it is possible to examine the homogeneity of the individual study-specific estimates relative to the combined estimate. A graphical display of the individual study-specific estimates and the combined estimate can be used to visually identify any results that stand out from the rest, i.e., those contributing to the heterogeneity, and a formal test can be conducted. In some instances, the study-specific estimates of the treatment effect can be quite heterogeneous, and in these cases the reporting of an overall estimate may not be appropriate.

Readers are referred to Whitehead (2002) for details of this homogeneity test and for some recommendations on how to handle the problem of heterogeneity should it arise.

9.11   EVALUATING ROBUSTNESS

Having calculated the result of a meta-analysis, it can be informative to assess the robustness of the analysis. In any meta-analysis some of the studies included will be larger than others, and sometimes a small percentage of included studies can be considerably larger than the majority of others. Because of the nature of the calculations performed,, the larger trials, i.e., those that have higher precision, will tend to dominate (Kay, 2007). Kay therefore suggested that it can be helpful to assess the robustness of the overall conclusion by performing the analysis without the data from the largest study or studies to see if the result remains qualitatively the same. As he noted, "If it does, then the result is robust. If it does not, then the overall result is undermined, as it is then giving a result that is driven by the largest trial or trials" (Kay, 2007, p. 236).

9.12   DISSEMINATION OF RESULTS AND CONCLUSIONS OF A META-ANALYSIS

The results of a completed meta-analysis typically include the following:

> ➢ The estimated treatment effect (a point estimate) for each individual study included in the analysis, and a 95% CI about each study's estimate.
> ➢ The overall estimated treatment effect and its 95% CI.

In both cases, the results can be reported on the measurement scale of the analysis (e.g., log odds ratio), the original scale (odds ratio), or both. This information can be displayed in tabular form or in a graphical form called a confidence interval plot.

As is true across all research methodology, if the correct study design has been employed and rigorous methodology has permitted the acquisition of optimum-quality data, the computational analysis itself is typically not difficult. The results of the meta-analysis are therefore not difficult to calculate. What is more difficult is the interpretation of the results and the appropriate degree of restraint needed to disseminate one's conclusions in a responsible manner. Given all of these considerations, the conduct and communication of a meta-analysis must be undertaken carefully, diligently, and responsibly. As Piantadosi (2005, p. 124) stated, "Despite high-profile instances of enhanced inferences arising from their use, *overviews* or *meta-analyses* remain a somewhat controversial tool for assessing evidence from multiple clinical trials."

9.13   AN ADDITIONAL CONSIDERATION

Finally, we address one other important issue in meta-analysis. This concerns the potential difficulty of determining how to deal with individual studies for which there are no events, i.e., no adverse events in our present context. In such cases, the estimate of the log relative risk or the log odds ratio is not (cannot be) defined, and the usual meta-analytic techniques may not be appropriate since the studies with no information are not included in the overall estimate of the treatment effect (Whitehead, 2002).

There are several approaches that could be considered in this case. One approach is to combine summary data over two or more similar studies (including the one with no events of interest) into a pooled group. The methods described previously for individual studies would still be applicable, including specification of the model and calculating weights. This approach would require pooling the data (e.g., the numerators and denominators) among the studies included in the group and then calculating a pooled estimate of the treatment effect and its variance. As we have seen, in the typical meta-analysis study is considered a source of variation. Since it is desirable not to dilute the effect of individual studies in the analysis, the pooling of data would require that the pooled studies be considered similar (e.g., used the same protocol and/or reporting conventions).

A second approach is to add 0.5 to the number of successes and failures in each study, where success is defined as the presence of Event A and failure is defined as the absence of Event B. Whitehead (2002) provided an example of using this approach when three studies do not have any events of interest. The result of using this method is that the estimates from the three studies have less bias but a greater standard error, and therefore less weight in the combined estimate.

A third approach is to use exact methods that do not rely so heavily on distributional assumptions. This problem can be potentially difficult to manage. As Whitehead (2002, p. 220) noted:

> In summary, when there are studies with no 'successes' or no 'failures' in both treatment arms, the usual meta-analysis methods which stratify by study may not be appropriate. These methods effectively ignore the data from such studies. Depending on the method used, problems may also be encountered when a study has either no 'successes' or no 'failures' in one treatment arm.

9.14   THE COCHRANE COLLABORATION

The Cochrane Collaboration was established in 1993. It is an international organization dedicated to helping people make well-informed decisions about health care. It does this by preparing, maintaining, and promoting the accessibility of systematic reviews, most (but not all) of which are based on randomized trials. Its web site is www.cochrane.org. As Clarke (2006, p. 39) noted:

> The Cochrane Collaboration is an international organisation dedicated to helping people make well-informed decisions about health care. It does this through preparing, maintaining and promoting the accessibility of systematic reviews of the effects of health care interventions. Most of these reviews are based on randomised trials but, in some circumstances, other types of study might be brought together, appraised, summarized and combined within the Cochrane review.

The Cochrane Collaboration is the largest single organization that prepares and maintains systematic reviews of the effects of health care interventions (Clarke, 2006). Systematic reviews of studies published in the literature are helpful in several ways. They can provide a succinct overview of a large number of individual papers. Physicians can therefore readily see the most salient points regarding a particular form of pharmacotherapy: such reviews bring together the findings from relevant research in as unbiased a way as possible and provide a key component in informed decision making. These reviews may also help clinical researchers to find the best experimental study design to provide additional and/or complementary information concerning the drug's safety and/or efficacy.

9.15   FURTHER READING

9.15.1   Therapeutic Use Trials

COMMIT (Clopidogrel and Metropolol in Myocardial Infarction Trial) Collaborative Group, 2005, Addition of clopidogrel to aspirin in 45,852 patients with acute myocardial infarction: Randomised placebo-controlled trial, *Lancet*, 366:1607–1621.

ISIS-4 (Fourth International Study of Infarct Survival) Collaborative Group, 1995, ISIS-4: A randomised factorial trial assessing early oral captopril, oral mononitrate, and intravenous magnesium sulphate in 58,050 patients with suspected acute myocardial infarction, *Lancet*, 345:669–685.

The ALLHAT Officers and Coordinators for the ALLHAT Collaborative Research Group, 2002, Major outcomes in high-risk hypertensive patients randomized to angiotensin-converting enzyme inhibitor or calcium channel blocker vs. diuretic. The Antihypertensive and Lipid-Lowering Treatment to Prevent Heart Attack Trial (ALLHAT), *Journal of the American Medical Association*, 288: 2981–2997. [This trial involved 33,357 participants.]

Yusuf, S., Held, P., Teo, K.K., and Toretsky, E.R., 1990, Selection of patients for randomized controlled trials: Implications of wide or narrow eligibility criteria, *Statistics in Medicine*, 9:73–86.

Yusuf, S., Sleight, P., Pogue, J., et al., 2000, The heart outcomes prevention evaluation study investigators: Effects of an angiotensin-converting enzyme inhibitor, ramipril, on cardiovascular events in high-risk patients, *New England Journal of Medicine*, 342:145–153.

9.15.2   Meta-analysis

Several meta-analyses are discussed in Chapter 12, and additional readings related to this statistical technique can therefore be found at the end of that chapter.

Normand, S-L.T., 1999, Meta-analysis: Formulating, evaluating, combining, and reporting, *Statistics in Medicine*, 18:321–359.

Stewart, L.A. and Clarke, M.J., 1995, Practical methodology of meta-analyses (overviews) using updated individual patient data, *Statistics in Medicine,* 14: 2057–2079.

Whitehead, A., 2002, *Meta-analysis of controlled clinical trials*, Hoboken, NJ: John Wiley & Sons.

9.15.3   Publication Bias in Meta-analysis

Rothstein, H.R., Sutton, A.J., and Borenstein, M. (Eds.), 2005, *Publication bias in meta-analysis: Prevention, assessment and adjustments*, Chichester, UK: John Wiley & Sons.
[This book provides a thorough exposition of this topic. One interesting aspect of the book is the Annotated Bibliography provided in Appendix B (Rothstein and Busing, pp. 331–346), which lists and describes a selection of articles that provide a detailed look at various aspects of publication bias.]

10

ASSESSMENT METHODOLOGIES IN NONEXPERIMENTAL POSTMARKETING SURVEILLANCE

10.1   INTRODUCTION

In the previous chapter we discussed experimental methods that can be used to gain information once a drug has been approved, and how therapeutic use trials can provide additional information to extend and complement that provided by preapproval clinical trials. Some therapeutic trials can be relatively small in size but provide useful information by including patients whose characteristics were not represented in the participants in preapproval clinical trials, e.g., those with hepatic impairment, older individuals, and those taking concomitant medications. Other therapeutic trials, large-scale trials, can be considerably larger in size than preapproval clinical trials: one such trial including 58,000 patients was listed in Section 9.8. We also discussed the analytical strategy of meta-analysis. Meta-analyses vary in the number of patients included, since this is dependent on the numbers in the individual trials combined in the new analysis. However, typical numbers are also in the (tens of) thousands (see examples in Chapter 12).

While these strategies are valuable and important for obtaining additional information about drug safety and effectiveness, there are additional approaches that can employ much greater numbers of patients. Assessment of effectiveness may provide information leading to changes in the formulation and/or dosing of the drug that subsequently provide greater therapeutic benefit to patients. It is also critical for meaningful assessments of safety as operationally defined in terms of the benefit-risk balance. Some of these additional approaches are discussed in this chapter.

10.2   USING INFORMATION FROM EXPERIMENTAL AND NONEXPERIMENTAL STUDIES

Assessing safety and the related benefit-risk balance in the postmarketing domain is more complex than assessing safety at the time of marketing approval. As we have seen, when marketing approval for a drug is requested by a sponsor, the regulatory agency relies mostly on data from preapproval controlled, randomized trials. However, in the postmarketing domain, relevant data from various sources need

Integrated Cardiac Safety: Assessment Methodologies for Noncardiac Drugs in Discovery, Development, and Postmarketing Surveillance. By J. Rick Turner and Todd A. Durham
Copyright © 2009 John Wiley & Sons, Inc.

to be considered. One of the primary resources here has been the Adverse Event Reporting System (AERS) database that contains spontaneous reports of adverse drug reactions from physicians, patients, and sponsors. The FDA has operated the AERS since 1998 (for an analysis of serious adverse drug reactions based on reports to the AERS see Moore et al., 2007). The FDA can now use other large databases. However, formal epidemiological studies are another potentially very informative source of relevant information. Just as nonclinical and preapproval clinical data should be considered complementary when making marketing decisions, data from postapproval randomized clinical trials (experimental studies) and epidemiological (nonexperimental) studies are complementary. As Avorn (2007, p. 2221) commented, both kinds of study are needed "to understand everything we should know about a drug."

Credit for the first randomized pharmaceutical clinical trial is most often given to Sir Austin Bradford Hill for his work in the late 1940s on the United Kingdom Medical Research Council's trial of the effects of the aminoglycoside antibiotic streptomycin on tuberculosis, which became the first antibiotic treatment for this disease. The criteria that Bradford Hill established have since become the standard by which epidemiologists and other postmarketing researchers determine causal links (e.g., see Bradford Hill, 1965). The criteria include evidence of the following:

> Strength of association.
> Specificity of association.
> Consistency of findings (can the findings be replicated and be found in varying conditions?).
> Temporality (does the cause precede the effect?).
> Dose-response or biological gradient (does increased exposure go along with increased effects?).
> Analogy (are the findings in other situations consistent?).
> Biological plausibility (is there a plausible mechanism of action for the effect?).
> Coherence (is the observed relationship consistent with other observations?).
> Experimental evidence (can a randomized blinded experiment be designed where control of the influence of interest—the cause—leads reliably to the observed changes, i.e., the effect?).

Matthews (1999, i) commented as follows:

> Over the last two to three decades randomised concurrently controlled clinical trials have become established as the method which investigators must use to assess new treatments if their claims are to find widespread acceptance. The methodology underpinning these trials is firmly based in statistical theory, and the success of randomised clinical trials perhaps constitutes

the greatest achievement of statistics in the second half of the
twentieth century.

However, it is fair to say that statistical methodology is currently less well
developed in the case of epidemiology studies than it is for randomized controlled
trials: this is not meant as a pejorative statement, but simply as a statement of the
current state of affairs that will very likely change as additional spotlights on and
developments in the field of pharmacoepidemiology increase (see also Shakir and
Layton, 2002; Perrio et al., 2007). As Avorn (2007, p. 2221) noted:

> We forget how difficult it was to establish the rules of the road
> for conducting randomized trials. In terms of design theory
> and public policy, drug-epidemiology research is now where
> randomized trials were in the 1950s. We have much to learn
> about methods, transparency, and protecting the public's interest.
> But that work can be done, and we often have no other way of
> gathering vital insights.

It should also be noted here that the term nonexperimental is not a pejorative one
compared with the term experimental. Piantadosi (2005) discussed two fundamental
types of study design, experimental and nonexperimental. As noted in Section
9.4.1, in experimental studies participants receive random treatment allocation,
and observations are made under conditions in which the influence of interest
is controlled by the research scientists. In nonexperimental studies the research
scientist also collects observations but does not exert control over the influence of
interest. Nonexperimental studies are often called observational studies, but this
term is inaccurate: it does not definitively distinguish between nonexperimental
studies and experimental studies, in which observations are also made. This
chapter reviews the nonexperimental methodologies employed in postmarketing
surveillance in general and in pharmacoepidemiology. Specific attention is drawn
to the various types of assessment, including experimental and nonexperimental
methods, as well as outlining future considerations and developments.

10.3   NOMENCLATURE CONSIDERATIONS

Three terms that are widely seen in the literature in the context of postmarketing
drug safety are pharmacovigilance, pharmacoepidemiology, and postmarking
surveillance. With regard to the first two terms, some sources suggest that
pharmacoepidemiological studies fall within the province of pharmacovigilance,
while others suggest that pharmacovigilance is one application of
pharmacoepidemiology, which also includes other applications such as
pharmacoeconomics, drug discovery, and drug development (see Arlett et al., 2005,
p. 105, Table 8.1). Before commencing our discussions in this chapter, therefore, it

may be helpful to provide an explanation for our choice of the term postmarketing surveillance in this book.

10.3.1 Pharmacovigilance

The term pharmacovigilance is a common and important term in drug safety investigations. The literature contains various definitions of pharmacovigilance by internationally acknowledged leaders in the field. However, as Stephens (2004) noted, unfortunately there is a degree of discrepancy between them. A definition provided by Mann and Andrews (2002: see also 2007a) regards pharmacovigilance as "the study of the safety of marketed drugs under the practical conditions of clinical usage in large populations." The wording of their 2007 definition is fractionally different, but the emphasis clearly remains on evaluating the safety of marketed drugs. In contrast, Shakir and Layton (2002, p. 467) offered a more encompassing definition, commenting as follows:

> Pharmacovigilance involves the monitoring, detection, evaluation and responding to drug safety hazards in humans during premarketing development and postmarketing. Drug safety signals or hypotheses are generated from several sources, including spontaneous reports of suspected adverse reactions, published case reports, clinical pharmacology, clinical trials and pharmacoepidemiological studies.

Stephens (2004, p. 2) listed the following related aims of pharmacovigilance, a list that effectively provides an agenda for many of our discussions in this book:

➢ Identification and quantification of previously unrecognized adverse drug reactions.
➢ Identification of patient subgroups at particular risk of adverse drug reactions (the risk being related to dose, age, sex, and underlying disease).
➢ Continued monitoring of a drug's safety throughout the duration of its use to ensure that its risks and benefits remain acceptable.
➢ Comparison of the adverse drug reaction profiles of drugs within the same therapeutic class.
➢ Detection of inappropriate prescription and administration.
➢ Further elucidation of a drug's pharmacological/toxicological properties and the mechanisms of action that lead to adverse drug reactions.
➢ Detection of significant drug-drug interactions between new drugs and co-therapy with agents already established on the market.
➢ Communication of appropriate information to health professionals.
➢ Refutation of "false positive" adverse drug reaction signals arising in the professional or lay media, or from spontaneous reports.

The terms signal (safety or adverse drug reaction signal) and spontaneous report are addressed in Section 10.6.

10.3.2   Pharmacoepidemiology

Strom (2005b, p. 3) defined pharmacoepidemiology as "the study of the use of and the effects of drugs in large numbers of people" and commented that the field of pharmacoepidemiology employs the methodology of chronic disease epidemiology to study the use and effects of drugs, including safety, effectiveness, utilization, and costs. Strom (2005b, p. 5) also noted that the primary application of these principles to date "has been in the context of postmarketing drug surveillance." More recently, the literature suggests that pharmacoepidemiological methods can also be usefully employed in preapproval clinical trials (see Guess, 2005). If pharmacoepidemiology continues to grow in its application to premarketing approval, its generally accepted meaning may also move in the all-encompassing direction.

10.3.3   Postmarketing Surveillance

As they are currently widely used, therefore, the terms pharmacovigilance and pharmacoepidemiology would both probably capture the contents of this chapter in a perfectly acceptable manner. We have simply chosen to use the term postmarketing surveillance in this book to unequivocally delineate this chapter's focus, and to differentiate the chapter's interest in drug safety from those in other stages of lifecycle drug development that we have discussed in previous chapters.

When we cite other authors' work in our discussions, their terminology is respected.

10.4   ADVERSE DRUG REACTIONS

The ICH Guidance E2A discusses adverse events observed during preapproval clinical trials and indicates that an adverse event can be considered an adverse drug reaction if there is evidence to suggest or support a causal relationship. Once a drug has been marketed, an adverse drug reaction is regarded as a response to a drug that is noxious and unintended and that occurs at doses usually used in man for prophylaxis, diagnosis, or therapy of disease or for modification of physiological function (see Arnold, 2004, p. 382; ICH Guidance E2A, 1995; ICH Guidance E6, 1997).

While modern medicines have changed the way in which diseases are managed and controlled, and provide tremendous benefits, considerable evidence continues to accumulate that adverse reactions to medicines are a common, yet often predictable and therefore preventable cause of illness, disability, and even death. In some countries, adverse drug reactions rank among the top 10 leading causes of mortality (WHO, 2004).

Many adverse drug reactions are predictable from the known pharmacology of the drug and the characteristics of the individual patient (see Routledge, 2004). This means that they are potentially avoidable. Two examples are particularly salient here. It is well documented in many cases that the interaction between two drugs that are being taken concomitantly, i.e., the drug-drug interaction, can be harmful. Therefore, if a patient is already receiving one of the drugs, he or she should not be prescribed the other drug. These deleterious interactions are likely in any patient who takes both of the drugs, and therefore patient characteristics are not the key factor here. In contrast, patient characteristics are extremely relevant in other cases. Again, it is well documented that certain drugs should not be prescribed for patients who exhibit certain characteristics, e.g., impaired hepatic function, heart failure. When adverse drug reactions occur for one of these avoidable reasons, they fall into the category of medication errors, a topic discussed in Chapter 13.

Other adverse drug reactions are unexpected. Some drugs appear to have intrinsic dangers associated with the products themselves, i.e., the vast majority of patients exposed to the drug experience the adverse drug reaction. For other drugs, most patients may experience beneficial effects, while a (very) small number exhibit unpredictable sensitivities. Reasons for this will be discussed in due course.

For other drugs, we are aware of the possibility that they may lead to a previously observed adverse drug reaction in a very small number of patients. This may be because the drug is very closely related chemically to a previously prescribed drug that resulted in the previously observed adverse drug reaction, or because preapproval clinical trials revealed that an unrelated drug displayed a (very small) tendency to induce a known adverse drug reaction, a liability that was noted by the regulatory agency but was not considered an important enough cause to tip the benefit-risk balance in the unfavorable direction.

Adverse drug reactions are a major cause of morbidity, and estimates suggest that they may account for up to 5% of all medical inpatient admissions (see Routledge, 2004), with a cost per hospital of approximately $5.6 million (Bates et al., 1995; Bates et al., 1997). Adverse drug reactions can also be fatal. While the percentage of patients who suffer an adverse drug reaction to a particular drug may be very small, very small percentages of very large numbers of patients can become significant concerns. Adverse drug reactions are therefore important clinical and public health issues (Routledge, 2004).

10.4.1   Type A Adverse Drug Reactions

Adverse drug reactions can occur in two forms, commonly called type A (or dose-related) and type B (or bizarre). Type A adverse drug reactions are accentuations of the normal effect of the drug. For example, an antihypertensive drug may be too effective in some patients and lead to hypotension. Type A reactions make up around 75% of adverse drug reactions. Their onset is typically gradual, which means that they may go unrecognized for some time, and they can lead to significant morbidity. Since these reactions are accentuations of normal pharmacodynamic activity, they can be understood in terms of the drug's pharmacology, i.e., their mechanisms of action can be determined and understood.

Type A adverse drug reactions, then, occur when the concentration of the drug at the site of action is increased above normal concentrations, and the mechanism of action for the adverse drug reaction is the same as the mechanism of action for normal pharmacotherapy. Reasons include:

➤ Pharmacokinetic activity is reduced.
➤ The target organ is particularly sensitive to a given drug concentration.

These pharmacokinetic and pharmacodynamic effects often occur together. Four groups of patients tend to be particularly susceptible:

➤ The young, particularly neonates.
➤ The elderly.
➤ Patients with hepatic impairment.
➤ Patients with renal impairment.

10.4.2 Type B Adverse Reactions

Type B reactions are unpredictable and often bizarre reactions to a drug. Their onset can be quick and can also be dramatic: both of these qualities tend to lead to quick recognition of the reactions. While type B reactions account for less of the overall total than type A reactions, they are more likely to have fatal consequences. Type B reactions can occur at very low concentrations, and they are not easily predicted from knowledge of the drug's mechanism of action.

Type B reactions are bizarre in that they cannot be predicted from the drug's known pharmacology. They include allergic reactions to drugs, and because of their often dramatic onset, they may be associated with a proportionately higher mortality than type A reactions even though they are less common. Hypersensitivity reactions can be severe. These reactions may only show up in 1 in 10,000, meaning that they would be probabilistically unlikely to have been seen in preapproval clinical trials, and they may show "a remarkable absence of a relationship between dose and severity" (Olsson and Meyboom, 2006, p. 231). The underlying mechanism for this reaction may be an inborn variation in metabolism, but in many cases the etiology is unknown.

10.5   THE NATURE OF POSTMARKETING SURVEILLANCE

Section 9.3 addressed the limitations of preapproval clinical trials, and noted that they cannot reasonably be expected to detect relatively rare adverse events since the occurrence of such events is probabilistically unlikely in the sample sizes employed. However, this situation changes when large numbers of patients start taking the drug in the months after marketing approval (or, strictly, product launch, since it is possible for there to be a delay between approval and launch). It is now probabilistically likely that such events will occur, and, unfortunately, they may be sensationalized by the media and others. Cobert (2007, pp. 11–12) captured such a scenario as follows:

> Should the AE [adverse event] in question be dramatic and rapidly discovered, such as torsades de pointes, aplastic anemia, or rhabdomyolysis (a severe skeletal muscle injury), there will be a torrent of recriminations about why this was not discovered earlier during the clinical testing. The correct response is that the testing of only 5,000 to 10,000 patients could not pick up such a rare event. This response is usually lost in the clamor.

A major focus of postmarketing surveillance is the identification and quantification of adverse drug reactions. Olsson and Meyboom (2006, pp. 229–230) observed that the ultimate goal of postmarketing surveillance is "the promotion of rational and safe use of medicines." Postmarketing surveillance requires surveillance for occurrences that have been identified in advance as potential safety concerns with a particular drug and also for new, unanticipated events. A regulatory agency may have approved the drug since its benefit-risk balance was judged to be favorable at the time of marketing approval, but made it clear that their view could change if certain adverse events suggested in the preapproval clinical data materialized to a concerning extent during postmarketing surveillance. In the case of cardiac adverse events, it is appropriate to monitor the occurrence (more correctly, the reports) of events such as TdP and myocardial infarctions, known potential cardiac adverse drug reactions, as well as monitoring for unexpected adverse reactions. The postmarketing surveillance paradigm can therefore be summarized as follows:

> - Quantification of any previously suspected and/or identified issues.
> - Detection of any new adverse reactions and/or other important drug-related problems (e.g., potential for abuse).
> - Conduct of benefit-risk assessments.
> - Dissemination of results to regulatory agencies with the necessary information to amend the recommendations on the use of the medicines.
> - Dissemination of information to health professionals to help them understand the benefit-risk balance of medicines that they prescribe.
> - Education of patients and the public on the benefits and risks of the medicines.

Since benefit-risk assessments must continue for the entire time that a drug is on the market, the pharmacovigilance process is an iterative one. It is also an extremely important process since it impacts many areas, including:

➢ National drug policy.
➢ The regulation of medicines.
➢ Clinical practice.
➢ Public health programs.

10.6   SPONTANEOUS REPORTING AND SAFETY SIGNALS

The spontaneous reporting system is the "fundamental underpinning" of postmarketing surveillance (Cobert, 2007, p. 12). Such systems are in place in over 50 countries, including the United States, Canada, Japan, Australia, New Zealand, and South Africa: they are also in place in the EU. In these systems all health care professionals are encouraged to spontaneously report adverse drug reactions to either the sponsor, the appropriate governmental health agency, or a third party. In some countries, including the United States, Canada, and the United Kingdom, patients are also encouraged to report such reactions. Cobert (2007, p. 12) made the following observation:

> What this means then is that the entire edifice of the drug safety system as it now stands depends on the good will and energy of nurses, pharmacists, physicians, and consumers to report AEs [adverse events]. Without them, no one would know of the AEs that are appearing as individual cases in isolated areas around the country or the world. These people must take time out of their day to report such events. The report will inevitably lead to a request for supplementary data (laboratory reports, cardiograms, hospital records, etc.) that are time and effort consuming. There is no evident or immediate gain to the reporter. The gain rather is to society at large, which is largely unaware of this noble effort.

Sponsors have particular responsibilities after a drug is marketed. They must review all safety data obtained from any source worldwide, including:

➢ Commercial marketing experience.
➢ Postmarketing clinical investigations.
➢ Postmarketing epidemiological/surveillance studies.
➢ Reports in published scientific literature.
➢ Reports in unpublished papers (as available).

10.6.1   Safety Signals

Safety signals can be detected from the information resulting from spontaneous reporting and also from other data collection methodologies. A safety signal constitutes an awareness of an excess of a particular adverse event. It is a comparative term, since "excess" occurrence of the event is judged against what would be expected in the absence of treatment with the drug, i.e., the background occurrence or incidence of the event. Safety signals are a common focus of interest in postmarketing surveillance, but they are not limited to the postmarketing arena: they can arise in nonclinical research, preapproval and postapproval clinical trials, and surveys of the published clinical literature. In postmarketing surveillance, a high background incidence of the event, e.g., cardiovascular disease in older adults in westernized countries, can make identification of excess events difficult (see discussions in Chapter 12).

Safety signals that may arise in postmarketing surveillance and that may warrant further investigation include (FDA, 2005b):

➢ Occurrence of serious events thought to be extremely rare in the general population.
➢ New unlabeled adverse events, especially if they are serious.
➢ An apparent increase in the severity of a labeled event.
➢ Identification of previously unrecognized at-risk subpopulations (e.g., groups of patients with specific genetic predispositions or specific comorbidities and those taking specific concomitant medications). It is unlikely that such occurrences would be picked up in preapproval clinical trials.
➢ New drug interactions (drug-drug, drug-medical device, drug-food, and drug-dietary supplement).
➢ Confusion about a drug's name, labeling, packaging, or use.
➢ Concerns arising from the way a drug is intended to be used (e.g., adverse drug reactions seen when higher than labeled doses have been administered or when the drug has been administered to populations for whom it is not indicated).
➢ Concerns arising from potential inadequacies of a currently implemented risk minimization action plan (RiskMAP): RiskMAPs are discussed in Chapter 14.

10.7   NONREGULATORY ORGANIZATIONS' INVOLVEMENT IN PHARMACOVIGILANCE

While much of the recent driving force behind postmarketing surveillance has come from international regulatory agencies, it is appropriate to note the activities of two other organizations.

10.7.1   The World Health Organization

The World Health Organization (WHO) has been influential in pharmacovigilance activities for the past 40 years. Much of the information in this section is synthesized from two of their reports (WHO, 2002, 2004).

As noted in Section 1.7, formalized drug safety monitoring can be traced to the thalidomide tragedy. The drug thalidomide, prescribed as a treatment for morning sickness and nausea, was introduced in 1956. It was subsequently linked to a congenital abnormality that caused severe birth defects in children of women who had been prescribed this medicine during pregnancy, a realization occurring in 1961. By 1965 it had been removed from the market in most countries (it is now on the market again for very limited indications). Following this tragedy, the first systematic international efforts were initiated to address drug safety issues. The WHO Pilot Research Project for International Drug Monitoring was created in 1968. Initially, 10 countries that already had established national reporting systems for adverse drug reactions took part. The purpose of this project

was to develop a system for detecting previously unknown or poorly understood adverse drug reactions that could be applicable internationally. This pilot project developed into the WHO Programme for International Drug Monitoring. As evidence of the success and growth of this project, the WHO 2004 report noted that, at the time of its preparation, 86 countries were participating, and the global database Vigibase had more than 3 million adverse drug reaction reports.

The WHO Collaborating Centre in Uppsala, Sweden, analyzes the reports in this database to:

> ➤ Identify early warning signals of serious adverse reactions to medicines.
> ➤ Evaluate the hazard.
> ➤ Study the mechanisms of action to aid the development of safer and more effective medicines.

10.7.2   The Council for International Organizations of Medical Sciences

In the early 1980s, in close collaboration with the WHO, the Council for International Organizations of Medical Sciences (CIOMS) launched its program on drug development and use. The CIOMS provided a forum for policy makers, pharmaceutical manufacturers, government officials, and academics to make recommendations on the communication of safety information between regulators and the pharmaceutical industry. The adoption of many of CIOMS' recommendations by the ICH in the 1990s has had a notable impact on international drug regulation.

10.8   THE SCIENCE OF PHARMACOVIGILANCE

Pharmacovigilance is not just a process, but a multidisciplinary and interdisciplinary science that is continuing to develop. Those involved in this discipline are charged with anticipating, describing, and responding to the continually increasing demands and expectations of many stakeholders, including health professionals, the public (including patients), health administrators, policy officials, and politicians.

Like other sciences, pharmacovigilance is an academic discipline replete with professional societies and professional journals. The creation of the European Society of Pharmacovigilance (ESOP, later ISoP, the International Society of Pharmacovigilance) in 1992 marked the formal introduction of pharmacovigilance to the research and academic worlds and its increasing integration into clinical practice.

As noted in Section 1.6, the benefit-risk assessment of a drug can become less favorable even if there is no decrease in safety (no increase in adverse drug reactions): this occurs when the effectiveness of the drug is not as great as originally estimated. Postmarketing evaluation of effectiveness as well as safety is therefore vital (e.g., see Lohr, 2007). A decrease in a drug's effectiveness is a potential reason for a drug to be withdrawn from the market. So too is the following reason. Consider two drugs that have been marketed for two years each. All available safety data suggest that the drugs are equally safe but that this equal safety actually represents sizable risks. If one drug demonstrates a high level of effectiveness, its benefit-risk assessment may well warrant its continued use. In contrast, if the other drug demonstrates a lower level of effectiveness, its benefit-risk assessment will be much less favorable. Even if the inferior level of effectiveness does not prompt twithdrawal of the drug from the market, it may be prescribed much less frequently. In this case, economic pressure may have an impact on the sponsor's future decisions regarding the continued marketing of this drug.

As the science of pharmacovigilance develops in the postmarketing arena, more systematic and robust epidemiological methods that take into account the limitations of spontaneous reporting will be required to address important safety issues such as the following:

> Improvement in patient care and safety in relation to the use of medicines, and all medical and paramedical interventions.
> Improvement in public health and safety in relation to the use of medicines.
> Contribution to the assessment of benefit, harm, effectiveness, and risk of medicines, encouraging their safe, rational, and more effective (including cost-effective) use.
> Promotion of understanding, education, and clinical training in pharmacovigilance and its effective communication to health professionals and the public.

10.9 ACTIVE POSTMARKETING SURVEILLANCE

While spontaneous reporting is a fundamental tool in postmarketing surveillance, and one that is vital for signal detection, it is also becoming increasingly clear that active surveillance can be beneficial and provide critical information too (e.g., see Wadman, 2007). Simply waiting to observe a certain number of safety signals in order to make evaluations is not sufficient. However, this methodological approach is not new. Inman (see Inman, 1981 a,b; Inman et al., 1986) was instrumental in founding prescription-event monitoring (PEM) at the University of Southampton (United Kingdom). PEM studies are prospective cohort studies in which "cohorts are established from prescription data and adverse events are solicited from prescribers using follow-up questionnaires" (Harrison-Woolrych and Coulter, 2007, p. 317). Inman's original goal in PEM was to recruit the first 10,000 patients who received a new drug to reliably identify any adverse drug reaction that occurred in more than 1 in 1,000 patients (see also Shakir, 2007).

10.10 EPIDEMIOLOGY AT THE U.S. FOOD AND DRUG ADMINISTRATION

The FDA's office formally known as the Office of Drug Safety (ODS) is now known as the Office of Surveillance and Epidemiology (OSE): accordingly, the acronym ODS/OSE is used here to avoid a very long full title. The ODS/OSE is comprised of a broad spectrum of health professionals from a variety of disciplines, including physicians, epidemiologists, pharmacists, nurses, project managers, social scientists, contract specialists, and technical information specialists. These persons are major contributors to many activities that impact on international public health activities, including those of the ICH, WHO, and CIOMS. The office is comprised of three divisions:

➤ Division of Surveillance, Research, and Communication Support.
➤ Division of Drug Risk Evaluation.
➤ Division of Medication Errors and Technical Support.

The Division of Surveillance, Research, and Communication Support provides critical safety data and risk communication resources to the ODS/OSE and to the CDER, and maximizes the Center's ability to:

➤ Utilize and interpret safety and epidemiological data resources.
➤ Effectively communicate risk information to health care professionals, patients, and international regulators.
➤ Evaluate risk management programs.

The ODS/OSE plays an important role in protecting public health and safety by performing several routine functions, including:

> Monitoring adverse experiences associated with marketed drug products.
> Working closely with the Office of New Drugs in developing and evaluating risk management plans designed to encourage the safe use of drug products.
> Answering important drug safety questions through the use of clinical databases.
> Tracking how drugs are used by patients and prescribed by physicians.

Under the third version of the Prescription Drug User Fee Act (PDUFA III: see the discussions in Chapter 14), which became effective on October 1, 2002, the ODS/OSE assumed an important new role in the review and evaluation of risk management plans and the need for postmarketing surveillance. It began to work closely with the Office of New Drugs in developing and evaluating risk management plans designed to encourage the safe use of drug products. This work addressed both preapproval and postmarketing drug safety. The ODS/OSE was charged with participation in pre-NDA (and pre-BLA) meetings to discuss preliminary risk management plans and to evaluate the success of these plans in the two- to-three year period following marketing approval. To produce guidance for industry on risk management activities, the ODS/OSE and the Office of New Drugs collaborated on the preparation of three concept papers. These led to three draft guidances that were circulated for public comment, culminating in the publication of three final guidance documents in March 2005. These guidances are discussed in Chapter 14.

10.11   ASSESSMENT METHODOLOGIES IN POSTMARKETING SURVEILLANCE

Postmarketing surveillance requires the reporting (passive) and collection (active) of relevant information, collating reports from all sources, analyzing these data and interpreting the results, and disseminating this information to health professionals. This process is crucial to public safety and public health. While data from preapproval trials that are presented in a newly approved drug's labeling are certainly of interest and help to prescribing physicians and their patients (recall the discussions in Chapter 8), data gathered once the drug has been marketed for some time and is in widespread use by large numbers of patients are likely to be considerably more useful, since they will come from a more heterogeneous population taking the drug in real-world conditions. Researchers, regulators, and industry representatives use experimental designs (randomized controlled trials) and nonexperimental designs (case reports, case series, and ecological, cross-sectional, case-control, and cohort studies) to conduct postmarketing surveillance.

10.11.1   Experimental Designs

Postmarketing surveillance conducted by industry investigators often employs experimental designs. The assessment of adverse events is continuously conducted in any FDA-mandated therapeutic use experimental trials and in randomized controlled trials conducted in the pursuit of new indications for the treatment and/or prevention of another disease or in a different population. Several significant adverse cardiovascular events have been identified through postmarketing surveillance of clinical trial data pursued for new indications. The cardiac event profile of rofecoxib was first made public through results of a randomized controlled trial conducted by the sponsor company in pursuit of a new indication (Bombardier et al., 2000). This drug is the central character in one of the case studies presented in Chapter 12.

10.11.2   Nonexperimental Studies

While experimental studies are an excellent source of postmarketing data, the main limitation of these designs is the relatively small number of individuals exposed to the drug: unless the sponsor pursues another indication or is mandated to conduct a trial, future trials may never occur. Nonexperimental epidemiological study designs then become the main research strategy in postmarketing surveillance and include the following:

- ➤ Case reports.
- ➤ Case series.
- ➤ Ecological studies.
- ➤ Cross-sectional studies.
- ➤ Case-control studies.
- ➤ Cohort studies.

While these methodologies are considered to follow a linear pattern of strength, with case reports being the least robust and cohort studies being the most robust (aside from the experimental designs), a recent FDA guidance noted that "FDA encourages sponsors to consider all methods to evaluate a particular safety signal" and recommended that "sponsors choose the method best suited to the particular signal and research question of interest" (FDA, 2005c, p. 12).

These studies can have formal protocols, control groups, and prespecified research hypotheses. However, because pharmacoepidemiological studies are nonexperimental in nature they may be subject to biases, making interpretation more difficult than for experimental designs (clinical trials). When performing a pharmacoepidemiological study, it is important to minimize bias and to account for possible confounding. Controlling (minimizing) bias is an issue in all types of studies, but it can be more problematic in nonexperimental studies than in experimental studies. Bias, confounding, and/or effect modification in pharmacoepidemiological studies evaluating the same hypothesis may provide different or even conflicting results. It is for this reason that pharmacoepidemiological studies employ various advanced statistical methods to reduce bias. It is almost always prudent to conduct more than one study, in more than one environment, and quite possibly to employ different designs. Agreement of the results from more than one study helps to provide reassurance that the observed results are robust.

Spontaneous Case Reports. Spontaneous case reports of adverse events are submitted to the sponsor and to the FDA by health care practitioners and by patients. These reports should be of high quality. In general, and especially in the case of serious events, follow-up by trained health care practitioners can enhance the quality, and hence the usefulness, of a report. Reports from the medical literature and clinical studies may also generate signals of adverse drug effects.

Case Series. When a signal is generated from postmarketing spontaneous reports, an initial careful review of the cases in conjunction with a search for additional cases is a useful strategy. Such additional cases may be identified from sources such as published literature, the sponsor's global adverse event databases, and other available databases such as the AERS.

It is inherently difficult to determine with a high level of certainty whether an identified event was caused by the drug in question on the basis of an individual case report. Addressing causality is a tricky issue. Three categories—probable, possible, and unlikely—are commonly used (but they are not mandated). When using these (or other) categories, it is useful to specify and describe them in sufficient detail that the regulatory agency can understand why a particular classification was made for a specific event. More information regarding the association (and potentially the causality) may be gained from later case-control studies and cohort studies with appropriate follow-up.

It is often more informative to consider information from several cases together. If one or more cases suggest the identification of a safety signal that warrants additional investigation, FDA recommends that a case series be assembled and descriptive clinical information be summarized to characterize the potential safety risk and, if possible, to identify risk factors.

Ecological Studies. One of the main limitations of spontaneously reported events is the lack of the at-risk population, i.e., the denominator, to be used to quantify the risk of the event. Ecological studies or analysis of secular trends is one approach to attempt to determine the nature and size of the population at risk of the event. This population denominator is devised in several ways and often assessed through multiple scenarios to include a best case and a worst case or, rather, the smallest and largest number of individuals likely to be exposed to the drug. Ecological studies can assess the rates of the adverse event in the population at a given time or over time. The time-dependent approach is often used to monitor the effectiveness of a risk management program in reducing the rate of exposure in a population.

Cross-sectional Studies. Studies designed to assess associations between event and exposure at a fixed time point are considered cross-sectional in nature due to limitations in determining temporal association, i.e., the occurrence of the event in relation to the time the drug was taken. These cross-sectional studies can be conducted using spontaneously reported event data paired with population-based exposure data or using drug exposure data from other sources such as administrative claims databases, registries, and clinical databases (electronic medical records).

Case-control Studies. Retrospective studies using previously collected data are termed case-control because they require identification of the event followed by a historical tracing to the exposure. Case-control studies can be used for postmarketing surveillance when a specific adverse event is rare. Modern availability of high-powered computers and informatics tools allow investigators to use the more robust nonexperimental method of a historical cohort design when retrospective data are available.

Cohort Studies. Nonexperimental studies that observe patients over time are termed cohort studies. Cohort studies are used widely in epidemiology and clinical epidemiology, and, as Haynes et al. (2006, p. 361) noted, "Evidence from cohort studies (also known as cohort analytical studies) is the next most powerful method after the controlled trial." (See also Fletcher and Fletcher, 2005, Webb et al., 2005; Woodward, 2005.) A group of individuals of particular interest in this context is patients who are receiving a specific drug. Postmarketing surveillance can be thought of as a type of cohort study involving patients receiving and not receiving a drug (perhaps a new drug) of particular interest (see Campbell and Machin, 2005). A widely used new drug may be monitored for any untoward medical event affecting patients receiving the drug. In addition to collecting this information, the incidence of adverse events with the new drug may be compared with the incidence in patients receiving alternatives to the new drug.

The cohort design can be current or historical in nature. Current cohort designs has characteristics similar to those of a randomized controlled trial, except that the patient's drug exposure is not dictated by a protocol but rather decided by the physician and patient in the same manner that would occur in clinical practice. Historical cohort designs require the employment of data that have already been collected on exposure and events. These historic cohort designs differ from current cohort designs in that the exposure and event data were collected in the past, allowing the investigator to start the cohort observation at some time period in the past and follow the cohort forward for observation of adverse events.

10.12   Methods for the Capture of Postmarketing Surveillance Data

There are several different data capture methods that are used to conduct nonexperimental pharmacoepidemiological study designs. These include prospective methods, such as patient interviews, surveys, and registries, and utilization of historical data such as administrative data and clinical databases/electronic medical records.

10.12.1   Patient Interviews

Patient interviews and assessments are conducted during a clinical trial, and a similar process can be used in the application of a nonexperimental study design. The only differences are that individuals are not randomized and the therapy they receive is not dictated by a protocol. Patient interviews in nonexperimental studies have documentation and coordination requirements similar to those ofclinical trials, and they can be very expensive.

10.12.2   Surveys

Surveys can be used to elicit specific details about the exposure and the event. This method is heavily dependent on survey respondent recall. The FDA has a recommended process for the development of a postmarketing surveillance survey that includes detailed development tracking and is grounded in patient response validation work prior to implementation. The use of appropriate psychometric techniques and translation methods is also recommended. The FDA has also stated that the sponsor should seek comments and review from the FDA to decrease threats to internal validity after data capture.

10.12.3   Registries

The FDA defines a registry as an organized system for the collection, storage, retrieval, analysis, and dissemination of information on individual persons exposed to a specific medical intervention who have either a particular disease, a condition (i.e., a risk factor) that predisposes them to the occurrence of a health-related event, or prior exposure to substances or circumstances known or suspected to cause adverse health effects. Registries allow for the capture of patient data through multiple sources of collection. They serve as a longitudinal database for a cohort of patients exposed to the drug. Registries often allow for the follow-up of a much larger number of patients than can be assessed through randomized controlled trials. One limitation of the registry methodology is that a non-xposed group is typically not enrolled, limiting comparisons that can be made to controls. The FDA has issued specific guidelines that recommend the appropriate development and use of registries, and sponsors are recommended to contact the FDA directly for guidance.

10.12.4 Administrative Databases

Administrative databases in the United States are often the result of a complex payment system for health care and health care services. Most of these databases are maintained at the organizational level, including health insurance plan carriers, hospitals and hospital network agencies, and pharmacy benefit management organizations. The databases allow for the tracking of adverse events in large populations through the use of coding schemes such as the *International Classification of Diseases, 9th Revision Clinical Modification* (ICD-9-CM) for diseases and procedures and the National Drug Code (NDC) list for drug exposures. Among the benefits of these databases are the large number of patients captured. For example, the Integrated Healthcare Information Services (IHCIS) database includes a base population of approximately 30 million covered persons and includes capture of all pharmacy, disease, and procedure claims. Other databases include Surveillance, Epidemiology, and End Results (SEER), Medicare, Medicaid claims, Canadian provincial claims databases, the Premier Inpatient Comparative Database, and large integrated health plan-health care organizations such as Kaiser Permanente.

10.12.5 Clinical/Electronic Medical Records

Electronic medical record or clinical databases are another source of patient data that can be used to conduct postmarketing surveillance. These databases differ from administrative databases in that they are primarily designed and maintained for the purposes of clinical information and record keeping rather than payment for services. Examples of such databases include the General Electric Medical database, a compilation of medical records of millions of patients recorded at the provider level. While very informative, these databases have limitations, such as missing data on service use such as hospitalizations or detailed drug exposure data.

10.13   DATA MINING

Systematic examinations of reported adverse events in large adverse event data-bases can prove informative in the overall process of risk identification and assessment. Such examinations, often called data mining, typically employ statistical or mathematical tools and can provide additional information about an excess number of adverse events reported for a given drug. Data mining can augment existing signal detection strategies and is especially useful for assessing patterns, time trends, and events associated with drug-drug interactions. However, it is important to note that data mining cannot establish causal relationships between drugs and adverse events.

10.14   THE ICH GUIDANCE E2E: *PHARMACOVIGILANCE PLANNING*

The ICH Guidance E2E, *Pharmacovigilance Planning*, was released in April 2005. This guidance noted that "The benefit-risk balance can be improved by reducing risks to patients through effective pharmacovigilance that can enable information feedback to the users of medicines in a timely manner" (ICH E2E, 2005, p. 2). Two key areas of discussion within this guidance are the safety specification and the pharmacovigilance plan.

10.14.1 The Safety Specification

The ICH E2E guidance discussed various areas within a safety specification that should be considered for inclusion for any drug. In the nonclinical arena, it is appropriate to include any nonclinical safety findings that have not been adequately addressed by clinical data. In the clinical arena, limitations to the clinical safety database (e.g., size of study samples, inclusion/exclusion criteria) and any implications with respect to predicting the safety of the drug in the marketplace should be discussed. The most important risks (adverse events and adverse drug reactions) should be identified and documented. This documentation should include "evidence bearing on a causal relationship, severity, seriousness, frequency, reversibility, and at-risk groups, if available" (ICH E2E, 2005, p. 15). Risks common to the drug's pharmacological class should be noted. The most important potential risks that require further characterization or evaluation should also be identified, and the evidence that led to the conclusion that there was a potential risk should be presented. Identified and potential interactions, including food-drug and drug-drug interactions, should also be presented.

Epidemiological evidence is also appropriate. The epidemiology of the drug's indication, including incidence, prevalence, mortality and relevant comorbidity, should be discussed. This discussion should take into account, whenever possible, stratification by age, sex, ethnic origin, and regional differences.

10.14.2 The Pharmacovigilance Plan

The safety specification is intended to help sponsors and regulatory agencies determine if there is a need for specific postmarketing surveillance data collection and to design the appropriate pharmacovigilance plan. The pharmacovigilance plan thus outlines the sponsor's strategy for postmarketing surveillance. This plan should pay particular attention to identified adverse events and adverse drug reactions to identify potential risks. To create a good plan, ICH E2E recommends that a sponsor's postmarketing surveillance experts get involved in this planning process early in product development, and that the sponsor a initiate dialog with regulatory agencies long before the marketing application is made.

Various methodologies can be used in the pharmacovigilance strategy detailed in this plan. These include:

➢ Passive surveillance.
  • Spontaneous reports.
  • Case series.
➢ Simulated reporting.
➢ Active surveillance.
  • Sentinel sites.
  • Drug event monitoring.
  • Registries.
➢ Comparative nonexperimental studies.
  • Cross-sectional study (survey).
  • Case-control study.
  • Cohort study.
➢ Targeted clinical investigations.
➢ Descriptive studies.
  • Natural history of the disease.
  • Drug utilization studies.

10.15   FUTURE METHODOLOGICAL DEVELOPMENTS

A significant number of methods are being developed to increase the efficiency and accuracy of postmarketing surveillance, including the integration of a national electronic medical record system and the use of molecular pharmacoepidemiology and pharmacogenetics.

10.15.1 The National Medical Record System

Recent advances have been made in information technology applications in the delivery of health care services. Congressional funding has streamlined the development of a national medical record system to increase the efficiency of health care and reduce the burden of disease progression. This system may represent the next step in postmarketing surveillance of drug exposures, allowing assessment of the entire U.S. population in real-time analyses. A considerable amount of work needs to be done before the implementation of this national system and its application to postmarketing surveillance. Nonetheless, with the application of pharmacoepidemiological study designs in large administrative databases, methods are continually being developed that will provide more unbiased estimates of exposure-event relationships.

10.15.2   Molecular Pharmacoepidemiology and Pharmacogenetics

The methods of molecular pharmacoepidemiology and pharmacogenetics continue to develop. These methods are dependent on gene identification, which has recently made significant advances following the work of the Human Genome Project (recall the discussions in Section 2.6). These methods may be able to better track specific candidates for adverse events that are linked to drug exposure. If genetic mapping techniques become widespread, they will be critical tools used in postmarketing surveillance.

10.16   ACKNOWLEDGMENT

The authors thank Christopher Blanchette for his contributions to this chapter. Dr. Blanchette is Associate Scientist and Director of the Center for Pharmacoeconomic and Outcomes Research at the Lovelace Respiratory Research Institute and Adjunct Professor of Clinical Research at the Campbell University School of Pharmacy.

10.17   FURTHER READING

10.17.1 Books

Fletcher, R.H. and Fletcher, S.W., 2005, *Clinical epidemiology: The essentials*, 4th edition, Philadelphia: Lippincott Williams & Wilkins.

Haynes, R.B., Sackett, D.L., Guyatt, G.H., and Tugwell, P., 2006, *Clinical epidemiology: How to do clinical practice research*, 3rd edition, Philadelphia: Lippincott Williams & Wilkins.

Jekel, J.F., Katz, D.L., Elmore, J.G., and Wild, D.M.G., 2007, *Epidemiology, biostatistics, and preventive medicine*, 3rd edition, Philadelphia: Saunders/ Elsevier.

Mann, R. and Andrews, E. (Eds.), 2007, *Pharmacovigilance*, 2nd edition, Chichester, UK: John Wiley & Sons.

Pearce, N., 2007, *Adverse reactions: The fenoterol story*, Auckland: Auckland University Press.

Strom, B.L. (Ed.), 2005, *Pharmacoepidemiology*, 4th edition, Chichester, UK: John Wiley & Sons.

Webb, P., Bain, C., and Pirozzo, S., 2005, *Essential epidemiology: An introduction for students and health professionals*, Cambridge, UK: Cambridge University Press.

Woodward, M., 2005, *Epidemiology: Study design and analysis*, 2nd edition, Boca Raton, FL: Chapman & Hall/CRC.

10.17.2 Journal Articles

Abraham, J. and Davis, C., 2005, A comparative analysis of drug safety withdrawals in the UK and the US (1971–1992): Implications for current regulatory thinking and policy, *Social Science Medicine*, 61:881–892.

Bate, A., Lindquist, M., and Edwards, I.R., 2008, The application of knowledge discovery in databases to post-marketing drug safety: Example of the WHO database, *Fundamental and Clinical Pharmacology*, 22:127–140.

Glasser, S.P., Salas, M., and Delzell, E., 2007, Importance and challenges of studying marketed drugs: What is a phase IV study? Common clinical research designs, registries, and self-reporting systems, *Journal of Clinical Pharmacology*, 47:1074–1086.

Hammond, I.W., Gibbs, T.G., Seifert, H.A., and Rich, D.S., 2007, Database size and power to detect safety signals in pharmacovigilance, *Expert Opinion in Drug Safety*, 6:713–721.

Harrison-Woolrych, M.L., 2007, Evaluating medicines: Let's use all the evidence, *Medical Journal of Australia*, 186:662.

Harrison-Woolrych, M.L., Garcia-Quiroga, J., Ashton, J., and Herbison, P., 2007, Safety and usage of atypical antipsychotic medicines in children: A nationwide prospective cohort study, *Drug Safety*, 30:569–579.

Hartford, C.G., Petchel, K.S., Mickail, H., et al., 2006, Pharmacovigilance during the pre-approval phases: An evolving pharmaceutical industry model in response to ICH E2E, CIOMS VI, FDA and EMEA/CHMP risk-management guidelines, *Drug Safety*, 29:657–673.

Hauben, M., Horn, S., and Reich, L., 2007, Potential use of data-mining algorithms for the detection of surprise adverse drug reactions, *Drug Safety*, 30:143–155.

Hughes, B., 2008, Spotlight on drug safety, *Nature Review Drug Discovery*, 7:5–7.

Kelly, W.N., Arellano, F.M., Barnes, J., et al. for the International Society for Pharmacoepidemiology and the International Society of Pharmacovigilance, 2007, Guidelines for submitting adverse event reports for publication, *Drug Safety*, 30:367–373. [Also published in *Pharmacoepidemiology and Drug Safety*, 2007, 16(5):581–587.]

Klein, D.F. and O'Brien, C.P., 2007, Improving detection of adverse effects of marketed drugs, *Journal of the American Medical Association*, 298:333–334.

Liu, J.P., 2007, Rethinking statistical approaches to evaluating drug safety, *Yonsei Medical Journal*, 48:895–900.

Lo Re, V. 3rd and Strom, B.L., 2007, The role of academia and the research community in assisting the Food and Drug Administration to ensure U.S. drug safety, *Pharmacoepidemiology and Drug Safety*, 16:818–825.

Mann, R.D., 2007, Multi-criteria decision analysis—A new approach to an old problem, *Pharmacoepidemiology and Drug Safety*, 16(S):S1.

Matsushita, Y., Kuroda, Y., Niwa, S., et al., 2007, Criteria revision and performance comparison of three methods of signal detection applied to the spontaneous reporting database of a pharmaceutical manufacturer, *Drug Safety*, 30:715–726.

Moore, T.J., Cohen, M.R., and Furberg, C.D., 2007, Serious adverse drug events reported to the Food and Drug Administration, *Archives of Internal Medicine*, 167:1752–1759.

Pearce, N., 2008, Corporate influences on epidemiology, *International Journal of Epidemiology*, 37:46–53.

Schneeweiss, S., 2007, Developments in post-marketing comparative effectiveness research, *Clinical Pharmacology and Therapy*, 82:143–156.

Schneeweiss, S., Patrick, A.R., Sturmer, T., et al., 2007, Increasing levels of restriction in pharmacoepidemiologic database studies of elderly and comparison with randomized trial results, *Med Care*, 45(S2):S131–S142.

Shakir, S.A. and Layton, D., 2002, Causal association in pharmacovigilance and pharmacoepidemiology: Thoughts on the application of the Austin Bradford-Hill criteria, *Drug Safety*, 25:467–471.

Stricker, B.H. and Psaty, B.M., 2004, Detection, verification, and quantification of adverse drug reactions, *British Medical Journal*, 329:44–47.

Strom, B.L., 2007, Methodologic challenges to studying patient safety and comparative effectiveness, *Med Care*, 2007, 45(S):S13–S15.

Sturmer, T., Rothman, K.J., and Avorn, J., 2008, Pharmacoepidemiology and "*in silico*" drug evaluation: Is there common ground? *Journal of Clinical Epidemiology*, 61:205–206.

Suissa, S., 2007, Immortal time bias in observational studies of drug effects, *Pharmacoepidemiology and Drug Safety*, 16:241–249.

Suissa, S., 2008, Immortal time bias in pharmacoepidemiology, *American Journal of Epidemiology*, 167:492–499.

Wadman, M., 2007, Experts call for active surveillance of drug safety, *Nature*, 446: 358–359.

Wysowski, D.K. and Swartz, L., 2005, Adverse drug event surveillance and drug withdrawals in the United States, 1969–2002: The importance of reporting suspected reactions, *Annals of Internal Medicine*, 165:1363–1369.

11

POSTMARKETING PROARRHYTHMIC CARDIAC SAFETY ASSESSMENTS

11.1 INTRODUCTION

This chapter provides a brief overview of marketing withdrawals that were the driving force behind the proarrhythmic cardiac safety evaluations now conducted under regulatory guidance in nonclinical and preapproval clinical studies. These evaluations were discussed in Chapters 6 and 7, respectively. In other potential organizational structures for this book, the current discussions could perhaps have preceded those in Chapters 6 and 7. However, we placed these discussions at this point so that they follow the introductions to postmarketing safety assessment methodologies provided in Chapter 10.

11.2 EXAMPLES OF RELEVANT DRUG WITHDRAWALS

The realization that drugs can have side effects is not new. The committee on Safety of Drugs in the United Kingdom was established after the thalidomide disaster to consider drug safety while the 1968 Medicines Act was being written. In its last report (for the years 1969 and 1970—some 40 years ago) the committee commented as follows (cited by Mann and Andrews, 2007b, p. 6):

> No drug which is pharmacologically effective is without hazard. Furthermore, not all hazards can be known before a drug is marketed.

Current interest lies with cardiac hazards. Shah (2007b, p. 109) commented as follows:

> Apart from drug-induced prolongation of the QT interval, and its subsequent degeneration into torsade de pointes, it is difficult to think of another type A pharmacological adverse drug reaction that has been responsible for the withdrawal of so many drugs from the market over the last two decades.

Postmarketing identification of QT prolongation, polymorphic ventricular tachycardia, TdP, and sudden cardiac death following the administration of noncardiac drugs to patients has been a significant impetus for cardiac safety becoming a major safety issue for sponsors and regulators, as evidenced by the discussions in Chapters 6 and 7.

Integrated Cardiac Safety: Assessment Methodologies for Noncardiac Drugs in Discovery, Development, and Postmarketing Surveillance. By J. Rick Turner and Todd A. Durham
Copyright © 2009 John Wiley & Sons, Inc.

Table 11.1, adapted from more extensive information provided by Talbot and Waller (2004), presents some examples of drugs that have been withdrawn from the U.K. and U.S. markets for cardiac safety reasons related to QT interval prolongation. The definition of 'withdrawal' used by Talbot and Waller was "any formulation, dose or indication withdrawn or suspended at any time" (Talbot and Waller, 2004, p. 667). The authors continued that "Although one reason may be given for withdrawal, presumably the decision was based on the overall balance of safety and efficacy with consideration of the other available alternatives." (It should be noted that the examples of market withdrawals provided in Table 11.1 took place before the publication of ICH S7B and ICH E14, discussed in Chapters 6 and 7, respectively: The nonclinical and preapproval clinical development programs for these drugs were therefore not officially guided by these documents.)

TABLE 11.1. Examples of Drug Market Withdrawals in the United Kingdom and the United States for Proarrhythmic Cardiac Safety Reasons.

Drug	Indication	Year Withdrawn
Prenylamine	Antianginal	1989 (UK)
Terodiline	Urinary incontinence	1991 (UK, US)
Sparfloxacin	Antibiotic	1996 (US)
Sertindole	Antipsychotic	1998 (UK)
Terfenadine	Antihistamine	1998 (US)
Astemizole	Antihistamine	1999 (US)
Grepafloxacin	Antibiotic	1999 (UK, US)
Cisapride	Gastroesophageal reflux	2000 (UK, US)
Droperidol	Schizophrenia	2001 (UK, US)
Levacetylmethadol	Opiate addiction	2003 (UK)

Source: Adapted from Talbot and Waller (2004, Appendix 1).

11.2.1 The Complexities of Drug Withdrawal

The complexities of drug withdrawal in general should be noted here. Drugs can be approved in different countries at different times and removed from different countries at different times (some removals are worldwide). They can also be removed, reintroduced, and removed again at a later time. Additionally, drugs that have been removed may be reintroduced at a later time with different labeling, restricted use, or restrictions of prescribers. As we have noted earlier, benefit-risk assessments can and should be continually made as new information becomes available throughout a drug's lifecycle.

11.3   CASE STUDIES

In this chapter and the following chapter, which discusses generalized cardiac safety, case studies are provided as a way of presenting examples of relevant postmarketing cardiac safety assessments and any regulatory consequences prompted by these investigations. In this chapter the two case studies concern the drugs terodiline and terfenadine, respectively.

11.3.1   Case Study I: Terodiline and UK Regulatory Activities

The following is a selection of notable dates and events in the terodiline case study's timeline:

1. Terodiline was marketed as an antianginal agent in Sweden in 1965.
2. Terodiline was first introduced in the United Kingdom in July 1986 (using a different brand name) for use in "urinary frequency, urgency, and incontinence in patients with detrusor instability and neurogenic bladder disorders" (Shah, 2007b, p. 111).
3. Some other countries in the EU approved the drug, but some did not. The primary markets were the UK, Sweden, and Japan. It is worth noting that, in general, the doses used in Sweden were lower than those used in the United Kingdom, and the doses approved in Japan were half of the recommended doses in the United Kingdom.
4. In 1987 one patient died suddenly and unexpectedly following an overdose of the drug.
5. Two proarrhythmic reactions to clinical doses were reported in each of the years 1987 and 1998.
6. Four reports of TdP occurred during the period 1998 to 1990.
7. These early cases were complicated by confounding factors, such as histories of ischemic heart disease and the use of concomitant medications. (Such complications are common, and a source of confounding influences, in many adverse reports.)
8. By May 1991 the marketing authorization holder (sponsor) was aware of 10 cases of TdP, and the UK regulatory authority (at that time called the Medicines Control Agency) was notified of this signal.
9. By July 21, 1991, there were a total of 21 adverse events, including 13 of TdP. None of these events was fatal.
10. The chairman of the Committee on Safety of Medicines reviewed these reports, and issued a "Dear Doctor" letter to all physicians and pharmacists in the United Kingdom warning them of the possibility of a fatal adverse drug reaction. Prescribers were advised that the drug should not be used in the presence of various risk factors.

11. Following this communication there was a rapid increase in reports of TdP, other arrhythmias, and other sudden unexplained deaths, and many of these were retrospective. By September 1991 there were almost 70 reports of drug-induced serious arrhythmias, the vast majority of which were from the United Kingdom.
12. While regulatory action was being considered, the marketing authorization holder withdrew the drug voluntarily from the worldwide market on September 13, 1991.

11.3.2 Case Study II: Terfenadine and U.S. Regulatory Activities

The following is a selection of notable dates and events in this case study's timeline:

1. Following initial identifications of TdP in patients who had overdosed, the first identification of TdP with therapeutic doses occurred in 1990.
2. In 1992 the drug received a black box labeling warning. Eighty-three cases of TdP and 15 deaths had been reported.
3. In January 1997 the FDA proposed removing the drug from the market.
4. In the same month the FDA gave marketing approval for the generic version of the drug.
5. In February 1998 the drug was removed from the market. A safer alternative drug was available at this time.
6. By the time the drug was removed from the market, about 100 million prescriptions had been written for 7.5 million patients, and approximately 350 deaths had been reported.

11.3.3 Discussion of Case Studies and Other Market Withdrawals

It is not uncommon for a drug to be introduced for one indication and then redeveloped for a quite different indication following the discovery of side effects that could be therapeutically beneficial. As noted, terodiline initially received marketing approval for another indication altogether, angina, in the mid-1960s in Sweden. While it was being used as an antianginal agent, side effects on the urinary bladder were noted (the drug has potent anticholinergic properties), which led to its later indication for urinary frequency, urgency, and incontinence.

It is appropriate to note that since the first published descriptions of TdP by Dessertenne (published in the French language) in 1966, it is "highly likely that any cases of [TdP] were simply not recognised, any emergent arrhythmias being attributed to the disease state" (Wild, 2007, p. 105).

It was noted in the previous chapter that underreporting of adverse drug reactions in the spontaneous reporting systems is a major problem. To illustrate the cardiotoxicity of terodiline, Shah (2007b) assumed a reporting rate of 20%, a rate he believed to be a generous estimation. It was estimated that 450,000 patients in the United Kingdom and 550,000 patients in other countries had been prescribed the drug at the time of its market withdrawal. The approximately 70 reports of cardiotoxicity in the United Kingdom at a rate of 20% would equate to 350 reports if all cases had been reported. Using the figures of 350 reports and 450,000 patients exposed to the drug results in an estimate of the incidence of risk of around 1 in 1,300. This revealed a "remarkably high cardiotoxic potential of terodiline" (Shah, 2007b, p. 112).

Layton et al. (2003) discussed pharmacoepidemiological studies conducted to investigate adverse drug reactions associated with another drug listed in Table 11.1, cisapride (their discussions are equally pertinent to other cases). Several pharmacoepidemiological studies were conducted investigating adverse drug reactions associated with cisapride use, including one that specifically examined the potential association with serious cardiac arrhythmias. While these nonexperimental studies were conducted using large population databases, they still failed to identify enough cases to establish a relationship. As the authors noted (Layton et al., 2003, p. 31):

> To estimate the risk of very rare adverse events, pharmacoepidemiological studies require very large numbers. Furthermore, the events in question need to be clinically recognisable by doctors and adequately documented in patients' notes, computer records, or on study questionnaires.

Future postmarketing evaluations of torsadogenic liability may benefit from the strategies discussed by these authors and those outlined in the previous chapter.

11.4   A BRIEF HISTORY OF THE DEVELOPMENT OF ICH GUIDANCES S7B AND E14

Having considered some examples of marketing withdrawals resulting from torsadogenic liability, it is perhaps useful at this point to briefly describe the development of ICH S7B and ICH E14. The approach represented by these guidances, which were developed in parallel, evolved over almost 10 years (and, as we have seen, it is still evolving: see also the discussions in Section 14.2).

As has been noted several times previously, the total number of participants in preapproval clinical trials is relatively small, and almost certainly too small to reliably identify rare side effects. Therefore, in the context of TdP, regulatory agencies sought approaches that could (would) identify torsadogenic liability as early as possible in lifecycle drug development. With regard to ICH S7B and ICH E14, the following is a selection of notable dates and events:

1. 1997: The EMEA's Committee of Proprietary Medicinal Products (CPMP) released a 'Points to Consider' document on the assessment of the potential

for QT interval prolongation by noncardiovascular medicinal products (CPMP/ SWP/986/96: see http://www.emea.europa.eu/htms/human/humanguidelines/ nonclinical.htm, accessed March 4, 2008).

2. June 1999: A policy conference entitled *The Potential for QT Prolongation and Proarrhythmia by Non-antiarrhythmic Drugs: Clinical and Regulatory Implications* was held by the European Society of Cardiology (see Haverkamp et al., 2000).

3. 1999: The FDA set up a working group and generated internal documents on QT assessment.

4. 2001: Health Canada submitted a Concept Paper to the FDA, and in 2003 a joint Health Canada/FDA Concept Paper was circulated and the ICH process initiated.

5. 2005: The ICH issued ICH S7B and ICH E14. These documents were adopted by the EMEA and the FDA in 2005 and by Health Canada in April 2006.

6. June 2006: The FDA established its QT Interdisciplinary Review Team (IRT). The IRT reviews study protocols and study reports for TQT studies and advises FDA review divisions. This team consists of a statistician, clinical pharmacologist, medical officer, data manager, and project manager.

7. November 2006: Health Canada released regional guidance documents to support the interpretation and implementation of ICH S7B and ICH E14. One of these is entitled *Guide for the Analysis and Review of QT/QTc Interval Data* (see http://www.hc-sc.gc.ca/dhp-mps/prodpharma/applic-demande/guide-ld/ qtqtc/qt_review_examen_e.html, accessed March 4, 2008). Another is entitled *Health Canada Question and Answer Document Regarding the ICH S7B and E14 Guidances* (see http://www.hc-sc.gc.ca/dhp-mps/prodpharma/applic-demande/guide-ld/ich/securit/qt_qa_qr_e.html, accessed March 4, 2008). On this date the web site contained four questions and answers concerning how Health Canada interprets the ICH guidances.

Guidance in this area is likely to continue evolving for some time.

11.5 Preapproval Identification of QT Liability Does Not Necessarily Mean That the Investigational Drug Will Not Be Approved

At the time of writing, the nonsedating H1 antihistamine ebastine has not been approved by the FDA because of its QT liability even though there are no documented reports of TdP associated with its extensive use in other markets. This is very likely because alternative drugs without QT liability are available, and so the overall benefit-risk balance is not favorable. On the other hand, determination that an investigational drug prolongs the QT interval, or even that it actually induces TdP or other ventricular tachyarrhythmias, does not mean that the drug is unmarketable. If the drug is thought likely to provide considerable therapeutic benefit for an unmet medical need, or to provide benefits that are judged as outweighing the risks, it is still possible that the drug will be approved. In such cases, the therapeutic benefit actually provided once the drug has been prescribed and administered to patients needs very careful assessment.

Torsadogenic liability is not an all-or-nothing characteristic of drugs. As Shah (2007b, p. 131) observed:

> Depending on the benefit offered by the drug, an incidence [of TdP] of 1 in 3,000 might be unacceptable, whereas an incidence of 1 in 500,000 might be considered acceptable, with a whole range of risk-benefit in between…Risk-benefit analysis in drug development and the regulatory approval process includes not only the alternatives already available, but also the seriousness of the condition under treatment. For relatively benign indications such as hay fever or gastroparesis, a risk of proarrhythmia even as low as 1 in 100,000 recipients is unlikely to be acceptable.

The approval of the drug arsenic trioxide is instructive here. This drug has a considerable QT liability resulting from its effects on KCNH2/hERG protein trafficking, and it has been shown to induce TdP. However, the therapeutic benefits of the drug in patients with acute promyelocytic leukemia are so marked that the benefit-risk balance has been considered favorable by regulatory agencies in the United States and the EU. (Recall the discussions in Section 4.7.2.)

Protease inhibitors used in antiretroviral therapy for HIV patients are another class of drugs with QT and torsadogenic liability. Anson et al. (2005) showed that lopinavir, nelfinavir, ritonavir, and saquinavir all caused *in vitro* dose-dependent block of KCNH2/hERG channels. However, it is considered that "their clinical benefits far outweigh their very small proarrhythmic risk" (Shah, 2007b, p. 131).

These drugs provide concrete examples of general discussions throughout the book regarding the need to assess both risk and benefit when making benefit-risk balance assessments. Benefit-risk considerations are discussed in several sections in Chapter 14, and Section 14.20, "Reflections on Central Themes in the Book," highlights the pervasiveness of these considerations throughout every stage of lifecycle drug development and therapeutic use.

12

GENERALIZED CARDIAC SAFETY

12.1 INTRODUCTION

Attention now turns to cardiac adverse events in the realm that we have called generalized cardiac safety. Events of interest in generalized cardiac safety include both cardiac and cardiovascular states, including occurrences of fatal myocardial infarctions, major irreversible morbidity (nonfatal myocardial infarctions, development of left ventricular dysfunction or heart failure), debilitating cardiovascular symptoms or events (e.g., transient ischemic attacks, marked fluid retention, and palpitations), and various pathophysiological characteristics that increase the likelihood of cardiac and cardiovascular events (see Borer et al., 2007).

Generalized cardiac safety is therefore a very broad field, and this chapter simply illustrates several aspects. First, three case studies are presented, concerning rofecoxib, rosiglitazone, and aprotinin. It should be noted that the issues and events surrounding these cases are complex, and these cases will likely continue to be discussed for some time. Therefore, in keeping with the approach taken throughout this book, we have provided introductory frameworks with some key events and dates: Additional material is listed in the chapter's Further Reading lists.

Following these case studies we address several other topics. The first topic concerns issues surrounding the long-term cardiotoxic implications of successful oncology treatments. Second, the paper by Borer et al. (2007) cited in the first paragraph in this section is addressed in more detail. Third, an approach for the prospective exclusion of unacceptable cardiovascular risk during drug development suggested by Brass et al. (2006) is considered. Finally, the topic of risk communication is discussed in further detail.

12.1.1 Some Examples of Market Withdrawals in this Arena

Table 12.1 on the following page notes some market withdrawals that fall in the domain of generalized cardiac safety investigations. The most recent of these examples forms the basis for the first of this chapter's case studies.

Integrated Cardiac Safety: Assessment Methodologies for Noncardiac Drugs in Discovery, Development, and Postmarketing Surveillance. By J. Rick Turner and Todd A. Durham
Copyright © 2009 John Wiley & Sons, Inc.

TABLE 12.1. Examples of Drugs Withdrawn from the Market in the European Union and the United States for Generalized Cardiac Safety Reasons.

Drug	Indication	Year Withdrawn	Major Safety Concerns
Fenfluramine	Appetite suppressant	1997 (EU, US)	Valvular heart disease
Dexfenfluramine	Appetite suppressant	1997 (EU, US)	Valvular heart disease
Amfepramone	Antiobesity	2000 (EU)	Primary pulmonary arterial hypertension
Phenylpropanolamine	Appetite suppressant	2000 (US)	Cerebral hemorrhage
Rofecoxib	Arthritis	2004 (EU, US)	Increased cardiovascular event risk

Source: Adapted from Talbot and Waller (2004, Appendix 1).

12.2   CASE STUDY I: ROFECOXIB

Rofecoxib is one of a group of drugs commonly referred to as COX-2 inhibitors, discussed in more detail in Section 12.2.3. These drugs seem to provide successful anti-inflammatory therapy without causing significant gastrointestinal toxicity.

12.2.1   Arthritis

Various medical disorders and injuries are characterized by pain and inflammation. Rheumatoid arthritis is an autoimmune disease whose etiology is unknown. This form of arthritis is the most common systemic inflammatory disease, affecting, for example, 2% to 3% of the U.S. population. Osteoarthritis, or degenerative joint disease, is the most common joint disease in the world, symptomatically affecting 10% of individuals over 60 years of age. In addition, radiographic evidence of osteoarthritis can be seen in most individuals over 65 years of age (Brenner and Stevens, 2006).

12.2.2   Nonsteroidal Anti-inflammatory Drugs

A relatively large group of drugs are classified as nonsteroidal anti-inflammatory drugs (NSAIDs), and these drugs are widely used to alleviate the symptoms of rheumatoid arthritis and osteoarthritis as well as to avoid (or lessen) the pain and fever associated with many arthritic condition drugs. The primary pharmacological action of NSAIDs is the inhibition of the action of an enzyme called cyclooxygenase (COX). COX is found in the lumen and membrane of the endoplasmic reticulum. This enzyme catalyzes the first step in the synthesis of prostaglandins. Prostaglandins amplify pain impulses and promote tissue inflammation. (Other mechanisms of action do occur, notably for aspirin, but the net effect of all NSAIDs is a decrease in prostaglandin production.)

12.2.3   Nonselective   Cyclooxygenase   and   Selective   Cyclooxygenase-2 Inhibitors

Nonselective COX inhibitors include aspirin, ibuprofen, and naproxen, drugs that are available without a prescription. Lower doses of NSAIDs are usually successful in treating mild to moderate pain and in treating fever. However, higher doses are usually needed to relieve the inflammation associated with arthritic disorders. While these drugs are effective pain relievers for chronic conditions, their consequent long-term use has been associated with a range of adverse events including gastrointestinal bleeding, peptic ulcers, and renal and hepatic dysfunction (Brenner and Stevens, 2006: see also Wolfe et al., 1999).

Selective cyclooxygenase-2 inhibitors, or COX-2 inhibitors (cyclooxygenase can exist as one of several isoforms), comprise a newer group of drugs that seem to provide successful anti-inflammatory therapy without causing significant gastrointestinal toxicity (see FitzGerald, 2003). This group includes celecoxib, rofecoxib, and valdecoxib, a group commonly referred to as the coxibs. In the United States, the first COX-2 inhibitor, celecoxib, was approved at the end of 1998, and the Celecoxib Arthritis Safety Study (CLASS) was the first large-scale randomized trial of a COX-2 inhibitor (see Silverstein et al., 2000). See also Chan and Jones (2007) for a discussion of the COX-2 inhibitors.

Rofecoxib and valdecoxib are no longer on the U.S. market. Valdecoxib was withdrawn from the market by the FDA in 2005 based on the occurrence of several side effects, both cardiac and noncardiac, some of which were fatal. Rofecoxib was voluntarily withdrawn from the worldwide market in 2004 following the analysis of data from a clinical trial investigating its effectiveness in the prevention of recurrence of colorectal polyps. This data analysis is discussed in the following section.

It should be noted that while celecoxib is on the market at the time of writing this book, an FDA warning indicates the drug's potential for increasing the risk of cardiovascular events. Brenner and Stevens (2006, p. 338) pondered on future developments with regard to this category of drugs:

> At the time of this writing, it is not clear if all COX-2 inhibitors share the same cardiovascular risk or if newer agents, still in development, will show less cardiovascular risk and make it to the market.

12.2.4   A Timeline of Events in this Case Study

The following is a selection of notable dates and events in this case study's timeline:

1. January 1999: The Vioxx Gastrointestinal Outcomes Research (VIGOR) trial was initiated.
2. May 1999: Rofecoxib was approved for marketing by the FDA.
3. October 1999: The Adenomatous Polyp Prevention On Vioxx (APPROVe) trial protocol was finalized. This trial was conducted to investigate the possible preventive influence of rofecoxib with regard to patients with a history of colorectal adenomas developing recurrent adenomatous polyps. Patients were randomized to receive rofecoxib or placebo for a three-year treatment period. Enrollment in the trial was completed in November 2001. The composite cardiovascular endpoint was "fatal and non-fatal myocardial infarction, unstable angina, sudden death from cardiac causes, fatal and non-fatal ischemic stroke, transient ischemic attack, peripheral arterial thrombosis, peripheral venous thrombosis, and pulmonary embolism" (Chan and Jones, 2007).
4. November 2000: The gastrointestinal and cardiovascular safety findings from VIGOR were published in the *New England Journal of Medicine* (Bombardier et al., 2000). The paper reported that treatment with rofecoxib was associated with significantly fewer clinically important upper gastrointestinal events than treatment with naproxen, a nonselective inhibitor. Three heart attacks were not included in this final version of the paper even though they had been reported to the FDA in October 2000.
5. February 2001: The FDA published compete data from VIGOR on their web site, including the final three heart attacks and data on additional cardiovascular events.
6. August 2001: A meta-analysis published in the *Journal of the American Medical Association* (Mukherjee et al., 2001) included data from the CLASS trial (8,059 patients) and the VIGOR trial (8,076 patients) as well as two smaller trials with approximately 1,000 patients each. Following

their analyses, the authors noted that "The available data raise a cautionary flag about the risk of cardiovascular events with COX-2 inhibitors. Further prospective trial evaluation may characterize and determine the magnitude of the risk" (Mukherjee et al., 2001).

7. April 2002: The U.S. labeling for rofecoxib was updated. The FDA followed an advisory panel's recommendation to require the sponsor to note a possible link to heart attacks and strokes.

8. October 2003: An analysis of pooled data from 23 studies published in the *American Heart Journal* (Weir et al., 2003) encompassed multiple disease states and included more than 14,000 patient-years at risk. The authors noted that "rofecoxib was not associated with excess CV thrombotic events compared with either placebo or nonnaproxen NSAIDs" (Weir et al., 2003). They concluded that "The totality of data is not consistent with an increased CV risk among patients taking rofecoxib."

9. September 2004: The External Data Safety Monitoring Board (DSMB) for the APPROVe trial recommended that the trial be ended. An interim analysis was conducted when 72 participants in the trial (46 in the rofecoxib treatment group and 26 in the placebo treatment group) had confirmed thrombotic events. The DSMB found an increased risk of cardiovascular events in the rofecoxib treatment arm: The relative risk was 1.92, with a 95% CI of 1.19 to 3.11 (Chan and Jones, 2007). The trial was terminated and the sponsor voluntarily withdrew rofecoxib from the worldwide market on September 30, 2004.

10. Since that date there have been several publications relevant to assessment of the benefit-risk balance of the coxibs, and readers are referred to Chan and Jones (2007) for summary of these papers. Benefit-risk assessments are likely to differ considerably among subgroups of patients defined by specific risk factors, and these authors concluded their chapter with the comment that additional systematic synthesis of all available data and quantitative benefit-risk assessments are needed for the nonselective NSAIDs and the COX-2 inhibitors.

12.2.5 Discussion

The sponsor requested a meeting with the FDA on September 27, 2004 to discuss issues surrounding rofecoxib and met with agency representatives the following day. During this meeting, the sponsor informed the agency of its decision to voluntarily withdraw the drug from the market worldwide. On September 30, 2004, the FDA released a statement addressing the withdrawal. Acting FDA Commissioner Dr. Lester Crawford commented as follows:

> Although the risk that an individual patient would have a heart attack or stroke related to Vioxx is very small, the study that was

halted [APPROVe] suggests that, overall, patients taking the drug chronically face twice the risk of a heart attack compared to patients receiving a placebo.

This comment highlights the issue of relative risk versus absolute risk. If the risks of two events are 1 in 10 and 2 in 10, respectively, it can be said that the probability of the event occurring in the second case is twice the probability of the event occurring in the first case. The same relative statement can be made for the probabilities of 1 in 1,000,000 and 2 in 1,000,000. However, the absolute risks are vastly different: 1 and 2 in 10, and 1 and 2 in 1 million. Hypothetically, suppose a drug that provided you with therapeutic benefit increased your risk of an adverse drug reaction from 1 in 10 to 2 in 10. Some individuals may feel that this is a risk they are not prepared to take. Now consider the hypothetical example of a drug that provided you with the same degree of therapeutic benefit and increased your risk of an adverse drug reaction from 1 in a million to 2 in a million. In contrast to the first scenario, some individuals may feel that, while the relative risk has doubled, the absolute risk has changed extremely slightly in the second scenario, and therefore may be willing to accept this increased risk to continue to receive the therapeutic benefit.

We noted in Chapter 8 that when providing physicians with information concerning the occurrence of adverse events during preapproval trials in an approved drug's labeling—information physicians and their patients can use to estimate the risks of adverse drug reactions if the patient takes the drug—it can be informative to provide both relative and absolute statements concerning the occurrence of adverse events in the drug treatment group versus the control group. (For many drugs, the control used in the therapeutic confirmatory trials contributing data to the labeling will be a placebo: the placebo information provides the best information on the background risk, i.e., the risk associated with not being treated with the approved drug, against which to judge the risk of the drug.) We feel the same way about information that is provided in other contexts concerning the relative likelihood of occurrences: both relative and absolute data are informative. As Gordon-Lubitz (2003, p. 95) noted, patients may make different decisions, depending on how risk information is communicated or 'framed:'

> Identical risk information may be presented in different ways, resulting in "framing bias." Perceptions of risk are particularly susceptible to framing effects. For example, patients are much more likely to favor radiation treatment over surgery when radiation is presented as having a 90% survival rate than when it is presented as having a 10% mortality rate. Although both numbers describe identical risks, the latter is perceived as more dangerous. Another common framing effect involves absolute and relative risks. For example, if a medication reduces an adverse outcome from 20% to 15%, then the absolute risk reduction is 5% and the relative risk reduction is 25%. Although the absolute and relative

risk estimates are derived from the same data, patients are more strongly persuaded by the larger changes in relative risk.

In a press release on November 5, 2004 (several weeks following the voluntary market withdrawal of rofecoxib by its sponsor) Acting FDA Commissioner Crawford commented as follows:

> Modern drugs provide unmistakable and significant health benefits, but experience has shown that the full magnitude of some potential risks [has] not always emerged during the mandatory clinical trials conducted before approval that evaluate these products for safety and effectiveness. Occasionally, serious adverse effects are identified after approval either in post-marketing clinical trials or through spontaneous reporting of adverse events...Detecting, assessing, managing and communicating the risks and benefits of prescription and over-the-counter drugs is a highly complex and demanding task. FDA is determined to meet this challenge by employing cutting-edge science, transparent policy, and sound decisions based on the advice of the best experts in and out of the agency.

Accordingly, Dr. Crawford authorized FDA's CDER to take the following measures:

> ➤ Sponsor an Institute of Medicine study of the drug safety system.
> ➤ Implement a program for adjudicating differences of professional opinion.
> ➤ Appoint a Director of the Office of Drug Safety (the position was vacant at the time of this statement).
> ➤ Conduct drug safety/risk management consultations.
> ➤ Publish risk management guidances.

Several of these measures and resulting initiatives are discussed in Chapter 14.

12.2.6 One of the Lessons Learned

We discussed nonclinical research in Chapter 6 and noted in Section 6.12 that, while nonclinical studies are informative, there are many nontrivial limitations of nonclinical development programs with regard to predicting the effects (desirable and undesirable) of the drug should it subsequently be administered in clinical trials. Greaves' (2007) observations with regard to the topic of this case study provide a strong example of this issue. He noted that reports of increased cardiovascular risks associated with COX-2 inhibitors have provided "a major lesson in drug safety and the limitations of animal studies" (Greaves, 2007, p. 294). He continued as follows:

While animal studies usually detect significant direct-acting toxicity of drugs on blood vessels, the levels of increase in cardiovascular risk reported with cyclooxygenase 2 inhibitors in patients would be difficult if not impossible to model in conventional toxicology studies performed in healthy animals.

Greaves' observations provide a powerful reminder that nonclinical studies are far from perfect when it comes to predicting potential human cardiotoxicity.

12.3   CASE STUDY II: ROSIGLITAZONE

Rosiglitazone is a member of a class of drugs called the thiazolidinediones, which are insulin-sensitizing agents used in the treatment of diabetes.

12.3.1   Diabetes Mellitus

Diabetes mellitus is a chronic disorder characterized by elevations in both basal and postmeal glucose levels. There are two major forms of diabetes, type I and type II. The typical age of onset of type I diabetes is less than 20 years of age, with a median of around 12 years of age (Brenner and Stevens, 2006). Type I diabetes is also known as insulin-dependent diabetes since patients with this disease do not produce enough insulin for healthy function. Multiple daily injections of insulin (i.e., exogenous insulin) are required to maintain life. Strict dietary rules, planned physical activity, and daily home glucose testing are also necessary.

   The characterization of type II diabetes has been changing in recent years. This form is sometimes called noninsulin-dependent diabetes. However, this is not strictly true, as some individuals with type II diabetes do require insulin. This form used to have a typical age of onset of 30 years of age or older, and the term adult-onset diabetes was commonly used. However, the epidemic of prediabetes and diabetes sweeping various Westernized countries is changing this situation: type II diabetes is now being seen in much younger individuals. It is characterized by decreased insulin secretion and insulin resistance and is often seen in obese individuals. Insulin resistance refers to the fact that insulin is not able to carry out its functions effectively: it cannot decrease plasma glucose levels through suppression of hepatic glucose production and stimulation of glucose use in skeletal muscle and adipose tissue (Raffa et al., 2005).

In individuals who do not need insulin, type II diabetes can be controlled with oral antidiabetic drugs in combination with dietary modifications and physical activity. Given that approximately 95% of diabetes is type II diabetes and that, for example, about 20 million individuals in the United States have diabetes, the need for oral antidiabetic drugs is considerable.

12.3.2   Insulin

The human hormone insulin is a protein comprised of two amino acid chains, A and B: the A chain has 21 amino acid residues and the B chain has 30 amino acid residues. Insulin plays a central role in regulating blood glucose levels within normal limits throughout the day. It lowers blood glucose levels by inhibiting production of glucose in the liver. Endogenous insulin is formed in a process consisting of several steps. Preproinsulin is synthesized in the endoplasmic reticulum of beta cells in the pancreas. Enzymatic activity then results in the creation of proinsulin. Proinsulin is then transported to the Golgi apparatus, where it is converted to insulin and C peptide (connecting peptide), the precise action of which is not known. Insulin is stored until it is released in response to rising glucose concentrations.

Recombinant DNA technology provides the ability to manufacture recombinant insulin. The insulin analog called insulin lispro is identical to human insulin except for amino acid substitutions at locations B29 and B30. Another insulin analog differs at just one location from human insulin. Insulin aspart has one amino acid substitution: the amino acid aspartic acid is substituted for the amino acid proline at location B28: the name insulin aspart reflects this substitution of aspartic acid. Insulin aspart provides an interesting example of how a small change in structure can have a significant impact on function (recall the discussions in Section 2.9.1). This single amino acid substitution in insulin aspart reduces the aggregation of insulin molecules, which means that this form of insulin dissociates rapidly and is absorbed rapidly (Brenner and Stevens, 2006).

12.3.3   Oral Antidiabetic Drugs

Oral antidiabetic drugs are used in the treatment of type II diabetes to maintain fasting and postmeal (postprandial) glucose concentrations in the normal range. There are two major classifications of these drugs, hypoglycemic agents and antihyperglycemic agents. Some of these drugs are presented in Table 12.2.

TABLE 12.2. Oral Antidiabetic Drugs.

Drug Category and Drugs	Mechanism(s) of Action
Hypoglycemic Drugs	
Sulfonylureas: glimepiride, glipizide, glyburide.	Increases insulin secretion, decreases secretion of glucagon.
Meglitinides: nateglinide, repaglinide	Increases insulin secretion during and immediately after a meal.
Antihyperglycemic Drugs	
Biguanides: metformin	Increases the number or affinity of insulin receptors in peripheral tissues (muscle and fat). Decreases hepatic glucose output.
α-Glucosidase Inhibitors: acarbose, miglitol	Competitively inhibits the enzyme α-glucosidase, leading via a chain of events to the reduction of postprandial hyperglycemia.
Thiazolidinediones: pioglitazone, rosiglitazone.	Acts as an agonist (i.e., activates) at the peroxisome proliferator-activated receptor-gamma (PPAR-γ) in skeletal muscle, adipose tissue, and the liver. Increases the number or affinity of insulin receptors in peripheral tissues (muscle and fat). Decreases hepatic glucose output.

12.3.4 A Timeline of Events in This Case Study

In this case study we have focused on the risk of myocardial infarction since two key studies reported data for this event. The studies also reported data for other events, some of them being composite endpoints, but these are not compared directly as easily as the data for the singular event of myocardial infarction. Our focus on myocardial infarction is not meant to imply a diminished importance of other cardiovascular events, and we recommend that you read the original papers and consider the other reported results too.

The following are a selection of notable dates and events in this case study's timeline:

1. 1999: Rosiglitazone was approved for marketing by the FDA.
2. May 21, 2007: The *New England Journal of Medicine* e-published a paper entitled "Effect of rosiglitazone on the risk of myocardial infarction and death from cardiovascular causes" (Nissen and Wolski, 2007). In this meta-analysis the odds ratio for myocardial infarction in the rosiglitazone group compared

with the control group was 1.43 (95% CI, 1.03 to 1.98, $p = 0.03$). This paper is discussed in Section 12.3.6 and commented on in Section 12.3.9.

3. May 23, 2007: The EMEA released a statement on the cardiac safety of rosiglitazone following the e-publication discussed in the previous point. This document is discussed in Section 12.3.5.

4. June 6, 2007: The U.S. Committee on Oversight and Government Reform held a "Hearing on FDA's Role in Evaluating Safety of Avandia®." (See http://oversight.house.gov/story.asp?ID=1325, accessed January 10, 2008.)

5. June 14, 2007: The *New England Journal of Medicine* published Nissen and Wolski's paper in the regular hardcopy format (Nissen and Wolski, 2007).

6. June 14, 2007: In the same issue of the *New England Journal of Medicine,* a paper was published by Home et al. (2007) describing interim analyses conducted on the data from the RECORD trial as a result of Nissen's paper.

7. July 30, 2007: A meeting of two FDA advisory committees, the Endocrinologic and Metabolic Drugs Advisory Committee and the Drug Safety and Risk Management Advisory Committee, was held to discuss the cardiovascular ischemic and thrombotic risks of the thiazolidinediones, with a particular focus on rosiglitazone, as presented by both the FDA and the sponsor. (See http://www.fda.gov/ohrms/dockets/ac/cder07.htm#gdac, and scroll to Drug Safety and Risk Management Advisory Committee listings for a comprehensive report of the meeting. See also an Executive Summary of the minutes from this meeting at http://www.fda.gov/ohrms/dockets/ac/07/minutes/2007-4308m1-final.pdf, accessed February 19, 2008.)

Data presented at the meeting by the sponsor are reflected by the data from the RECORD trial discussed in the subsection of Section 12.3.7 entitled "RECORD."

The results of the FDA meta-analysis of 42 randomized trials comparing rosiglitazone with placebo or other drugs (e.g., see Rosen, 2007) included the following result for the odds ratio for myocardial infarction, cardiovascular death, or stroke: 1.2 (95% CI, 0.70 to 1.8, $p = 0.40$). For a PowerPoint® presentation of the FDA meta-analysis, see http://www.fda.gov/ohrms/dockets/ac/07/slides/2007-4308s1-05-fda-mele.ppt, accessed February 19, 2008).

Two votes were taken at the advisory committees' meeting. First, the committees voted 20–3 that rosiglitazone increases the cardiac risk in patients with type II diabetes, although, as Krall (2007) noted, "many members of the committee made statements accompanying their votes that drew a distinction between the risk as compared with placebo and the risk as compared with other antidiabetic drugs." Second, the committees voted 22–1 that rosiglitazone should not be removed from the market, and should hence remain available to physicians and their patients.

8. September 12, 2007. Singh et al. (2007) published a paper in the *Journal of the American Medical Association*. They reported a meta-analysis in which the relative risk of myocardial infarction for rosiglitazone compared with a control group was 1.42 (95% CI, 1.06 to 1.91, $p = 0.02$).
9. October 18, 2007. The EMEA released a statement entitled "European Medicines Agency confirms positive benefit-risk balance for rosiglitazone and pioglitazone." This document is discussed in Section 12.3.5.
10. November 19, 2007. The FDA announced that the sponsor had agreed to add new information to the existing boxed warning strengthened August 14, 2007 (the text of which concerned heart failure) about potential increased risk for heart attacks.

12.3.5   Regulatory Perspectives

Three regulatory statements cited in the previous section, two press releases by the EMEA and the revised labeling, are provided here.

On May 23, 2007, the EMEA released the following statement (Doc Ref. EMEA/230057/2007):

> An article published in the *New England Journal of Medicine* (*NEJM*) has raised concern about a small increased risk of myocardial infarction and cardiovascular death in patients with type 2 diabetes treated with rosiglitazone. The article, based on an analysis of data retrieved from 42 clinical studies, showed a small increased risk for myocardial infarction and cardiovascular death among approximately 15,500 patients treated with rosiglitazone. However, death from all causes was not significantly increased.
>
> When rosiglitazone was first authorised in the EU in 2000, it was contraindicated in patients with a history of cardiac failure. Since then, the European Medicines Agency's Committee for Medicinal Products for Human Use (CHMP) has kept rosiglitazone under close surveillance for cardiovascular effects (cardiac failure and other cardiac disorders including myocardial infarction). The majority of the studies included in the NEJM paper have already been assessed by the CHMP. The EU product information was updated in September 2006 with information about the risk of cardiac ischaemic events.
>
> Some of the studies in the NEJM paper included patients who were not treated in line with the indication approved in the EU. Prescribers are reminded to adhere to the restrictions for use in patients with cardiac disease as set out in the product information.

Patients are advised not to stop treatment with rosiglitazone and to discuss the medication with their doctor at their next regular visit.

On October 18, 2007, the EMEA issued a statement (Doc. Ref. EMEA/484277/ 2007) entitled "European Medicines Agency confirms positive benefit-risk balance for rosiglitazone and pioglitazone." The text was as follows:

Finalising a review of the benefits and risks of the thiazolidinediones rosiglitazone (Avandia) and pioglitazone (Actos), the European Medicines Agency has concluded that the benefits of these antidiabetic medications continue to outweigh their risks in the approved indications. However, the Agency recommended changing the product information for rosiglitazone and agreed [on] further initiatives to increase scientific knowledge on the safety of both medicines.

The Agency's Committee for Medicinal Products for Human Use (CHMP) carried out this review as part of its continuous monitoring of the safety of medicines, because of new information on these medicines' side effects. This included information on the risk of bone fractures in women, and, in patients taking rosiglitazone, a possible risk of ischaemic heart disease (reduced blood supply to the heart muscle). This raised concerns over the benefit-risk balance of both rosiglitazone and pioglitazone.

Having assessed all available data, the CHMP concluded that the benefits of both rosiglitazone and pioglitazone in the treatment of type 2 diabetes continue to outweigh their risks. However, the prescribing information should be updated to include a warning that, in patients with ischaemic heart disease, rosiglitazone should only be used after careful evaluation of each patient's individual risk. In addition, the combination of rosiglitazone and insulin should only be used in exceptional cases and under close supervision.

These changes will be introduced in forthcoming regulatory procedures for rosiglitazone-containing medicines. No changes to the prescribing information for medicines containing pioglitazone were considered necessary. The Committee will review the results of currently ongoing studies. It also recommended that further studies be performed in order to increase the level of scientific knowledge on the two medicines.

Part of the new text agreed to on November 19, 2007, by the FDA and the sponsor for rosiglitazone read as follows:

> A meta-analysis of 42 clinical studies (mean duration 6 months; 14,237 total patients), most of which compared Avandia to placebo, showed Avandia to be associated with an increased risk of myocardial ischemic events such as angina or myocardial infarction. Three other studies (mean duration 41 months; 14,067 patients), comparing Avandia to some other approved oral antidiabetic agents or placebo, have not confirmed or excluded this risk. In their entirety, the available data on the risk of myocardial ischemia are inconclusive.

12.3.6   NISSEN AND WOLSKI'S (2007) META-ANALYSIS

For this meta-analysis the authors screened 116 therapeutic exploratory, therapeutic confirmatory, and therapeutic use trials. Forty-eight met the predefined inclusion criteria of having a randomized comparator group, a similar duration of treatment in all groups, and more than 24 weeks of drug exposure. Of these 48 trials, 6 did not report any myocardial infarctions or deaths from cardiovascular causes and therefore could not be included in the form of analysis chosen by the meta-analysts (recall discussions in Section 9.13 concerning approaches to this potential difficulty in meta-analysis). Forty-two trials were therefore included in this meta-analysis, and the combined total number of participants was almost 28,000.

The odds ratio for myocardial infarction in the rosiglitazone group compared with the control group was 1.43 (95% CI, 1.03 to 1.98, $p = 0.03$). These figures indicated a statistically significance difference: since the lower limit of the 95% CI is above 1.00 (unity), a statistically significant difference is indicated, and the level of this significance is provided by the accompanying p-value). These data are compatible with as little as a 3% increase and as much as a 98% increase in the odds for myocardial infarction. Since the risks of myocardial infarction are low, the odds ratio can be interpreted as a relative risk. Compared to the control, treatment with rosiglitazone is associated with 1.03 to 1.98 times the risk of a myocardial infarction.

In addition to this statement of relative risk, it is instructive to look at the absolute numbers of events: we have noted on several occasions that we believe that a risk can be best communicated by using both relative and absolute statements. In the rosiglitazone group (approximately 15,600 patients) there were 86 myocardial infarctions, and in the comparator group for this analysis (approximately 12,300 patients) there were 72 myocardial infarctions. If one makes the reasonable assumption that the results for the control group reflect the general background incidence of myocardial infarction in patients with type II diabetes who are not treated with rosiglitazone, the increase in the absolute number of myocardial infarctions is small (14 events).

12.3.7   Trials Conducted with Rosiglitazone

Three trials of interest in this case study are ADOPT (A Diabetes Outcome Progression Trial), the DREAM (Diabetes Reduction Assessment with Ramipril and Rosiglitazone Medication) trial, and the RECORD (Rosiglitazone Evaluated for Cardiac Outcomes and Regulation of Glycaemia in Diabetes) trial. The information below is based on the sponsor's Advisory Committee Briefing Document for the advisory committees meeting detailed in point 7 in Section 12.3.4 (accessed February 19, 2008).

ADOPT. ADOPT directly compared the clinical profile of three commonly used oral antidiabetic agents in long-term therapy: rosiglitazone, glyburide/glibenclamide, and metformin. Approximately 4,300 individuals participated in the trial, which was a double-blind, randomized, international, parallel group study in which patients received treatment for between four and six years. The trial was conducted to fulfill a postmarketing commitment to the FDA to conduct a long-term evaluation of rosiglitazone's safety and effectiveness. The primary endpoint was time to monotherapy failure. In addition to other measurements, the occurrence of cardiovascular events was monitored. Myocardial ischemic events included reported events of angina, coronary artery disease, and myocardial infarction. The sponsors noted several results in their summary of the study's results, including the following:

➢ The overall incidence of myocardial ischemia was low in all treatments and was comparable over the duration of the trial.
➢ In summary, the ADOPT study does not suggest that rosiglitazone was associated with an increased risk of myocardial ischemia relative to the other two commonly used antidiabetic agents.

DREAM. The DREAM trial was a double-blind, randomized, placebo-controlled, large international multicenter study designed to test if rosiglitazone and/or ramipril (an angiotensin converting enzyme [ACE] inhibitor) reduced the development of type II diabetes in nondiabetic participants with impaired glucose tolerance or impaired fasting glucose. Approximately 5,300 individuals participated and were recruited in 21 countries. The primary outcome was a composite endpoint including the development of diabetes or death. Cardiovascular and renal events were monitored: a secondary study objective was the assessment of a composite cardiorenal endpoint. An Events Adjudication Committee was responsible for the adjudication (determining the occurrence or nonoccurrence of an event based on available reports) of all primary and secondary endpoints. The sponsors noted that there was no statistical difference between rosiglitazone and placebo treatment in the incidence of the composite endpoint, myocardial infarction, or any of the individual components with the exception of heart failure (see Section 12.3.8) (see also Gerstein et al., 2006).

RECORD. RECORD was an ongoing trial at the time that the sponsor submitted their advisory committee briefing document on July 3, 2007. It is still ongoing at the time of completing this chapter. The "last patient last visit" will be in December 2008, and final study results will be available in 2009 (subsequent to this book's publication in late 2008). The RECORD trial is a six-year, randomized, open-label, noninferiority study in type II diabetic patients with inadequate blood glucose control on metformin or sulphonylurea alone. The primary outcome is the occurrence of cardiovascular death or cardiovascular hospitalization. The primary analysis is the time to the first occurrence of one of these outcomes (see Home et al., 2005).

Following the meta-analysis conducted by Nissen and Wolski (2007), Home et al. (2007) conducted an unplanned interim analysis on available data for 4,447 participants with a mean follow-up of 3.75 years, figures that translate into 16,675 patient-years of follow-up. At the time the analysis was conducted not all events had been adjudicated, so the authors provided results for adjudicated events alone and for events where adjudication was pending (i.e., counting the pending events as actual events). For acute myocardial infarctions the difference between the rosiglitazone and the control group was not statistically significant. Using only adjudicated events, the reported hazard ratio was 1.16 (95% CI, 0.75 to 1.81). Addition of the pending events increased the hazard ratio somewhat to 1.23 (95% CI, 0.81 to 1.86). In both cases, the lower limit of the 95% CI was below 1.00 (unity). Using the CIs associated with the higher point estimate, the data for myocardial infarction are compatible with as much as 19% less risk and as much as 86% greater risk.

The Data Monitoring Safety Board for this study considered all interim analyses, as well as that for myocardial infarction, and recommended that the trial continue.

12.3.8 Heart Failure

In Home et al.'s (2007) interim analysis of data from the RECORD trial, there was statistically significant evidence of a higher risk of congestive heart failure in the rosiglitazone treatment group. Looking at adjudicated events only, there were 38 events in the rosiglitazone treatment group and 17 in the control treatment group.

These figures resulted in a hazard ratio of 2.24 (95% CI, 1.27 to 3.97). The data for adjudicated events plus events pending adjudication were 47 and 22 events, respectively. These data resulted in a hazard ratio of 2.15 (95% CI, 1.30 to 3.57). These data are compatible with an excess risk of heart failure in the rosiglitazone group of 3.0 (95% CI, 1.0 to 5.0) events per 1,000 patient-years of follow-up.

The concept of events per patient-years is a way of presenting incidence data. Incidence is a rate calculated as the number of new events occurring per unit of time. In this instance the unit of time is patient-years of follow-up, which is obtained by multiplying the number of patients with each length of follow-up by the length of follow-up in years. For example, if 100 patients were followed for 2 years, these patients will have had 200 patient-years of follow-up. If another 100 patients were followed for 5 years, these patients will have had 500 patient-years of follow-up. Finally, between the two groups of patients (total of 200), the total patient-years of follow-up is 700 patient-years. The scale used in the statement "3.0 events per 1,000 patient-years of follow-up" is used to aid the interpretation. An additional three events in 1,000 patient-years of follow-up is equivalent to an additional 0.3 event in 100 patient-years of follow-up, but the former statement, expressed in terms of whole events rather than fractions of events, is typically interpreted more readily than the latter.

This finding of an increased risk of heart failure was not unexpected. It is consistent with previous evidence regarding heart failure and the thiazolidinediones (e.g., Nesto et al., 2003; Dormandy et al., 2005; Kahn et al., 2006; Singh et al., 2007). It is again worth noting that both relative and absolute data are meaningful here. First, the absolute excess risk of heart failure in the rosiglitazone treatment group was small. Second, the relative risk was more than twice that for the control treatment group. Home et al. (2007) therefore noted that "this finding is of concern and reinforces advice that patients should be warned of the risk and that thiazolidinediones should not be started or continued in patients with heart failure." As noted in Section 12.3.5, rosiglitazone was contraindicated in patients with a history of cardiac failure when first approved for marketing in the EU in 2000. On August 14, 2007, the FDA announced that the sponsor had agreed to add a stronger warning on the risk of heart failure in the drug's labeling in the form of a "boxed" warning, the FDA's strongest form of warning. The upgraded warning emphasizes that the drug may cause or worsen heart failure in certain patients (see http://www.fda.gov/bbs/topics/NEWS/2007/NEW01683.html, accessed February 19, 2008). (It should be noted that the only other thiazolidinedione currently on the market at the time of writing is pioglitazone. The sponsor of pioglitazone also agreed to add this warning. See also Section 12.3.11.)

12.3.9   Discussion

In this section, we first present limitations of the Nissen and Wolski (2007) meta-analysis and the Home et al. (2007) meta-analysis as noted by the authors themselves. Then, given that the Nissen and Wolski (2007) analysis can be regarded as the seminal event in this case study, we present some observations published by other authors.

Limitations Noted by the Respective Authors. Nissen and Wolski (2007) noted limitations of their study that included the following:

> ➤ The meta-analysis pooled the results of a group of trials that were not originally intended to explore cardiovascular outcomes.
> ➤ Most of the trials included in the analysis did not centrally adjudicate cardiovascular outcomes, and the definitions of myocardial infarction were not available.
> ➤ Many of the trials were small and short-term, resulting in few adverse cardiovascular events or deaths.
> ➤ Since the results of the analysis were based on a relatively small number of events, the odds ratios "could be affected by small changes in the classification of events."
> ➤ The confidence intervals for the odds ratios are wide, "resulting in considerable uncertainty about the magnitude of the observed hazard."
> ➤ The meta-analysts did not have access to original source data for any of the trials included in the meta-analysis (i.e., they did not have participant-level data). This precluded the use of time-to-event analysis.
> ➤ The researchers also noted that "A meta-analysis is always considered less convincing than a large prospective trial designed to assess the outcome of interest."

Related to the second bullet point here, noting the importance of definition and adjudication of events, trials indicating higher rates of heart failure are sometimes difficult to interpret unless criteria for how heart failure is defined are given. It is important to evaluate whether these events differentiated between fluid overload, a heart failure hospitalization, and new-onset heart failure.

Home et al. (2007) noted limitations of their study that included the following:

> ➤ The interim analysis conducted was an unplanned analysis conducted as a result of Nissen and Wolski's (2007) meta-analysis.
> ➤ Because the trial had not proceeded to its conclusion and because of withdrawal of participants from their assigned treatment and losses to follow-up, the analyses had limited statistical power to detect treatment differences, and the authors noted that the data "were insufficient to determine whether the drug was associated with an increase in the risk of myocardial infarction."

- ➤ RECORD is an open-label trial.
- ➤ The primary composite endpoint reflects the study's objective, which is an assessment of overall cardiovascular safety. However, because of this, it includes "some hospitalizations (e.g., for valvular disease) that no observer would consider potentially related to treatment." Since this favors the achievement of noninferiority (the study is a noninferiority trial, so this favors finding what is hoped for), the authors noted that "sensitivity analyses will be performed at the end of the study that include only events related to atherosclerotic arterial disease."

Limitations Noted in Publications by Other Authors. Several publications by other authors have addressed the meta-analytic methodology employed by Nissen and Wolski (2007). Pignone's (2007) commentary on this meta-analysis included some of the limitations detailed by Nissen and Wolski themselves, and also noted others, including the following:

- ➤ Lack of participant-level data limits the assessment of the role of important covariates such as age and sex, as well as precluding time-to-event analysis.
- ➤ A fixed effects model was used to combine information from the studies included in the analysis.

We discussed the methodology of fixed effects models and random effects models in general terms in two subsections of Sections 9.10.2, along with the ramifications of the choice made between them when conducting a specific meta-analysis. The observations made by Pignone (2007) in the specific case of the Nissen and Wolski (2007) meta-analysis provide a concrete example of the general points made by Whitehead (2002) and Kay (2007) as presented in Chapter 9. Nissen and Wolski (2007) chose to use a fixed effects model for combining studies. As Pignone (2007) commented:

> A fixed-effect model assumes that all of the trials included drew their participants from the same underlying patient pool, an assumption that is difficult to support. It would have been more appropriate to use a random-effects model, which accounts for both within- and between-study variability. Fixed-effects models usually produce narrower confidence intervals for their summary estimates, which leads to overestimation of the precision of the data.

As noted in the first subsection of Section 9.10.2, Whitehead (2002, pp. 153–154) expressed the final sentence of this Pignone quote in equivalent terms:

One advantage of the random effects model is that it allows the between-study variability in the treatment difference estimates to influence the overall estimate and, more particularly, its precision. Therefore, if there is substantial variability this will be reflected in a wide confidence interval.

What might be the consequences of the wider confidence intervals that would likely have resulted had Nissen and Wolski (2007) employed the random effects model suggested by Pignone (2007)? Before answering this question, we will remind ourselves of Nissen and Wolski's result: the odds ratio for myocardial infarction in the rosiglitazone group compared with the control group was 1.43 (95% CI, 1.03 to 1.98, $p = 0.03$). These figures indicated a statistically significance difference: since the lower limit of the 95% CI is above 1.00 (unity), a statistically significant difference is indicated. These data are compatible with as little as a 3% increase and as much as a 98% increase in the odds for myocardial infarction. Returning to our question concerning the consequences of a wider CI resulting from the use of a random effects model, consider first the impact on the upper limit of the CI. This would increase from the reported value of 1.98 that resulted from the use of a fixed effects model. Therefore, the results would be compatible with as much as an X% increase in odds for myocardial infarction (the exact value, one that is greater than 98%, would be reported here). However, and much more importantly given the attention typically afforded to the lower CI in such analyses, the reported value of 1.03 resulting from the use of a fixed effects model would have decreased. If it decreased but still did not fall below 1.00 (unity) a statement would be made that the data are compatible with as little as a Y% increase in odds for myocardial infarction (the exact value, one that is less than 3%, would be reported here). If the lower confidence limit decreased to a value below 1.00 (unity), there would be two related consequences. First, a claim of a statistically significant result at the traditional $\alpha = 0.05$ level could not be made. Also, the second statement concerning the data's compatibility would need to be changed to include the word "decrease," and it would be expressed as follows: "The data are compatible with as much as a Z% decrease (the exact value would be reported here) in the odds for myocardial infarction."

In fairness, the authors of this book certainly acknowledge and agree that, as a general statement, clinically significant (clinically important) effects can certainly be found in situations where a traditional level of statistical significance is not observed: that is, blind adherence to characterizing a result as either significant or not significant using a $\alpha = 0.05$ level is not necessarily a clinically meaningful strategy in every case. However, applying equal fairness in the other direction, general acceptance of the $\alpha = 0.05$ level does at least provide a line in the sand in such situations (as do the regulatory thresholds of concern related to drug-induced QTc prolongation, discussed in detail in Chapter 7). When researchers report a level of statistical significance that is slightly above 0.05, the statement is often made that the result "approached" statistical significance. However, when researchers report a level of statistical significance that is just below 0.05, it is exceedingly unlikely that they made the statement that their result "only just made it." Indeed, in the latter context, achieving statistical significance is typically, if implicitly, regarded as an all-or-none phenomenon, while in the former case it is not.

Returning to the specific case at hand, Diamond et al. (2007, p. 578) also commented on the limitations of the Nissen and Wolski (2007) meta-analysis:

> The meta-analysis was not based on a comprehensive search for all studies that might yield evidence about rosiglitazone's cardiovascular effects. Studies were combined on the basis of a lack of statistical heterogeneity, despite substantial variability in study design and outcome assessment. The meta-analytic approach that was used required the exclusion of studies with zero events in the treatment and control groups. Alternative meta-analytic approaches that use continuity corrections show lower odds ratios that are not statistically significant. We conclude that the risk for diabetic patients taking rosiglitazone is uncertain: Neither increased nor decreased risk is established.

The authors discussed the justification for pooling data from studies that were heterogeneous on the basis of a lack of statistically significant evidence of heterogeneity as indicated by the Cochran Q test, a test that has "limited ability to detect variation across studies with sparse [event] data" (Diamond et al., 2007). [To the authors of this book, this appears to illustrate an argument similar to that made a couple of paragraphs ago: that is, authors regard the absence of statistically significant evidence of something as an all-or-none statement of its complete absence. Despite reasonable evidence of heterogeneity, the fact that the Cochran Q test did not attain statistical significance was regarded as justification to disregard this reasonable evidence altogether.]

Diamond et al. (2007) also noted that Nissen and Wolski (2007) used a single methodological approach called the Peto fixed effects model, an approach that requires the exclusion of studies with zero events. Diamond et al. presented illustrations of the use of alternate models, some alternate fixed effects models and some random effects models, and analyses that circumvented this exclusion difficulty, and demonstrated "the fragility of effect sizes" for the risk of myocardial infarction. Odds ratio point estimates were typically of lesser magnitude, and CIs typically contained unity (Diamond et al., 2007).

It is of concern in such situations when the results obtained by different models are qualitatively different from each other as well as quantitatively different (a certain degree of numerical, or quantitative, difference is to be expected in the results). This occurrence makes it problematic to pick a certain model, to the exclusion of all others, and make powerful interpretations and statements on the basis of the single result obtained. In contrast, qualitatively similar results obtained with various analytical approaches produce a much greater degree of confidence in the eventual conclusion. A particularly clear example of this phenomenon is seen in the analysis of efficacy data in preapproval clinical trials. Data from two analysis populations, the intent-to-treat (ITT) population and the per-protocol population, are typically used in two separate sets of efficacy analyses. The ITT population comprises all participants in a clinical trial who were randomized to a treatment group, regardless of the extent of their subsequent involvement in the trial. The per-protocol population is a subset of the ITT population comprising participants whose involvement in the trial was compliant with requirements and activities detailed in the study's protocol. As far as regulatory agencies are concerned, when reviewing a marketing application, it is encouraging if the results from the ITT and per-protocol analyses are qualitatively similar (see Turner, 2007, pp. 166–168 for discussion of how and why qualitative dissimilarity between the two sets of analyses can reduce the overall confidence placed in the trial's findings).

Following a discussion of the ramifications of many factors and limitations in the conduct of a meta-analysis, Diamond et al. (2007) observed that "In the end, we believe that only prospective clinical trials designed for the specific purpose of establishing the cardiovascular benefit or risk of rosiglitazone will resolve the controversy about its safety." Their paper was e-published by the *Annals of Internal Medicine* on August 6, 2007, and subsequently published in the regular hard-copy format on October 16, 2007. Their conclusion concerning the current status of knowledge about the cardiovascular risk of rosiglitazone is in agreement with, and preceded, the conclusion reached by the FDA and indicated in the revised labeling for rosiglitazone released on November 19, 2007 (recall the discussion in Section 12.3.5): "In their entirety, the available data on the risk of myocardial ischemia are inconclusive."

12.3.10   Current Marketing Status of Rosiglitazone

The events in this case study are many and complex. How, then, are we to provide some empirical conclusion here? The simplest may be the following: At the time of preparing the final text of this book, rosiglitazone remains on the market in both the US and the EU.

12.3.11   Rosiglitazone and Pioglitazone

As noted in Section 12.3.8, rosiglitazone and pioglitazone are the only thiazolidinediones on the market at the time of writing. While this case study has focused on rosiglitazone, the following references are examples of articles that provided discussion of both of these thiazolidinediones: Balkrishnan et al. (2007); Norris et al. (2007); Berneis et al. (2008); and Doggrell (2008).

12.4   CASE STUDY III: APROTININ INJECTION

This case study is brief and was added to the chapter during the final stages of its preparation following a segment on the television program "60 Minutes," aired on February 17, 2008. This segment discussed events surrounding the drug aprotinin, a drug that has been used to limit blood loss in at-risk patients during heart surgery.

In the January 26, 2006 edition of the *New England Journal of Medicine* Mangano et al. (2006) reported that the "the use of aprotinin was associated with a dose-dependent doubling to tripling in the risk of renal failure requiring dialysis among patients undergoing primary or complex coronary-artery surgery." They also noted that, for the majority of patients, damage to other organs (the heart and the brain) accompanied the damage to the kidneys, "suggesting a generalized pattern of ischemic injury" (Mangano et al., 2006). The authors noted one limitation of their study: it was an observational (nonexperimental) study, not a randomized, controlled clinical trial. Given this lack of randomization, the investigators reviewed and employed more than 200 covariates per patient that were then used on a patient-by-patient level when conducting a multivariate statistical analysis called propensity scores analysis to obtain their results.

Karkouti et al. (2006) also used propensity scores analysis in a case-controlled comparison of aprotinin and another drug, tranexamic acid, in high-transfusion-risk cardiac surgery. They concluded that "Within the confines of propensity score matching, our results suggest that aprotinin may be associated with renal dysfunction."

Randomized trials may be difficult to conduct when investigating certain drugs in certain patients, and sufficiently large and comprehensive nonexperimental studies may provide "the best information available about side effects" (Avorn, 2006). However, Avorn (2006) continued as follows:

> Propensity scores and other multivariable techniques applied to epidemiologic research cannot always control for all the inevitable selection bias, making the transparency of methods and raw data even more important than in randomized trials.

Vlahakes (2006) commented on Mangano et al.'s (2006) study, as did Hiatt (2006). At the time his article was published, Dr. Hiatt was the chair of the FDA's Cardiovascular and Renal Drugs Advisory Committee, and his article describes how this committee examined relevant data (Dr. Hiatt noted that the opinions expressed were his and not necessarily those of the FDA or this FDA advisory committee).

12.4.1   FDA Announcements

The following is a selection of dates and events in this case study's timeline:

1. February 8, 2006: Following the e-publication of the Karkouti et al. (2006) article on January 20, 2006, and the January 26, 2006 publication of the Mangano et al. (2006) article, the FDA announced that it was evaluating these studies, along with other studies in the literature and reports submitted to the FDA through the MedWatch program, to determine if labeling changes or other actions were warranted (see http://www.fda.gov/cder/drug/advisory/aprotinin.html, accessed February 18, 2008). The FDA noted that, while it conducted its evaluations, physicians using this drug should carefully monitor patients for the occurrence of toxicity, particularly to the kidneys, heart, or central nervous system, and promptly report adverse event information to the sponsor or to the FDA MedWatch program. They also noted that physicians should consider limiting the use of the drug to those situations where the clinical benefit of reduced blood loss is essential to medical management of the patient and outweighs the potential risks.

2. December 15, 2006: The FDA approved revised labeling for aprotinin "to strengthen its safety warnings and to limit its approved usage to specific situations." The purpose of the label change was to inform physicians and patients about the risks associated with the drug and "to ensure they understand the new warnings and use the product as directed by the label" (see http://www.fda.gov/bbs/topics/NEWS/2006/NEW01529.html, accessed February 18, 2008).

3. November 5, 2007: The FDA announced that, at the agency's request, the sponsor had agreed to a marketing suspension of aprotinin (see http://www.fda.gov/bbs/topics/NEWS/2007/NEW01738.html, accessed February 18, 2008). As noted in this press release, the marketing suspension was requested by the FDA pending "detailed review of preliminary results from a Canadian study that suggested an increased risk for death. FDA requested the suspension in the interest of patient safety based on the serious nature of the outcomes suggested in the preliminary data."

Given the brief nature of this final case study, readers who are using this book as a course text may wish to conduct a more detailed literature review and prepare a more thorough case study report (see several papers in Section 14.24).

12.5   ONCOLOGY TREATMENT AND CARDIOTOXICITY

The assessment of benefit-risk balances associated with pharmacotherapy is an ongoing theme in our discussions. Consideration of oncology pharmacotherapy illustrates how benefit-risk balances can differ in different circumstances. Consider the scenario in which an individual oncology patient's diagnosis is that his or her cancer is likely to be terminal in several months. Some patients may be prepared to take a sizable risk in an attempt to prolong their life by a relatively short but personally significant time and/or to improve their quality of life for their remaining time: In this scenario the risk of cardiotoxicity several years in the future may not seem at all significant since the patient's life is likely to end much sooner.

However, a paradox has arisen in this therapeutic area. Pharmacotherapy (sometimes in conjunction with surgery and/or radiation therapy) has proved very successful in many cases: disease states have gone into remission and patients have lived for considerable periods of time following their treatment. While the prolongation of life can be considered a great success, an unfortunate corollary in some cases is that cardiotoxicity can be experienced by such patients years after the cessation of their treatment. Some of these patients may have exhibited cardiac/cardiovascular symptoms at the time of pharmacotherapy, and others may not. Cardiotoxicity following cancer chemotherapy and thoracic radiotherapy is therefore a special situation that remains a significant problem in long-term survivors. The following discussions are based on a presentation given by Polina Voloshko, MD, at the CBI Second Annual Cardiac Safety Assessment Summit, in Alexandria, Virginia, in January 2008.

At therapeutic doses some cytotoxic anticancer drugs, particularly anthracyclines, can produce myocardial damage by direct damage to subcellular systems within cardiac myocytes. Cardiovascular manifestations of cancer chemotherapy include:

> ➢ Heart failure.
> ➢ Cardiomyopathy.
> ➢ Pericardial/pleural effusion.
> ➢ Myocardial ischemia.
> ➢ Arterial hypotension and hypertension.
> ➢ Myocarditis.
> ➢ Bradycardia.
> ➢ Thromboembolism.
> ➢ QT interval prolongation (recall the earlier discussions of arsenic trioxide).

The time course of various cardiotoxicities can differ considerably following chemotherapy and radiation therapy. Acute concerns can arise, e.g., immediately after a single dose of anthracycline therapy. Others can develop slowly after completion of therapy (perhaps during the following 12 to 48 months), and some surface up to 12 years following radiation therapy or multiple chemotherapies.

Various noninvasive methodologies have been used to monitor cardiotoxicity, including radionuclide ventriculography, ECG and stress myocardial perfusion imaging (ischemic complications), and 24-hour Holter monitoring (arrhythmias). Currently, Doppler echocardiography is the most widely used noninvasive method. This method allows the identification of several forms of cardiac/cardiovascular complications (including subclinical diagnoses), including left ventricular dysfunction, valvular heart disease, pericarditis and pericardial effusion, and carotid artery lesions. Echocardiographic evaluations are therefore useful for oncological patients before, during, and long after therapy.

Echocardiography has several characteristics that make it particularly useful: as well as being noninvasive, it is widely available in many countries and is a relatively cheap procedure. Echocardiography provides good and widely used measures, it can be conducted by all sonographers, and the interrater correlations are relatively high. However, when large multicenter trials are conducted, a core echocardiography lab can be extremely valuable. A properly designed study protocol, thoroughly trained staff at all investigational sites, and the reproducibility of analysis that results from the employment of a small number of trained experts at the core lab contribute enormously to optimum-quality data acquisition.

Measurement parameters that can be used as an index of systolic function include left ventricular ejection fraction, left ventricular systolic dimension, left ventricular diastolic dimension, and left ventricular endocardial fraction shortening. Indices of diastolic function include early peak mitral inflow velocity (represented as E), atrial peak mitral inflow velocity (represented as A), and the E/A ratio.

Finally, here, while echocardiography is widely used to assess cardiotoxicity in oncological cases, it can also be used in other therapeutic areas.

12.6   GENERAL DISCUSSIONS

Borer et al. (2007) published a paper entitled *Cardiovascular safety of drugs not intended for cardiovascular use: Need for a new conceptual basis for assessment and approval* that addresses many key issues in generalized cardiac safety. The following commentary is based upon their paper.

Borer et al. (2007, p. 1905) noted that there is general consensus on the nature of major cardiovascular risks, and that these risks comprise three broad categories:

➢ Cardiovascular death or major irreversible morbidity (e.g., nonfatal myocardial infarction and stroke).
➢ Debilitating but reversible cardiovascular symptoms or events (e.g., fluid retention sufficient to cause dyspnoea, palpitations, lightheadedness, syncope due to nonlethal arrhythmias, angina, and transient ischemic attacks).
➢ Pathophysiological characteristics that increase the likelihood of cardio-vascular adverse events (e.g., hypertension, accelerated thrombogenesis, and asymptomatic arrhythmogenesis).

Their paper also addressed TdP and the need for nonclinical and clinical preapproval proarrhythmic liability testing, but having discussed this topic in Chapters 6 and 7, we do not address it in this chapter.

12.6.1   Challenges of Spontaneous Cardiac Event Reporting

The detection of cardiac events in preapproval trials of noncardiac drugs generally relies on "spontaneous reporting of adverse events by investigators not trained in cardiology, who may not recognize subtle cardiovascular complaints" (Borer et al., 2007, p. 1905). A similar situation arises in postapproval detection of cardiac events: this detection "depends on spontaneous cardiac event reporting by practitioners (largely non-cardiologists), a notoriously insensitive and inefficient approach" (Borer et al., 2007, p. 1905). Obtaining reliable cardiac event data both pre- and postapproval is therefore challenging.

12.6.2   Changing the Nature of Preapproval Clinical Trials

The limitations of preapproval trials were discussed earlier, and it has been noted that the probability of observing occurrences of rare (drug-related) side effects is very small in such trials as they are currently conducted. Given these limitations, two theoretically advantageous strategies are:

> ➢ Increase the length of preapproval trials.
> ➢ Increase the sample sizes employed in preapproval trials. The relatively small number of participants in preapproval trials provides limited statistical power to detect differences in the rates of infrequent events between the investigational drug and a comparator drug. This limitation is even more salient if the pretreatment cardiovascular risk is low. Given the exhaustive exclusion criteria used in most preapproval trials, this is more likely than not to be the case.

However, these strategies have "potentially important drawbacks" (Borer et al., 2007, p. 1905) as well as potential advantages. Cost is a factor in both cases. The costs of trials can increase markedly as they increase in duration, and there are also substantial costs of increasing the sample size while maintaining the duration: such costs relate to additional participant evaluation and to accelerated recruitment. Moreover, in the case of increased trial duration, if the patent life of the drug were to remain the same, the manufacturer would have less time to recoup the cost of bringing a drug to market. (Related to this point, Hondeghem et al. [2007] suggested that the potential benefits of patent life prolongation should be considered.)

12.6.3   Changing the Approach to Cardiovascular Risk Assessment

Following initial nonclinical assessment of drug effects on cardiac physiology and pharmacology, Borer et al. (2007) observed that human pharmacology and therapeutic exploratory trials of noncardiac drugs should evaluate prespecified parameters including, but not limited to:

➢ Body weight.
➢ Blood pressure.
➢ Blood lipid concentrations.
➢ Coagulation profiles.
➢ Cardiac dimensions.
➢ Left ventricular size and function.
➢ To the extent feasible, interactions between drug effects and specific genomic or proteomic characteristics.
➢ QT intervals and other ECG parameters.

Data from these assessments can then provide the information upon which therapeutic confirmatory trials of noncardiac drugs can be based and designed. The study protocols for such trials should contain related information and instruction, including:

➢ Prespecification of the measurement of cardiovascular events of interest and associated precise statements of the diagnostic criteria to be used in the identification of these events.
➢ Regular measurement of variables to detect clinically silent events (this should be mandated).
➢ Definition of a method for pooling adverse events in the drug development program. This strategy would enhance the statistical power to identify any problems that exist. (This could also appear in a statistical analysis plan associated with the protocol.)

The size of therapeutic confirmatory trials for drugs for noncardiac indications is typically on the order of several thousand participants (of whom half will be exposed to the investigational drug if participants are randomized 1:1 with the drug and a control treatment). From an ethical perspective, it can be argued that the appropriate size of a trial should be the smallest number that reasonably permits the testing of the hypothesis of interest (e.g., in a preapproval superiority trial, this may be that the investigational drug displays statistically significantly more efficacy than the control treatment). In addition, the extensive exclusion criteria often employed in such trials may mean that participants are at low cardiovascular risk. Taken together, these characteristics of therapeutic confirmatory trials mean that "the capacity to detect cardiovascular adversity is inherently limited even if such events truly are associated with therapy" (Borer et al., 2007, p. 1906).

Brass et al. (2006) have proposed an approach that may be useful in some instances. In discussions of the TQT study in Chapter 7, we saw that confidence intervals about the mean QTc effect (the indicator for torsadogenic liability employed in this study) are used to exclude a threshold effect of regulatory concern. Brass et al. (2006) proposed a similar approach that could be used to investigate the relative risk of cardiovascular adverse events during drug development programs where surrogate efficacy endpoints related to functional capacity or symptoms are being employed (versus development programs using clinical outcomes such as death or myocardial infarction). The authors commented as follows (Brass et al., 2006, p. 166):

> From a public health perspective, we propose that the most relevant safety issue concerning a new drug is not the specific, quantitative estimation of the risk associated with the drug, but rather defining with a reasonable degree of certitude that the risk does not exceed some predefined unacceptable level. Specifically, in the context of a clinical development program, the point estimate of any absolute or relative risk associated with a drug is less important than the upper limit of the 90% confidence interval (or other numeric boundary) associated with that estimate.

Implementation of this approach in drug development would require identification, or at least a quantitative operational definition, of an unacceptable level of cardiovascular risk given the expected extent of the therapeutic benefit. Unlike the definitions provided in ICH E14 concerning the regulatory threshold of concern with regard to QTc prolongation, to our knowledge there are currently no equivalent regulatory statements for the other events listed earlier in this section.

If the test treatment and placebo are truly equal in terms of the risk of an adverse event, the sample estimates of the relative risk from a study will be around 1.00 (unity) but will have an upper confidence bound greater than 1.00. Increasing the sample size will have the effect of narrowing the width of a CI and thus excluding values of the relative risk that are of concern. A greater risk of an adverse event may be considered acceptable for a new drug associated with a larger therapeutic benefit than for a drug with a lesser degree of benefit. Once an upper bound for the regulatory threshold of concern has identified (e.g., an upper bound of 1.25 for the relative risk of a significant cardiovascular event), the sponsor could prospectively plan studies that were large enough and long enough to exclude the upper bound. At the time of a regulatory submission the sponsor could then conclude, with 90% confidence, that the true relative risk of a cardiovascular event did not exceed 1.25.

A practical suggestion presented by Brass et al. (2006) on the implementation of their approach is to extend the length of therapeutic exploratory and confirmatory trials past the time at which statistically significant evidence for the efficacy outcome is obtained. This would provide the opportunity to accrue the patient-years of follow-up needed to exclude the threshold of importance.

To our knowledge, this approach is unique in that it prospectively and proactively considers the role of risk in the consideration of the benefit-risk trade-off. However, Brass et al. (2006) noted the following limitations:

> ➤ The approach would not be effective in target populations with low background rates of the event, or when relative risks less than 1.5 were to be excluded, because the sample size requirements would be too great.
> ➤ This approach would increase the costs and duration of studies. Adjudication of cardiovascular events is costly and time-consuming in any study.
> ➤ Participants may be reluctant to enroll in studies with long periods of observation, given the chance of being randomized to a placebo treatment group.
> ➤ It is essential to identify precisely which adverse outcome is relevant. While some indications can be provided by knowledge of previously approved drugs in the same chemical class (if they exist), sponsors cannot always know which adverse outcome is the target for intensive monitoring during development. For example, an unacceptably high cardiovascular risk may be excluded by this approach, while unacceptably high hepatotoxicity may not be detected because effects on the liver may not have been monitored as closely.
> ➤ Identifying an unacceptable risk threshold is difficult and must consider a number of factors: the seriousness of the adverse event; the size of the population which may be exposed; the background incidence; potential uncertainty concerning the benefit of the new drug; and availability of other therapies. In addition, a *single* threshold of regulatory concern may not be appropriate.

We would like to expand on this last point, i.e., the appropriateness of the threshold, since it illustrates a point addressed again in Section 14.2. In reference to this point, Brass et al. (2006, p. 170) noted that:

> Unfortunately, population risk estimates do not easily translate into risk-benefit judgments for individual patients. In particular, it has been suggested that patients with severely debilitating symptoms and decreased quality of life may be willing to accept some increased risk in exchange for the possibility of symptomatic relief. For example, 40% of patients with mild to moderate congestive heart failure indicated a willingness in one study to accept an absolute 5% increase in risk of death associated with the therapy if they might regain some physical function. Thus, if the upper bound for the confidence interval can be defined, patients and physicians might find relative risks for morbid events of 1.5 or even 2.0 (with point estimates well below these levels) acceptable if the pharmacotherapy provides meaningful symptomatic relief for a debilitating symptom complex and the absolute risks are not excessive.

Identifying and quantifying risks so that they can be readily and meaningfully provided to prescribing physicians and their patients can be difficult. The risks quantified during lifecycle drug development pertain to a study population or multiple populations, but the consumer (and assumer) of the risk information and the actual risk for the single individual patient is the patient him- or herself. In regard to the clinical communication of risk, Bogardus et al. (1999, p. 1040) noted as follows:

> The biggest challenge may be to help patients reconcile averages derived from populations and their meaning at an individual level. For example, although lower serum cholesterol levels result in a reduction in the number of myocardial infarctions in a large population of patients, an individual patient may be chagrined to learn that he is paying a lot of money and possibly experiencing a reduction in his quality of life for a very small chance of individual benefit. Or, a patient may face a given treatment with the reassuring advice from a physician that the chances of a serious complication are only 1 in 100, but he/she may remain very concerned about whether he/she will be that 1 in 100. The angioplasty patient does not experience a 4% myocardial infarction complication; for each individual patient, the outcome is an all-or-none phenomenon. Thus, even if we can identify and describe risks, the information must ultimately be expressed in terms that are meaningful to individual patients and must allow them to make decisions with which they are comfortable.

12.7 FURTHER READING

12.7.1 Paper of Particular Interest

Shah, R.R., 2007, Cardiac repolarisation and drug regulation: Assessing cardiac safety 10 years after the CPMP guidance, *Drug Safety*, 30:1093–1110. [This paper was cited in Chapter 7 since it addresses both acquired QT interval prolongation and QT interval shortening. In addition, it addresses "Cardiac Safety in Broader Context," and the paper is highly recommended to readers.]

12.7.2 Journal Articles Related to the Case Study I

Andersohn, F., Schade, R., Suissa, S., et al., 2006, Cyclooxygenase-2 selective nonsteroidal anti-inflammatory drugs and the risk of ischemic stroke: A nested case-control study, *Stroke*, 37:1725–1730.

Arellano, F.M., 2005, The withdrawal of rofecoxib, *Pharmacoepidemiology and Drug Safety*, 14:213–217.

Aw, T.J., Haas, S.J., Kiew, D., et al., 2005, Meta-analysis of cyclooxygenase-2 inhibitors and their effects on blood pressure, *Archives of Internal Medicine*, 165:490–496.

Chan, A.T., Manson, J.E., Albert, C.M., et al., 2006, Nonsteroidal anti-inflammatory drugs, acetaminophen, and the risk of cardiovascular events, *Circulation*, 113: 1578–1587.

Depont, F., Fourrier, S., Merliere, Y., et al. for the CADEUS Team, 2007, The CADEUS study: Methods and logistics, *Pharmacoepidemiology and Drug Safety*, 16:571–580. [The acronym CADEUS represents the COX-2 Inhibitors and NSAIDs: Description of Users trial.]

Drazen, J.M., 2005, COX-2 inhibitors: A lesson in unexpected problems, *New England Journal of Medicine*, 352:1131–1132.

FitzGerald, G.A., 2004, Coxibs and cardiovascular disease, *New England Journal of Medicine*, 351:1709–1711.

Furberg, C.D., Psaty, B.M., and FitzGerald, G.A., 2005, Parecoxib, valdecoxib, and cardiovascular risk, *Circulation*, 111:249.

Harrison-Woolrych, M., Herbison, P., McLean, R., Ashton, J., and Slattery, J., 2005, Incidence of thrombotic cardiovascular events in patients taking celecoxib and rofecoxib: Interim results from the New Zealand Intensive Medicines Monitoring Programme, *Drug Safety*, 28:435–442.

Konstam, M.A., Weir, M.R., Reicin, A., et al., 2001, Cardiovascular thrombotic events in controlled, clinical trials of rofecoxib, *Circulation*, 104:2280–2288.

Moore, R.A., Derry, S., and McQuay, H.J., 2007, Cyclo-oxygenase-2 selective inhibitors and nonsteroidal anti-inflammatory drugs: Balancing gastrointestinal and cardiovascular risk, *BMC Musculoskeletal Disorders*, 8:73.

Mukherjee, D., Nissen, S.E., and Topol, E.J., 2001, Risk of cardiovascular events associated with selective COX-2 inhibitors, *Journal of the American Medical Association*, 286:954–959.

Psaty, B.M. and Furberg, C.D., 2005, COX-2 inhibitors: Lessons in safety, *New England Journal of Medicine*, 352:1133–1135.

Urquhart, J., 2005, Some key points emerging from the COX-2 controversy, *Pharmacoepidemiology and Drug Safety*, 14:145–147.

Velantgas, P., West, W., Cannuscio, C.C., et al., 2006, Cardiovascular risk of selective cyclooxygenase-2 inhibitors and other non-aspirin non-steroidal anti-inflammatory medications, *Pharmacoepidemiology and Drug Safety*, 15: 641–652.

Weir, M.R., Sperling, R.S., Reicin, A., and Gertz, B.J., 2003, Selective COX-2 inhibition and cardiovascular effects: A review of the rofecoxib development program, *American Heart Journal*, 146:591–604.

12.7.3   Journal Articles Related to Case Study II

Diamond, G.A., Bax, L., and Kaul, S., 2007, Uncertain effects of rosiglitazone on the risk for myocardial infarction and cardiovascular death, *Annals of Internal Medicine,* 147:578–581.

Home, P.D., Pocock, S.J., Beck-Nielsen, H., et al. for the RECORD Study Group, 2007, Rosiglitazone evaluated for cardiovascular outcomes: An interim analysis, *New England Journal of Medicine*, 357:28–38.

McCullough, P.A. and Lepor, N.E., 2007, The rosiglitazone meta-analysis, *Reviews in Cardiovascular Medicine*, 8:123–126.

Nesto, R.W., Bell., D., Bonow, R.O., et al., 2003, Thiazolidinedione use, fluid retention, and congestive heart failure: A consensus statement from the American Heart Association and the American Diabetes Association, *Circulation*, 108: 2941–2948.

Nissen, S.E. and Wolski, K., 2007, Effect of rosiglitazone on the risk of myocardial infarction and death from cardiovascular causes, *New England Journal of Medicine*, 356:2457–2471.

Psaty, B.M. and Furberg, C.D., 2007, The record on rosiglitazone and the risk of myocardial infarction, *New England Journal of Medicine*, 357:67–69.

Richter, B., Bandeira-Echtler, E., Bergerhoff, K., Clar, C., and Ebrahim, S.H., 2007, Rosiglitazone for type 2 diabetes mellitus, *Cochrane Database Systematic Reviews*, July 18; 3:CD006063.

Toth, P.P., 2007, Editorial: Avandia and risk for acute cardiovascular events: Science or sabotage? *The Journal of Applied Research*, 7, 147–149.

12.7.4   Papers Related to Case Study III

Deanda, A., Jr., 2008, Aprotinin and cardiac surgery, *Journal of Thoracic and Cardiovascular Surgery*, 135:492–494.

Liu, C.M., Chen, J., and Wang, X.H., 2008, Requirements for transfusion and postoperative outcomes in orthotopic liver transplantation: A meta-analysis on aprotinin, *World Journal of Gastroenterology*, 14:1425–1429.

Mouton, R., Finch, D., Davies, I., Binks, A., and Zacharowski, K., 2008, Effect of aprotinin on renal dysfunction in patients undergoing on-pump and off-pump cardiac surgery: A retrospective observational study, *Lancet*, 371:475–482.

Ranucci, M., 2008, Aprotinin and microvascular thrombosis in cardiac surgery, *Intensive Care Medicine*, February 27 [e-publication ahead of print].

Ray, W.A., 2008, Learning from aprotinin—Mandatory trials of comparative efficacy and safety needed, *New England Journal of Medicine*, 358:840–842.

Schetz, M., Bove, T., Morelli, A., et al., 2008, Prevention of cardiac surgery-associated acute kidney injury, *International Journal of Artificial Organs*, 31: 179–189.

Westaby, S., 2008, Aprotinin: Twenty-five years of claim and counterclaim, *Journal of Thoracic and Cardiovascular Surgery*, 135:487–491.

12.7.5   Papers Related to Oncology, Cardiotoxicity, and Echocardiography

Adams, M.J., Lipsitz, S.R., Colan, S.D., et al., 2004, Cardiovascular status in long-term survivors of Hodgkin's disease treated with chest radiotherapy, *Journal of Clinical Oncology*, 22:3139–3148. [While our main focus is on pharmacotherapy, radiotherapy is of interest in its own right and also because it may be administered in conjunction with pharmacotherapy.]

Arbel, Y., Swartzon, M., and Justo, D., 2007, QT prolongation and torsades de pointes in patients previously treated with anthracyclines, *Anticancer Drugs*, 18:493–498.

Arques, S., Roux, E., and Luccioni, R., 2007, Current clinical applications of spectral tissue Doppler echocardiography (E/E ratio) as a noninvasive surrogate for left ventricular diastolic pressures in the diagnosis of heart failure with preserved left ventricular systolic function, *Cardiovascular Ultrasound*, 5:16.

Bryant, J., Picot, J., Levitt, G., et al., 2007, Cardioprotection against the toxic effects of anthracyclines given to children with cancer: A systematic review, *Health Technology Assessment*, 11:iii, ix–x, 1–84.

Dranitsaris, G., Rayson, D., Vincent, M., et al., 2008, The development of a predictive model to estimate cardiotoxic risk for patients with metastatic breast cancer receiving anthracyclines, *Breast Cancer Research and Treatment*, 107: 443–450.

Gorcsan, J., 3rd, 2008, Role of echocardiography to determine candidacy for cardiac resynchronization therapy, *Current Opinion in Cardiology*, 23:16–22.

Horacek, J.M., Pudil, R., Jebavy, L., et al., 2007, Assessment of anthracycline-induced cardiotoxicity with biochemical markers, *Experimental Oncology*, 29: 309–313.

Horacek, J.M., Pudil, R., Tichy, M., et al., 2007, Biochemical markers and assessment of cardiotoxicity during preparative regimen and hematopoietic cell transplantation in acute leukemia, *Experimental Oncology*, 29:243–247.

Jannazzo, A., Hoffman, J., and Lutz, M., 2008, Monitoring of anthracycline-induced cardiotoxicity, *Annals of Pharmacotherapy*, 42:99–104.

Jones, R.L. and Ewer, M.S., 2006, Cardiac and cardiovascular toxicity of nonanthracycline anticancer drugs, *Expert Review of Anticancer Therapy*, 6: 1249–1269.

Lipshultz, S.E., 2006, Exposure to anthracyclines during childhood causes cardiac injury, *Seminars in Oncology*, 33:S8–S14.

Ng, R., Better, N., and Green, M.D., 2006, Anticancer agents and cardiotoxicity, *Seminars in Oncology*, 33:2–14.

Pai, V.B. and Nahata, M.C., 2000, Cardiotoxicity of chemotherapeutic agents: Incidence, treatment and prevention, *Drug Safety*, 22:263–302.

Sereno, M., Brunello, A., Chiappori, A., et al., 2008, Cardiotoxicity: Old and new issues in anti-cancer drugs, *Clinical and Translational Oncology*, 10:35–46.

Towns, K., Bedard, P.L., and Verma, S., 2008, Matters of the heart: Cardiac toxicity of adjuvant systemic therapy for early-stage breast cancer, *Current Oncology*, 15:S16–S29.

van Dalen, E.C., van den Brug, M., Caron, H.N., and Kremer, L.C., 2006, Anthracycline-induced cardiotoxicity: Comparison of recommendations for monitoring cardiac function during therapy in paediatric oncology trials, *European Journal of Cancer*, 42:3199–3205.

Yeh, E.T.H., 2006, Cardiotoxicity induced by chemotherapy and antibody therapy, *Annual Review of Medicine*, 57:485–498.

Youssef, G. and Links, M., 2005, The prevention and management of cardiovascular complications of chemotherapy in patients with cancer, *American Journal of Cardiovascular Drugs*, 5:233–243.

Yuan, X.P., White, J.A., and Drangova, M., 2007, Tissue Doppler imaging of mitral annular motion is an effective surrogate of left ventricular dyssynchrony and predicts response to resynchronization therapy, *Journal of the American Society of Echocardiography*, 20:1186–1193.

12.7.6   Other Papers Related to Generalized Cardiac Safety

Graham, J. and Coghill, D., 2008, Adverse effects of pharmacotherapies for attention-deficit hyperactivity disorder: Epidemiology, prevention and management, *CNS Drugs*, 22:213–237.

Nissen, S.E., 2006, ADHD drugs and cardiovascular risk, *New England Journal of Medicine*, 354:1445–1448.

Pliszka, S.R., 2007, Pharmacologic treatment of attention-deficit/hyperactivity disorder: Efficacy, safety and mechanisms of action, *Neuropsychology Review*, 17:61–72.

Prasad, S., Furr, A.J., Zhang, S., Ball, S., and Allen, A.J., 2007, Baseline values from the electrocardiograms of children and adolescents with ADHD, *Child and Adolescent Psychiatry and Mental Health*, 1:11.

Wolraich, M.L., McGuinn, L., and Doffing, M., 2007, Treatment of attention deficit hyperactivity disorder in children and adolescents: Safety considerations, *Drug Safety*, 30:17–26.

Young, D., 2006, FDA ponders cardiovascular risks of ADHD, *American Journal of Health-System Pharmacy*, 63:492–494.

13

MEDICATION ERRORS, ADHERENCE, AND CONCORDANCE

13.1 INTRODUCTION

In the previous parts of this book, the main protagonists have been professionals involved directly in drug design and development and physicians who make treatment decisions in partnership with their patients. These have included researchers and clinicians who work at (or for, in the case of contract research organizations and other subcontractors) a sponsor company, a regulatory agency, or a government agency or academic institution involved in postmarking surveillance. Investigational sites are also crucial to clinical research. Physicians can participate in clinical trials as Principal Investigators, functioning in this context as clinical research professionals running clinical trials. We have noted the work of physicians when considering the benefit-risk assessments they must make in deciding upon an appropriate treatment regimen on a patient-by-patient basis when they are functioning as clinicians treating individual patients. We have also discussed patients to a certain extent in that we have acknowledged that the ideal patient-physician relationship is that of a patient health management team. The physician is an expert in biology, medicine, and each patient's medical and family history: the patient is an expert in his or her own life circumstances and hopes for his or her future, including improving and/or maintaining health and well-being.

In this chapter, our discussions turn first to the work of physicians, pharmacists, and nurses in providing care to patients and errors that are made during this care. In keeping with the focus of this book, our attention centers on pharmaceutical health care. Given this book's primary interest in cardiac adverse drug reactions, it should be noted that it is not always easy to partition out data specifically addressing the occurrences of cardiac adverse drug reactions when looking at overall estimates of medication errors, and therefore the majority of this chapter addresses behavioral drug safety in general. However, medication errors undoubtedly lead to cardiac adverse drug reactions.

While they are not the only medical errors that occur (e.g., issues can arise with medical devices, and inappropriate operations have been conducted on patients), medication errors have been studied extensively for several pragmatic reasons (Institute of Medicine, 2000):

Integrated Cardiac Safety: Assessment Methodologies for Noncardiac Drugs in Discovery, Development, and Postmarketing Surveillance. By J. Rick Turner and Todd A. Durham
Copyright © 2009 John Wiley & Sons, Inc.

> ➤ They are one of the most common types of error, and substantial numbers of patients are affected. From a methodological point of view, it is easy to identify an adequate sample size of individuals who experience adverse drug effects to be included in research studies.
> ➤ They account for a substantial increase in health care expenditures.
> ➤ The drug-prescribing process provides good documentation of medical decisions. The majority of these data are readily accessible.
> ➤ Deaths attributable to medication errors are indicated on death certificates.

It should also be noted at this point that many of the statistics cited in this chapter are drawn from studies conducted using data from inpatient or institutional settings. This certainly does not imply that these are the only settings in which errors occur. They undoubtedly occur in ambulatory care and community care settings too, and given that the number of patients receiving pharmaceutical treatment in hospitals is likely much less than the number of nonhospitalized patients receiving treatment at any given time, the impact of errors in ambulatory settings may be considerably greater (Institute of Medicine, 2000). The focus on inpatient (hospital) settings is simply indicative of the fact that earlier research was conducted in these settings.

Outpatient research is certainly being conducted too. Consider as one example the study conducted by Lasser et al. (2006), which assessed how frequently patients at 51 outpatient practices received prescriptions in violation of black box warnings for drug-drug, drug-laboratory, and/or drug-disease interactions during one year (2002). Of the 324,548 outpatients receiving a medication, 2,354 (0.7%) received a prescription in violation of a black box warning. While less than 1% of patients had an adverse drug event as a result of a prescribing violation, adverse drug events did occur (see the discussions in Section 13.3.1 about small percentages of large numbers being nontrivial).

The number of adverse drug reactions that result from medication errors is staggering, and the fundamental issues of concern in this field are behavioral, hence the title of this chapter, "Medication Errors, Adherence, and Concordance." First, the behaviors of individual health care practitioners (physicians, pharmacists, nurses, care givers in residential homes, etc.) need to be considered. Second, their interactions with health care systems need attention. While these systems can be (and need to be) examined in their own right, it is the human interaction with them that is of principal interest. These systems need to be engineered to promote optimum interfacing between the systems and multiple health care providers.

Discussions in the second part of this chapter turn to the role of patients in their own health care and how well they adhere to prescribed therapeutic regimens. As for medication errors, the fundamental issues in the domain of adherence to medication regimens are behavioral in nature. This chapter therefore reviews both of these areas of behavioral concern, highlighting some major concerns and potential solutions as identified by leading authorities in these fields. It is appropriate to note here that both aspects of behavioral cardiac safety discussed in this chapter occur in the postmarketing arena. While it is certainly possible for pharmaceutical errors to occur before a drug receives marketing approval (e.g., for an inappropriate drug substance to be used in the preparation of drug products used in preapproval clinical trials or for the wrong dose of a drug to be used in such trials), the vast majority occur once the approved drug is prescribed for patients.

13.2   THE "FIVE RIGHTS" OF SAFE MEDICATION USE

In the first chapter of Cohen's (2007a) book *Medication Errors* (2nd Edition), Leape (2007, p. 3) observed the following:

> An error can be defined as an unintended act (either of omission or commission) or as an act that does not achieve its intended outcome. Until recently, medical errors were seldom discussed. The public preferred to believe that errors in medical practice were rare. Health professionals, fearing loss of trust and impaired reputation, sought to perpetuate that misconception. The adversarial climate produced by the threat of malpractice litigation exacerbated this "see nothing, do nothing" approach.
>
> All this has changed in the past 10 years. A new "movement" for patient safety began in 1995, when a series of apparently egregious errors resulting in death or inappropriate surgery were widely publicized. Hospitals began to recognize that they could do more to prevent patient injuries by using a nonpunitive approach to errors. The result has been substantial increases in both research on the causes of medical error and implementation of preventive mechanisms.

Cohen has addressed medication errors at the level of the individual health care professional and also at the systems level. He commented as follows (Cohen, 2007b, p. 55):

> Most health care professionals have learned the "five rights" of safe medication use: the right patient, right drug, right time, right dose, and right route of administration. Yet even when practitioners believe they have verified these "rights," errors, including fatal ones, occur.

He continued with the following observation (Cohen, 2007b, p. 55):

> The five rights focus on individual performance and overlook crucial system components that contribute to errors. For example, poor lighting, inadequate staffing patterns, poorly designed medical devices, handwritten orders, doses with trailing zeroes,

and ambiguous drug labels can prevent health care professionals
from verifying the five rights, despite their best efforts.

The professionals working in health care are among the most educated and dedicated
in any industry. However, while many other industries (notably the aviation industry)
have long histories of designing, developing, and constantly improving safety-
focused systems, the health care industry has been very slow to adopt such practices.
Consequently, error rates have been disturbingly high. Humans make mistakes, no
matter how diligent, trained, and dedicated they may be: this is simply a fact of
life. As noted in Chapter 1, we should expect human errors. The best approach to
preventing (or reducing) errors is to put systems in place that maximize the likelihood
of correct outcomes and minimize the likelihood of incorrect outcomes. As noted in
the Institute of Medicine's 2000 report *To Err Is Human: Building a Safer Health
System*, "The problem is not bad people: the problem is that the system needs to be
made safer" (Institute of Medicine, 2000, p. 49).

13.3   THE INSTITUTE OF MEDICINE'S 2000 REPORT *TO ERR IS HUMAN*

The first part of this chapter takes a historical perspective on the subject of
medication errors by reviewing several major publications from the Institute of
Medicine over the last several years that have focused on improving safety in health
care. Because the first report discussed was published in 2000, some of the figures
cited are from studies conducted some years ago, but they are indicative of the
information that was available at that time. (It should be noted here that the Institute
of Medicine's reports are typically released before they are officially published in
book format. At times, therefore, their release dates can be a year earlier than their
publication dates. When sources are cited in this chapter, the dates of the books'
publication are used.)

The Institute of Medicine's 2000 report *To Err Is Human: Building a Safer
Health System* noted that patient safety problems of many kinds occur during the
course of providing health care, including (Institute of Medicine, 2000, p. 35):

- Adverse drug reactions.
- Transfusion errors.
- Surgical injuries.
- Wrong-site surgeries.
- Preventable suicides.
- Restraint-related injuries or death.
- Hospital-acquired or other treatment-related infections.
- Falls.
- Burns.
- Pressure-related ulcers.
- Mistaken identity.

Our primary interest in this book is adverse reactions to drugs that are correctly prescribed and correctly taken, and our discussions of proarrhythmic and generalized cardiac safety reflect this interest. This situation changes in the present chapter: interest lies with adverse drug reactions that are the result of incorrectly prescribed, dispensed, and/or administered drugs or drug doses, i.e., the result of medication errors. We leave other authors to address the other 10 sources of health care-related problems just listed.

13.3.1   Small Percentages of Very Large Numbers

Reading *To Err Is Human* is an eye-opening experience, since it cites a litany of studies revealing disturbing statistics on medication errors. Before reviewing some of these, it is worth noting that very small percentages of a total number of events can represent a considerable number of events if the total number is sufficiently large. One percent of 100 events represents just one event, but 1% of 1 million events represents 10,000 events. Consider now the fact that in 1998 nearly 2.5 billion prescriptions were dispensed to patients in U.S. pharmacies (Institute of Medicine, 2000, p. 32). One percent of 2.5 billion is 25 million. One-hundredth of 1% (0.01%) of 2.5 billion is 250,000. Even one-thousandth of 1% (0.001%) of 2.5 billion represents a considerable number, i.e., 25,000. So, when talking about very large numbers of events, even small percentages of these numbers represent a large number of occurrences.

Davis and Cohen (1981, cited by Institute of Medicine, 2000, p. 39) reviewed published literature and other sources of evidence and found an error rate of 12% to be common in the preparation and administration of medications in hospitals. First, calculating 12% of the 1998 estimated number of drug administrations in U.S. hospitals, i.e., 3.75 billion (Institute of Medicine, 2000, p. 32) reveals the number 450 million. Second, consider the following statement (Institute of Medicine, 2000, p. 34): "Current estimates of the incidence of medication errors are undoubtedly low because many errors go undocumented and unreported." As noted in Section 13.1, the numbers here are staggering.

It is certainly true that not every error causes an adverse drug reaction. However, imagine that just 1 in every 100 errors (1% of errors) were to lead to an adverse drug reaction: using the figures cited in the previous paragraph, that would add up to 4,500,000 adverse drug reactions caused by medication errors. It is also true that not every adverse drug reaction is serious. Similarly, imagine that only 1% of adverse drug reactions caused by medication errors were serious: this scenario still results in 45,000 serious adverse drug reactions. These calculations are presented here to reinforce the statement made earlier in this section: very small percentages of a total number of events can represent a considerable number of events if the total number is sufficiently large.

13.3.2   The Structure of *To Err Is Human*

To Err is Human is the first of two reports from the Institute of Medicine's Quality of Health Care in America Committee. This committee's mandate was to develop a strategy that would lead to a threshold improvement in quality over the subsequent decade. From this perspective, there are three quality domains:

> ➢ Patient safety: freedom from accidental injury.
> ➢ Provision of services consistent with current medical knowledge.
> ➢ Customization of care.

Additionally, quality problems can be categorized into three areas:

> ➢ Misuse: avoidable complications that prevent patients from receiving the full potential benefit of a health care service.
> ➢ Overuse: the potential for harm that results from the provision of service that exceeds the possible benefit.
> ➢ Underuse: the failure to provide a health care service that would have produced a favorable outcome for the patient.

The first of these problems, issues of misuse, are most likely to be addressed under safety concerns, the focus of this report.

The *To Err Is Human* report has eight chapters and five appendices. The recommendations made occur in specific chapters, and the number associated with each recommendation first reflects the chapter in which it is presented and then the order in which it is presented within that chapter. The respective chapters provide detailed background information related to each recommendation. These recommendations are summarized in the following section. While acknowledging that no single activity can offer a complete solution, the report commented that, taken together, its recommendations provided "a roadmap toward a safer health system" (Institute of Medicine, 2000, p. 15). The report also noted that progress in this regard should be evaluated after five years.

13.4   RECOMMENDATIONS IN *TO ERR IS HUMAN*

This section presents a summary of the nine recommendations made in *To Err Is Human*.

13.4.1   Recommendation 4.1

Congress should create a Center for Patient Safety within the Agency for Healthcare Research and Quality. This Center should:

> Set national goals for patient safety, track progress made, and issue an annual report to the President and Congress on patient safety.
> Develop knowledge and understanding of errors in health care by developing a research agenda for evaluating methods for identifying and preventing errors, funding Centers of Excellence, and funding the dissemination of information to improve patient safety.

Specific initial areas of focus for the Center for Patient Safety should be:

> Enhancing understanding of the impact of various management practices (e.g., maximum work hours and overtime) on the likelihood of errors.
> Applying safety methods and technologies from other industries to health care, especially human factors and engineering principles.
> Increasing understanding of errors in different settings (ambulatory, home care) and for vulnerable populations (children, the elderly).
> Establishing baseline rates of particular errors and monitoring trends.
> Monitoring error rates that accompany the introduction of new technologies.
> Increasing understanding of the use of information technology to improve patient safety (e.g., automated drug order or entry systems, reminder systems).

13.4.2 Recommendation 5.1

It is important to establish a nationwide mandatory reporting system that facilitates the collection of standardized information by state governments about adverse events that result in death or serious harm. Hospitals should be the first institutions to be required to conduct such reporting, and eventually it should be required of other institutions and ambulatory care delivery settings. Congress should:

> Designate the National Forum for Health Care Quality Measurement and Reporting as the body responsible for establishing a core set of reporting standards to be used by states.
> Provide funds and technical expertise for state governments to adapt their current error reporting systems to the standardized one, or to establish one where necessary. States should analyze the standardized information collected and conduct follow-up action as needed with a health care organization.

13.4.3 Recommendation 5.2

The development of voluntary reporting efforts should be encouraged. The Center for Patient Safety should:

> Formulate and disseminate information on external voluntary reporting programs, fund and evaluate pilot projects for reporting systems, track the development of new reporting systems as they form, and encourage greater participation in them.
> Convene meetings between sponsors and users of external reporting systems to evaluate what works and what does not work well in the programs, and evaluate methods to make them more effective.
> Periodically assess whether and where additional efforts are necessary.

Recommendations 5.1 and 5.2, then, call for both mandatory and voluntary reporting systems that should be operated separately. These are regarded as complementary, and both serve specific and important purposes. The focus of mandatory systems is on the reporting of serious errors or deaths, and the purpose is to hold health care providers accountable. These systems are operated by state regulatory bodies, and these have investigational authority and the power to issue penalties or fines for wrongdoing. These systems create, and make visible, a minimum level of protection for the public. They also provide an incentive to health care organizations to improve patient safety to avoid potential penalties and public exposure. Having said this, there is an extremely small percentage of health care providers who need to be censured for demonstrably careless or egregious errors. Most errors are truly accidental and occur as professionals do their best in good faith. Indeed, it is critical to remove the culture of blame and replace it with a culture where safety is the paramount concern.

The purpose of voluntary reporting systems is to focus on less serious errors or on near misses, cases where an adverse drug reaction could have occurred but an additional intervention or pure good luck meant that it did not. Studying such errors is extremely beneficial in developing systems that enhance the likelihood of successful outcomes and minimize the likelihood of adverse outcomes. There are no penalties associated with actions that are reported: reports are usually submitted in confidence. The aim of voluntary reporting systems is to "identify and remedy vulnerabilities in systems before the occurrence of harm" (Institute of Medicine, 2000, p. 87).

This report also notes that simply implementing reporting systems and collecting data is not enough: analysis, interpretation, and follow-up action are required. This requires additional resources on top of those that were initially required to implement the reporting procedure, and appropriate budgetary considerations are therefore critical.

13.4.4 Recommendation 6.1

Congress should pass legislation to extend peer review protections to data related to patient safety and quality improvement that are collected and analyzed by health care organizations for internal use or shared with others solely for purposes of improving safety and quality.

13.4.5   Recommendation 7.1

Performance standards and expectations for health care organizations should focus greater attention on patient safety.

➢ Regulators and accreditors should require health care organizations to implement meaningful patient safety programs with defined executive responsibility.
➢ Public and private purchasers should provide incentives to health care organizations to demonstrate continuous improvement in patient safety.

13.4.6   Recommendation 7.2

Performance standards and expectations for health professionals should focus greater attention on patient safety.

➢ Health professional licensing bodies should implement periodic reexaminations and relicensing of key health care providers with regard to both knowledge and competent implementation of safety practices. Unsafe providers should be identified in collaboration with certifying and credentialing and action taken.
➢ Professional societies should make a visible commitment to patient safety by establishing a permanent committee dedicated to safety improvements.

13.4.7   Recommendation 7.3

The FDA should focus more attention on the safe use of drugs in both preapproval and postmarketing processes, as suggested below:

➢ Develop and enforce standards for the design of drug packaging and labeling that will maximize safe use.
➢ Develop FDA-approved methods that pharmaceutical companies must use to test proposed drug names to identify and eliminate potential confusion with existing names that look similar (written format) and sound similar (verbal format).
➢ Work with physicians, pharmacists, consumers, and other stakeholders to develop appropriate responses to problems identified in postmarketing surveillance.

13.4.8   Recommendation 8.1

Health care organizations and affiliated professionals should declare their serious commitment to continuously improved patient safety, and demonstrate this by establishing patient safety programs that have defined executive responsibility.

To be most effective, the implementation of patient safety programs must be championed and supported by the highest levels of the organization, such as chief executive officers (CEOs) and boards of directors/trustees. Senior level management should monitor the outcomes and results of defined program objectives and report regularly to the CEOs and board members. A critical component of these endeavors is to cultivate a culture of safety, not a culture of blame. A culture of blame leads to reluctance to report errors, and the organization is therefore not aware of errors that do occur. Summarizing, classifying, and addressing the root causes of these errors is therefore not possible. Nonpunitive environments within health care organizations are of the greatest importance.

13.4.9   Recommendation 8.2

Health care organizations should implement proven medication safety practices. Strategies and systems for reducing human errors and improving safety have been well demonstrated in other fields, and they should be strongly considered by health care environments and organizations including hospitals, long-term care facilities, ambulatory settings and other health care delivery sites, and outpatient and community pharmacies. Methodologies that are beneficial here include:

> Reducing reliance on memory.
> Reducing reliance on vigilance.
> Simplification and standardization.
> Using constraints and forced functions.
> Appropriate use of protocols and checklists.
> Differentiating between products that sound or look alike.

Human factors research (the study of the interrelationships between humans, their use of tools, and their environments) has been successfully used in other industries and warrants consideration in health care settings. A key component here is improving the human-system interface by designing better systems and processes. Improvements include:

> Simplifying and standardizing procedures.
> Building in redundancy to provide backup and opportunities for recovery.
> Improving communications and coordination within teams.
> Redesigning equipment to improve the human-machine interface.

13.4.10   Summary of the Report's Message

The authors of the *To Err Is Human* report were fully aware that, while regulation is important, it alone is not sufficient for achieving a significant improvement in patient safety: multi-faceted solutions are necessary. It is necessary to balance regulatory/ legislative influences and the influences of economic and other incentives. As the authors of the report noted (Institute of Medicine, 2000, p. 21):

> The committee's strategy for improving patient safety is for the external environment to create sufficient pressure to make errors so costly in terms of ability to conduct business in the marketplace, market share, and reputation that the organization *must* take action. The cost should be high enough that organizations and professionals invest the attention and resources necessary to improve safety. Such external pressures are virtually absent in health care today. The actions of regulatory bodies, group purchasers, consumers and professional groups are all critical to achieving this goal. At the same time, investments in an adequate knowledge base and tools to improve safety are also important to assist health care organizations in responding to this challenge.

13.5   THE INSTITUTE OF MEDICINE'S 2001 REPORT *CROSSING THE QUALITY CHASM*

The Institute of Medicine's 2001 report *Crossing the Quality Chasm: A New Health Care System for the 21ˢᵗ Century* was the second and final report published by the Committee on Quality of Health Care in America. It took a broader approach to quality-related issues than the *To Err Is Human* report discussed in Section 13.4, providing "a strategic direction for redesigning the health care delivery system of the 21ˢᵗ century" (Institute of Medicine, 2001, p. xi). While the *To Err Is Human* report on safety is sobering, it does not by any means address all aspects of quality in the U.S. health care system. As the *Crossing the Quality Chasm* report noted, "Other defects are even more widespread and, taken together, detract still further from the health, functioning, dignity, comfort, satisfaction, and resources of Americans" (Institute of Medicine, 2001, p. 2). Americans need to receive health care that is:

➢ Safe.
➢ Effective.
➢ Patient-centered.
➢ Timely.
➢ Efficient.
➢ Equitable.

Unfortunately, the *Crossing the Quality Chasm* report made it very clear that the health care delivery system at that time did not meet these criteria, observing that "Health care today harms too frequently and routinely fails to deliver its potential benefits," and that "Quality problems are everywhere, affecting many patients. Between the health care we have and the care we could have lies not just a gap, but a chasm" (Institute of Medicine, 2001, p. 1). This report envisions the 21st century's health care system having three central characteristics:

> ➤ Evidence-based.
> ➤ Patient-centered.
> ➤ Systems-oriented.

Since this book's focus is on drug safety we do not discuss *Crossing the Quality Chasm* in as much detail as other reports that address drug safety specifically. However, this report merits inclusion in this chapter since the other topics it discussed also impinge on safety considerations. The following subsections therefore represent a sampling of observations cited in this report.

13.5.1 Translating Knowledge into Practice

Knowledge gained from clinical research will not benefit patients unless that knowledge is translated into clinical practice. The term translational research reflects the interest in, and the need for, rapid translation of acquired knowledge into advances in clinical practice. [For an additional example of translational research discussions, see http://www.cancer.gov/aboutnci/trwg/executive-summary.pdf (accessed October 1, 2007) for the Executive Summary of the June 2007 report from the Translational Research Working Group of the National Cancer Advisory Board, National Cancer Institute, National Institutes of Health.]

13.5.2 Lack of Information Technology Capabilities

The present health care delivery system is fragmented, with patients often being seen by several clinicians at several locations during the course of evaluation and treatment for a single condition. The lack of even rudimentary clinical information capabilities results in care processes that are poorly designed (if designed is the right word here: evolution via happenstance may be a more accurate descriptor) and that result in unnecessary duplication of services, delays, and long waiting times. The automation of administrative, financial, and clinical transactions is essential for both preventing errors and improving efficiency. As the report noted (Institute of Medicine, 2001, p. 15):

The meticulous collection of personal health information throughout a patient's life can be one of the most important inputs to the provision of proper care. Yet for most individuals, that health information is dispersed in a collection of paper records that are poorly organized and often illegible, and frequently cannot be retrieved in a timely fashion, making it nearly impossible to manage many forms of chronic illness that require frequent monitoring and ongoing patient support.

13.5.3   Lack of Integrated Clinical Care Programs

This observation relates to the previous one. The predominant need from the health care delivery system is not for clinical programs for acute disease states but rather for programs for chronic diseases. Chronic conditions (including, among many, heart disease, diabetes, and asthma) are the leading cause of illness, disability, and death, affecting almost 50% of the U.S. population. Despite this situation, one that did not arise overnight but developed over several decades, there are few clinical programs with the infrastructure necessary to provide the full complement of services needed by patients with heart disease and other common chronic conditions.

13.5.4   Six Aims for the 21st Century Health Care System

As noted early in the report (Institute of Medicine, 2001, pp. 5–6), the report's position was that health care should be:

➢ Safe—avoiding injuries to patients from the care that is intended to help them.
➢ Effective—providing services based on scientific knowledge to all who could benefit from them (avoiding underuse) and refraining from providing services to those not likely to benefit from them (avoiding overuse).
➢ Patient-centered—providing care that is respectful of, and responsive to, individual patient's preferences, needs, and values, and ensuring that each individual patient's values guide all respective clinical decisions.
➢ Timely—reducing waits and delays that can sometimes be harmful to patients. Waiting time should also be reduced for those who give care as well as those who receive it.
➢ Efficient—avoiding waste. This including waste of equipment, supplies, ideas, and energy.
➢ Equitable—providing care that does not vary in quality according to sex, ethnicity, geographical location, and socioeconomic status.

The report recommended that all health care organizations, professional groups, and private and public purchasers should pursue these six aims. It also recommended that care systems should be redesigned. Health care must be delivered by health care delivery systems that have been carefully and consciously designed to facilitate provision of care that meets all of these six aims. These systems need to make full use of available information technology to support both administrative and clinical processes.

The fourth recommendation in this report provided 10 principles to guide the redesign of health care processes by private and public purchasers, health care organizations, clinicians, and patients working together (see Institute of Medicine, 2001, pp. 8–9 for more details):

➢ Care based on continuous healing relationships, not just at face-to-face meetings.
➢ Customization based on patient needs and values.
➢ The patient as the source of control. Patients should be involved in care-related decision making to the degree that each individual patient chooses to be.
➢ Shared knowledge and free flow of information between patients and clinicians.
➢ Evidence-based decision making (see the following section).
➢ Safety as an inherent property of health care delivery systems.
➢ Transparency, including providing patients and their families with information describing health care delivery systems' safety performance, degree of evidence-based practice, and patient satisfaction.
➢ Anticipation of needs, rather than reactions to events.
➢ Continuous decrease in waste.
➢ Cooperation among clinicians and medical institutions to ensure an appropriate exchange of information and a coordination of care.

13.6   THE INSTITUTE OF MEDICINE'S 2004 REPORT *PATIENT SAFETY*

The Institute of Medicine's 2004 report *Patient Safety: Achieving a New Standard for Care* was prepared by the Institute's Committee on Data Standards for Patient Safety. As noted in the preface to this report (p. ix):

> Unintended harm arising from medical management is not limited to the hospital setting; nor is it limited to acts of commission. The Committee on Data Standards for Patient Safety believes that patient safety should be a new standard for quality care—care that is free of unintended injury from acts of commission or

omission, in any setting in which it is delivered. Consequently, data standards needed to support patient safety go well beyond the needs of adverse event and near-miss reporting.

Development of the health care delivery system that is needed requires "first, a commitment by all stakeholders to a culture of safety and, second, improved information systems" (Institute of Medicine, 2004, p. 1). Accordingly, this report provided seven recommendations, a selection from which is summarized in the following sections.

13.6.1 Recommendation 1

All patients deserve safe care in all health care settings, e.g., hospitals, doctors' offices, and nursing homes. All health care organizations should establish comprehensive patient safety systems that achieve the following objectives: the provision of immediate access to complete patient information and decision support tools for clinicians and their patients, and the capture of information on patient safety as a by-product of care. Additionally, the information collected should be used to design even safer care delivery systems.

13.6.2 Recommendation 2

The federal government should facilitate the development of a national health information infrastructure. This facilitation should include provision of targeted financial support for the establishment and maintenance of standards for data that support patient safety. In addition, individual health care providers should invest in electronic health record systems that possess certain key capabilities, including those necessary to provide safe and effective care and to enable the continuous improvement of care processes designed to improve patient safety.

13.6.3 Recommendation 5

All health care settings should establish comprehensive patient safety programs operated by trained personnel within a culture of safety. These programs should encompass aspects that will facilitate the following:

> ➤ Identification of system failures.
> ➤ An understanding of the factors that contribute to system failures.
> ➤ System redesign to prevent errors in the future.

13.6.4 Recommendation 6

The federal government should pursue "a robust applied research agenda on patient safety, focused on enhancing knowledge, developing tools, and disseminating results to maximize the impact of patient safety systems" (p. 19).

13.7 THE INSTITUTE OF MEDICINE'S 2007 REPORT *PREVENTING MEDICATION ERRORS*

This report was prepared by the Institute's Committee on Identifying and Preventing Medication Errors. The report's preface opens in the following manner (Institute of Medicine, 2007a, p. ix):

> In 2000, the Institute of Medicine (IOM) report *To Err Is Human: Building a Safer Health System* raised awareness about medical errors and accelerated existing efforts to prevent such efforts. The present report makes clear that with regard to medication errors, we still have a long way to go. The current medication-use process, which encompasses prescribing, dispensing, administering, and monitoring, is characterized by many serious problems and issues that threaten both the safety and positive outcomes of the process. Each of the steps in the process needs improvement and further study.

Despite the powerful nature and calls to action of the previous reports discussed in this chapter, there is still much that needs to be done.

Consider the following statistics. It has been estimated that the extra cost of inpatient care for a preventable adverse drug reaction incurred while in the hospital was $5,857, and this value is in 1993 dollars. If we then assume conservatively that the annual incidence of in-hospital preventable adverse drug reactions is around 400,000 and that each incurs $5,857 in extra hospital costs in 1993 dollars, we get an annual cost of $2.3 billion in 1993 dollars, a figure that translates into $3.5 billion in 2006 dollars (see Institute of Medicine, 2007a, p. 5). Just as one comparator, consider that the Human Genome Project cost around $3 billion. Each year, then, the cost of in-hospital preventable adverse drug reactions incurred in extra hospital expenses could have funded a similar project: just imagine the phenomenal benefits to medicine alone of this hypothetical scenario.

This report contains seven recommendations, a selection from which is summarized here. Readers are encouraged to read these recommendations in full in the original report.

13.7.1   Recommendation 1

Specific measures should be instituted to strengthen patients' capacities for sound medication self-management, including:

> ➢ Patients (or their surrogates) should create and constantly update a list of all prescription drugs, over-the-counter drugs, and dietary supplements they are taking and the reasons for which they are taking them. Additionally, all known drug allergies should be recorded. Every provider involved in the medication use for a patient should have access to this list.
> ➢ Providers should take definitive action to educate patients (or their surrogates) about the safe and effective use of medications.
> ➢ Consultations regarding their medications should be available to patients at key points in the medication-use process: during clinical decision making in inpatient and ambulatory care settings, at hospital charge, and at the pharmacy.

13.7.2   Recommendation 2

Government agencies such as the FDA and the National Library of Medicine should enhance the resource base for consumer-oriented drug information and medication self-management support systems. These efforts require:

> ➢ Standardization of pharmacy medication information leaflets.
> ➢ Improved online medication resources.
> ➢ The establishment of a national drug information telephone helpline.
> ➢ The development of personal health records.

13.7.3   Recommendation 3

All heath care organizations should immediately make complete patient-information and decision-support tools available to clinicians and patients. Additionally, to improve the safety of their care delivery systems, health care systems should capture and use information on medication safety.

13.7.4   Recommendation 6

The Agency for Healthcare Research and Quality should work with other government agencies such as the FDA and the National Library of Medicine to coordinate a far-reaching research agenda on the safe and appropriate use of medications across all care settings. Furthermore, Congress should allocate the funds necessary to carry out this agenda.

13.7.5 Concluding Quotations Regarding Medication Errors

Before moving on to discuss the topic of adherence to pharmaceutical treatment regimens in the next section, two thought-provoking quotes are presented here. The first quote is from Smetzer's chapter entitled "Managing medication risks through a culture of safety" (2007, p. 605):

> Health care is a highly complex, error-prone industry. From emergency departments to high-volume pharmacies, providing patient care involves nonstop activity and intricate, interdisciplinary processes in which the slightest mistake could spell catastrophe. Other industries, such as chemical manufacturing, nuclear power production, and aviation, are equally prone to errors with potentially dire consequences, yet many of them have better safety records than health care.

The second quote is from the Institute of Medicine's report *Preventing Medication Errors* (Institute of Medicine, 2007a, p. 53). It is particularly salient since it addresses general drug safety and quality of patient care and captures many of the topics that have been discussed in this book:

> Building safety and quality into the system starts with rational ideas for new drug products, followed by sound scientific research; reliable clinical testing; rigorous regulatory reviews; appropriate labeling; use of good manufacturing processes; proper distribution techniques; adequate supplies; ethical marketing practices; competent prescribing, dispensing, and administration of medications; and finally suitable monitoring of the patient, reporting of errors, and measurement of outcomes (Martin, 1978). If standards do not exist, are inadequate, have not been met, or are not enforced at any point along this chain, patient safety and quality of care can be compromised.

13.8 ADHERENCE TO PHARMACEUTICAL TREATMENT REGIMENS

Attention now turns to the second of our behavioral safety considerations, adherence to pharmaceutical treatment regimens. It is possible to think of adherence issues as a subset of medication errors, but this chapter addresses the subject in its own right.

Lack of adherence in taking properly prescribed and dispensed drugs as indicated is a major problem in drug therapy. A given patient's lack of adherence can be accidental (unintentional) or intentional (e.g., see Kim et al., 2007), and there are complex behavioral, cultural, and psychological issues surrounding adherence: indeed, adherence is addressed in the literature of many disciplines, bearing witness to the need for a truly interdisciplinary approach to this issue.

It can be much more difficult than might naively be assumed to adhere to even the simplest medication regimen (e.g., one tablet once a day). Two immediate problems are remembering to take the tablet and remembering whether one took the tablet or not. The former scenario can result in a day's medication not being taken. The latter scenario may result in an incorrect memory—not taking the tablet when in fact the tablet was taken—which could result in the person taking a second tablet and therefore receiving an inappropriate dose. Many systems have been developed with the goal of improving adherence. One of these involves the seven-day dispenser. Such a dispenser can be prepared at the beginning of a week, and it can be placed in a prominent place to aid with the first problem, i.e., remembering to take each day's medication, and the second problem, i.e., providing evidence that a day's medication has or has not been taken. This system is certainly fallible, however, in that, for example, the dispenser must be filled correctly and on a regular schedule, and it must be remembered when traveling or otherwise breaking one's usual routine.

There are considerable challenges to conceptualizing and measuring adherence in this context (Bosworth et al., 2006). Accordingly, research reviews find widely ranging rates of adherence. An average figure of 50% adherence is not unreasonable (Bosworth et al., 2006), but there are certainly much lower estimates in the literature. In a meta-analysis of seven studies, Sullivan et al. (1990) estimated that 5.5% of hospital admissions can be attributed to drug therapy noncompliance, amounting to almost 2 million admissions and $8.5 billion in hospital expenditure in 1986. Lack of adherence is a major problem that crosses therapeutic boundaries. As examples, articles addressing adherence in HIV/AIDS (Marino et al., 2007; Simoni et al., 2007; Weaver et al., 2005) and in psychiatric conditions (Ascher-Svanum et al., 2006; Byerly et al., 2007; Clatworthy et al., 2007) are provided in the reference section at the end of the book, along with articles addressing adherence in pediatric populations (Simons and Blount, 2007) and older populations (De Smet et al., 2007).

13.8.1   Financial Considerations in the Domain of Adherence

While adherence and lack of adherence have direct implications for patients' health, the implications extend to a wider circle. Examples of other areas of investigation within this domain concern medical sociology, social policy analysis, and health economics. As one example of the last, consider what may happen if a patient's health is not helped by a drug therapy regimen because the patient is very nonadherent to the regimen. This scenario may involve additional visits to the patient's physician, additional medications being prescribed, and/or hospital visits and even hospital admittance. When this individual scenario is extended to large numbers of patients, the general health economic considerations quickly escalate.

Consider also a second example of the interaction between adherence and economics. Chernew et al. (2008) described an intervention whereby an employer reduced copayments for several chronic medication classes in the context of a disease management program. Copayments for generic medications were reduced from $5 to $0, and copayments for branded drugs were reduced by 50%. Adherence was then compared with a control employer using the same program (without reducing copayments). There was a statistically significant improvement in adherence for heart disease, diabetes, and high cholesterol. As Osterberg and Blaschke (2005) observed, poor adherence to regimens employed in chronic diseases can lead to increasing health care costs as well as worsening of disease, complications, and death. Improving adherence is indeed a much needed goal.

In lieu of detailed discussions here in the text, Section 13.11 provides a collection of further readings on adherence, with Section 13.11.2 dealing specifically with issues relating to cardiac and cardiovascular health.

13.9 CONCORDANCE

In 2004, an edited volume entitled *Concordance* was published (Bond, 2004). The editor noted that the concept of concordance "can be used with respect to both the process and the outcome of a discussion or consultation between a patient and healthcare professional," and that it embodies "a new way of looking at medicine-taking" that promotes the patient's beliefs and rights, and accords them equal weight to those of the healthcare professional" (Bond, 2004, p. xi). Horne and Weinman (2004, p. 122) noted that "The terms 'adherence' and 'compliance' reflect different perspectives of the same phenomenon: the degree to which the patient's behaviour matches medical advice: for many purposes the terms are interchangeable." While the terms adherence and compliance describe the behavior of one individual, the patient, concordance is "a much more complex and less well-defined term that relates to the process and outcomes of prescribing" (Horne and Weinman, 2004, p. 122). As Britten and Weiss (2004, p. 9) noted, in compliance and adherence models "a patient who does not take medicine as prescribed is seen as being willfully disobedient to the prescriber's wishes." On the other hand, "The model of concordance overtly recognises that the patient makes the final decision about whether or not to take medicines. It aims to make explicit any differences between patient and professional, and to promote decision-making processes that respect these differences" (Britten and Weiss, 2004, p. 9). Marinker (2004, p. 7) also captured the spirit of concordance well: "The aim is to achieve for each patient an optimum balance between the best that medical science can offer and the health-enhancing benefits of personal enablement."

The origins of research on concordance can in some ways be traced to a 1995 meeting arranged by the Royal Pharmaceutical Society of Great Britain in partnership with Merck Sharp & Dohme, at which discussions took place concerning what was known about the difficulties patients have in taking medicines as they are prescribed. Marinker (2004, p. 2) provided the following personal reflections on this work:

> I had long regarded non-compliance as something more than a procedural accident—the result of misunderstood instructions, or of the patient's physical, social, or psychological inability to follow them. Without knowing as much as I ought to have done about how patients feel about taking medicines, I had long sensed that non-compliance was often a positive act—albeit not always consciously reasoned. All medicine-taking involves a balance of risk between the damage of the disease process, unmodified by medication, on the one hand, and the potential damage which might be inflicted by the medicine, on the other. Intentional non-compliance therefore simply represents a particular choice—a defense mechanism against a perceived (and sometimes an actual) iatrogenic threat.

Stevenson (2004, p. 30) addressed these sentiments in this manner: "Patients have complex sets of beliefs, drawn from their own and their families' experiences, and any advice that they are given has to pass through a filter of these beliefs. These beliefs may be internally consistent but often contradict biomedical theories."

Mead and Bower (2000: cited by Britten and Weiss 2004, pp. 12–13) discusses a patient-centered process and detailed five conceptual dimensions in such a process:

➤ Adopting a biopsychosocial perspective.
➤ Understanding the individual's experience or illness or seeing the patient as a person.
➤ Sharing power and responsibility in the encounter.
➤ Developing a therapeutic alliance in which the importance of the doctor-patient relationship is recognized.
➤ Acknowledging the doctor as a person, in which doctor subjectivity and a greater awareness of the influence of the doctor's emotional responses are seen as an inherent, and potentially valuable, part of the patient-centered process.

Finally, in this section, it is fitting to quote again from Marinker (2004, p. 5):

> The clinical encounter is concerned with two sets of contrasted but equally cogent health beliefs—that of the patient, and that of

the doctor. The task of the patient is to convey her or his health beliefs to the doctor; and of the doctor, to enable this to happen. The task of the doctor or other prescriber is to convey his or her (professionally informed) health beliefs to the patient; and of the patient, to entertain these. The intention is to assist the patient to make as informed a choice as possible about the diagnosis and treatment, about benefit and risk, and to take full part in a therapeutic alliance. Although reciprocal, this is an alliance in which the most important determinations are agreed to be those that are made by the patient.

13.10 FURTHER READING: MEDICATION ERRORS

13.10.1 Books (Arranged Chronologically)

Institute of Medicine of the National Academies, 2000, *To err is human: Building a safer health system,* Washington, DC: National Academies Press.

Institute of Medicine of the National Academies, 2001, *Crossing the quality chasm: A new health system for the 21ˢᵗ century*, Washington, DC: National Academies Press.

World Health Organization, 2003, *Adherence to long-term therapies: Evidence for action*, Geneva: World Health Organization.

Harman, R.J., 2004, *Development and control of medicines and medical devices*, London: Pharmaceutical Press.

Institute of Medicine of the National Academies, 2004, *Patient safety: Achieving a new standard for care*, Washington, DC: National Academies Press.

Cohen, M.R. (Ed.), 2007, *Medication Errors,* 2ⁿᵈ edition, Washington, DC: American Pharmacists Association.

Institute of Medicine of the National Academies, 2007, *Preventing medication errors*, Washington, DC: National Academies Press.

13.10.2 Journal Articles and Book Chapters (Arranged Chronologically)

Fortescue, E.B., Kaushal, R., Landrigan, C.P., et al., 2003, Prioritizing strategies for preventing medication errors and adverse drug events in pediatric inpatients, *Pediatrics*, 111:722–729.

Bobb, A., Gleason, K., Husch, M., et al., 2004, The epidemiology of prescribing errors: The potential impact of computerized prescriber order entry, *Archives of Internal Medicine*, 164:785–792.

Shulman, R., Singer, M., Goldstone, J., and Bellingan, G., 2005, Medication errors: A prospective cohort study of hand-written and computerised physician order entry in the intensive care unit, *Critical Care*, 9:R516–R521.

Cullen, G., Kelly, E., and Murray, F.E., 2006, Patients' knowledge of adverse reactions to current medications, *British Journal of clinical Pharmacology*, 62: 232–236.

Aimette, S.A., Tuohy, N.R., and Cohen, M.R., 2007, The patient's role in preventing medication errors. In Cohen, M.R. (Ed.), *Medication Errors,* 2nd edition, Washington, DC: American Pharmacists Association, 289–313.

Bendavid, E., Kaganova, Y., Needleman, J., Gruenberg, L., and Weissman, J.S., 2007, Complication rates on weekends and weekdays in U.S. hospitals, *American Journal of Medicine*, 120:422–428.

Burkhardt, M., Lee, C., Taylor, L., Williams, R., and Bagian, J., 2007, Root cause analysis of medication errors. In Cohen, M.R. (Ed.), *Medication Errors,* 2nd Edition, Washington, DC: American Pharmacists Association, 67–86.

Offner, P.J., Heit, J., and Roberts, R., 2007, Implementation of a rapid response team decreases cardiac arrest outside of the intensive care unit, *Journal of Trauma*, 62:1227–1228.

Wang, J.K., Herzog, N.S., Kaushal, R., et al., 2007, Prevention of pediatric medication errors by hospital pharmacists and the potential benefit of computerized physician order entry, *Pediatrics*, 119:e77–e85.

Weant, K.A., Cook, A.M., and Armitstead, J.A., 2007, Medication-error reporting and pharmacy resident experience during implementation of computerized prescriber order entry, *American Journal of Health-system Pharmacy*, 64:526–530.

13.11   FURTHER READING: ADHERENCE AND CONCORDANCE

13.11.1 Books and Book Chapters (Arranged Chronologically)

McGavock, H., 1996, *A review of the literature on drug adherence*, London: Royal Pharmaceutical Society of Great Britain/Merck Sharp & Dohme.

World Health Organization, 2003, *Adherence to long-term therapies: Evidence for action*, Geneva: World Health Organization.

Bond, C. (Ed.), 2004, *Concordance*, London:Pharmaceutical Press.

Bosworth, H.B., Oddone, E.Z., and Weinberger, M. (Eds.), 2005, *Patient treatment adherence: Concepts, interventions, and measurement*, Mahwah, NJ: Lawrence Erlbaum Associates.

Fincham, J.E., 2005, *Taking your medication: A guide to medication regimens and compliance for patients and caregivers*, New York: Pharmaceutical Products Press.

O'Donohue, W.T. and Levensky, E.R. (Eds.), 2006, *Promoting treatment adherence: A practical handbook for health care providers*, Thousand Oaks, CA: Sage Publications.

Shea, S.C., 2006, *Improving medication adherence: How to talk with patients about their medications* (with a Foreword by C. Everett Koop, MD), Baltimore, MD: Lippincott Williams & Wilkins.

Park, D.C. and Liu, L.L., (Eds.), 2007, *Medical adherence and aging: Social and cognitive perspectives*, Washington, DC: American Psychological Association.

Urquhart, J. and Vrijens, B., 2007, Introduction to Pharmionics: The vagaries in ambulatory patients' adherence to prescribed drug dosing regimens, and some of their clinical and economic consequences. In Mann, R. and Andrews, E. (Eds.), *Pharmacovigilance*, 2nd edition, Chichester, UK: John Wiley & Sons, 603–618.

13.11.2 Journal Articles

Hobden, A., 2006a, Concordance: A widely used term, but what does it mean? *British Journal of Community Nursing,* 11:257–260.

Hobden, A., 2006b, Strategies to promote concordance within consultations, *British Journal of Community Nursing,* 11:286–289.

O'Connor, P.J., 2006, Improving medication adherence: Challenges for physicians, payers, and policy makers, *Archives of Internal Medicine,* 166:1802–1804.

13.11.3 Journal Articles Related to Cardiac and Cardiovascular Health

Brookhart, M.A., Patrick, A.R., Schneeweiss, S., et al., 2007, Physician follow-up and provider continuity are associated with long-term medication adherence: A study of the dynamics of statin use, *Archives of Internal Medicine,* 167:847-852.

Brunenberg, D.E., Wetzels, G.E., Nelemans, P.J., et al., 2007, Cost effectiveness of an adherence-improving programme in hypertensive patients, *Pharmacoeconomics,* 25:239–251.

Domino, F.J., 2005, Improving adherence to treatment for hypertension, *American Family Physician,* 71:2089–2090.

Frishman, W.H., 2007, Importance of medication adherence in cardiovascular disease and the value of once-daily treatment regimens, *Cardiology Reviews,* 15: 257–263.

Gehi, A., Ali, S., Na, B., and Whooley, M.A., 2007, Self-reported medication adherence and cardiovascular events in patients with stable coronary heart disease: The heart and soul study, *Archives of Internal Medicine,* 167:1798–1803.

Gehi, A., Haas, D., Pipkin, S., and Whooley, M.A., 2005, Depression and medication adherence in outpatients with coronary heart disease: Findings from the heart and soul study, *Archives of Internal Medicine,* 165:2508–2513.

Gerbino, P.P. and Shoheiber, O., 2007, Adherence patterns among patients treated with fixed-dose combination versus separate antihypertensive agents, *American Journal of Health Systems Pharmacy,* 64:1279–1283.

Gonzalez, J.S., Safren, S.A., Cagliero, E., et al., 2007, Depression, self-care, and medication adherence in type 2 diabetes: Relationships across the full range of symptom severity, *Diabetes Care*, 30:2222–2227.

Hallas, J., Haghfelt, T., Gram, L., Grodum, E., and Damsbo, N., 1990, Drug related admissions to a cardiology department: Frequency and avoidability, *Journal of Internal Medicine*, 228:379–384.

Harmon, G., Lefante, J., and Krousel-Wood, M., 2006, Overcoming barriers: The role of providers in improving patient adherence to antihypertensive medications, *Current Opinion in Cardiology*, 21:310–315.

Jolly, K., Taylor, R., Lip, G.Y., et al., 2007, The Birmingham Rehabilitation Uptake Maximisation Study (BRUM). Home-based compared with hospital-based cardiac rehabilitation in a multi-ethnic population: Cost-effectiveness and patient adherence, *Health Technology Assessment*, 11:1–18.

Kim, E.Y., Han, H.R., Jeong, S., et al., 2007, Does knowledge matter? Intentional medication nonadherence among middle-aged Korean Americans with high blood pressure, *Journal of Cardiovascular Nursing*, 22:397–404.

Krantz, M.J., Baker, W.A., Estacio, R.O., et al., 2007, Comprehensive coronary artery disease care in a safety-net hospital: Results of Get With the Guidelines quality improvement initiative, *Journal of Managed Care Pharmacy*, 13:319–325.

Lee, J.K., Grace, K.A., and Taylor, A.J., 2006, Effect of a pharmacy care program on medication adherence and persistence, blood pressure, and low-density lipoprotein cholesterol: A randomized controlled trial, *Journal of the American Medical Association*, 296:2563–2571.

Lehane, E. and McCarthy, G., 2007, An examination of the intentional and unintentional aspects of medication non-adherence in patients diagnosed with hypertension, *Journal of Clinical Nursing*, 16:698–706.

Lin, P.H., Appel, L.J., Funk, K., et al., 2007, The PREMIER Intervention helps participants follow the Dietary Approaches to Stop Hypertension Dietary Pattern and the Current Dietary Reference Intakes recommendations, *Journal of the American Dietetic Association*, 107:1541–1551.

Lowry, K.P., Dudley, T.K., Oddone, E.Z., and Bosworth, H.B., 2005, Intentional and unintentional nonadherence to antihypertensive medication, *Annals of Pharmacotherapy*, 39:1198–1203.

Mann, D.M., Allegrante, J.P., Natarajan, S., Halm, E.A., and Charlson, M., 2007, Predictors of adherence to statins for primary prevention, *Cardiovascular Drugs Therapy,* 21:311–316.

Morgan, A.L., Masoudi, F.A., Havranek, E.P., et al., for the Cardiovascular Outcomes Research Consortium (CORC), 2006, Difficulty taking medications, depression, and health status in heart failure patients, *Journal of Cardiac Failure,* 12:54–60.

Morrow, D.G., Weiner, M., Steinley, D., Young, J., and Murray, M.D., 2007, Patients' health literacy and experience with instructions: Influence preferences for heart failure medication instructions, *Journal of Aging and Health,* 19:575-593.

Nelson, M.R., Reid, C.M., Ryan, P., Willson, K., and Yelland, L., 2006, Self-reported adherence with medication and cardiovascular disease outcomes in the Second Australian National Blood Pressure Study (ANBP2), *Medical Journal of Australia,* 185:487–489.

Schedlbauer, A., Schroeder, K., and Fahey, T., 2007, How can adherence to lipid-lowering medication be improved? A systematic review of randomized controlled trials, *Family Practice,* 24:380–387.

14

FUTURE DIRECTIONS IN DRUG SAFETY

14.1 INTRODUCTION

At the start of this concluding chapter it is appropriate to briefly review our journey to this point. Following a general introduction to the book's topic in Chapter 1, Chapters 2 through 4 provided fundamental biological and physiological information relevant to integrated cardiac safety. Chapters 5 through 12 then discussed proarrhythmic and generalized cardiac safety. Chapter 13 addressed behavioral cardiac safety and also behavioral drug safety in general: Medication errors still lead to far too many adverse drug reactions, and lack of adherence to drug regimens compromises optimum therapeutic benefit for far too many patients.

Initial discussions in this chapter return to proarrhythmic cardiac safety, addressing potential future developments in this field. There are two reasons for this. First, this field of investigation is evolving rapidly, and discussions here provide references to work published shortly before this chapter was written. Second, this field provides a useful model for other areas of drug safety investigation. It is a fully integrated lifecycle model, one in which the information gained in several domains is regarded as complementary. It is also one in which an explicit threshold of regulatory concern is stated. Leaving aside discussions of whether or not the actual value specified is optimal, the existence of such a threshold provides a certain degree of uniformity to activities and occurrences within this field. It is likely that thresholds of regulatory concern will be usefully specified in other fields within drug safety in the future.

This chapter then follows the lead of the previous chapter by widening the scope of our discussions to drug safety in general. It provides an overview of various regulatory guidances addressing drug safety, a report released by Institute of Medicine in September 2006 on the future of drug safety, the Food and Drug Administration Amendments Act (FDAAA) of 2007, and the release of the FDA's Sentinel Initiative in May 2008. The FDAAA and the Sentinel Initiative will play major roles in drug safety activities for years to come.

We then discuss the process of decision making, a topic met in several earlier chapters, and introduce a quantitative method called decision analysis. We also consider several areas of investigation within precision medicine, where scientific advances may prove of considerable benefit in providing individual patients with drugs that safely achieve their intended therapeutic benefit. Finally, we conclude our discussions by highlighting some themes that have recurred throughout the

Integrated Cardiac Safety: Assessment Methodologies for Noncardiac Drugs in Discovery, Development, and Postmarketing Surveillance. By J. Rick Turner and Todd A. Durham
Copyright © 2009 John Wiley & Sons, Inc.

book. Among these themes are the importance of ongoing benefit-risk assessments and adopting an integrated approach to drug safety.

While regulatory discussions here focus primarily on the FDA's drug safety activities, many issues discussed can be generalized to other agencies' deliberations, in spirit if not always in precise operational implementation. Additionally, several relevant web sites providing information about European drug safety activities are provided towards the end of our discussions.

14.2   Future Developments in Torsadogenic Liability Assessment

Chapter 7 discussed the TQT study as presented in ICH Guidance E14. At the time of writing this chapter, ICH E14 is the dominant regulatory document in the field of clinical proarrhythmic liability assessment, and therefore the strategies described therein are the recommended means of assessing torsadogenic liability as indicated by QT/QTc interval prolongation. However, it is appropriate to remind ourselves here that we are not interested in QT interval prolongation *per se*, but rather in the likelihood that a marketed drug will induce TdP in patients prescribed the drug. These two items—QT/QTc prolongation and drug-induced TdP—are not identical entities.

The incidence of drug-induced TdP is typically estimated to fall within a wide range of 1:10,000 to 1:1,000,000. (As we noted in Section 9.3, events this rare are probabilistically not likely to be picked up in preapproval trials, and hence the need for postmarketing surveillance.) Many authors have noted that when drug-induced TdP does occur, it is often the result of a perfect storm scenario, i.e., multiple risk factors are present at the same time (e.g., see Simko et al., 2008). These risk factors include (but are not limited to) advanced age, female sex, a drug regimen involving many drugs, impaired drug metabolizing capacity, a genetic predisposition, electrolyte abnormalities, and existing structural heart disease. It is important to note that while TdP is always associated with QT prolongation, the converse is not true.

The TQT study thus uses QT/QTc prolongation as a risk indicator. It should be noted that there is widespread acknowledgment that QT interval prolongation is not the most accurate predictor of, i.e., the best indicator for, torsadogenic liability. Indeed, some researchers have commented that if it were not relatively easy to measure (at least theoretically: precise identification of the offset of the T-wave can be very difficult for some waveforms), it might be discarded all together. The remaining subsections in this section address alternate assessment methodologies for torsadogenic liability. However, as noted at the beginning of this section, ICH E14 currently needs to be given due attention, as does ICH S7B. In the future, revisions to these guidance documents and/or the release by other regulatory agencies of "Questions and Answers" documents similar to those released by Health Canada (discussed in Section 11.4) may be of benefit.

14.2.1 Correcting for Heart Rate Is More Complex than It Initially Seems

Sections 6.9 and 7.5 described procedures for correcting for heart rate by calculating QTc from QT and concurrent heart rate. In addition to the difficulties of determining which correction formula is most appropriate in any given circumstance, the phenomenon of hysteresis also presents a problem.

While QT is related to heart rate (albeit in an imperfect nonlinear manner), a further complication is that the change in QT lags behind the change in heart rate that leads to it. The delay can be up to a couple of minutes. This delay in the accompanying QT change has the following effect: the same QT is not always associated with the same heart rate, hence, using the same heart rate to correct different QT values leads to more than one associated QTc value. Consider as an example a case where heart rate increases from 60 bpm to 80 bpm over a period of time. At the point where the heart rate is 70 bpm the QT interval will not have adapted, in this scenario shortened, as much as it would if the heart rate had been at a steady rate of 70 bpm for some time. Now consider a case where the heart rate decreases from 80 bpm to 60 bpm over a period of time. At the point where the heart rate is 70 bpm, the QT interval will not have adapted, in this scenario lengthened, as much as it would if the heart rate had been at a steady rate of 70 bpm for some time. Using the value of 70 bpm to correct the two QT values measured at a heart rate of 70 bpm in these two cases, i.e., two different QT values, will therefore result in two different QTc values for the same heart rate, which defeats the point of correcting for heart rate in the first place.

Another fundamental problem with QTc measurements is that there is a lot of variation, i.e., considerable differences of values within a given data set. As Mason (2008) noted in this context, variance makes it more difficult to determine if an observed change in QTc is actually due to a drug effect. Biological sources of variance in QTc include autonomic influences, circadian influences, disease states, food, environmental influences, and gene mutations and gene variants. The correction procedure itself can also lead to variance due to inadequate correction formulae and hysteresis, and also due to measurement-induced variance by both the methodology employed and the readers determining QT values from the ECGs (Mason, 2008). Anything that can be done to reduce variance leads to improved statistical power, which in turn means that fewer participants in the TQT study are needed (if the same number of ECGs are obtained per participant), or fewer ECGs per participant.

One ideal scenario is one in which heart rate does not change, so that no correction for heart rate is required. However, this is not always possible or practical: some drugs may have an effect on heart rate, and maintaining a precisely level heart rate in humans is difficult (although heart rate pacing may be possible in some animal models). Because of these difficulties, it may be helpful to find an index of torsadogenic liability that is independent of heart rate, i.e., one where the heart rate at the time of the index's measurement does not need to be known.

14.2.2 Holter Monitoring

Another approach that represents a departure from those discussed previously is to use the entire Holter datastream, which may contain on the order of 100,000 beats per day. This is a much bigger number than the number of beats (ECGs) used in the TQT study, on the order of 100 beats. While this approach has certain advantages, an immediate problem is the time it would take for a human reader to analyze 100,000 beats and the cost of this service. This therefore suggests the potential utility of semi-automated or automated approaches.

A number of algorithms have been proposed that might be used to identify the end of the T-wave as part of an automatic measurement of the QT interval, but the use of automated methods for assessing QT prolongation in drug-safety studies is not yet well accepted (Couderc and Zareba, 2005). Mortara (2005) emphasized that continued development in the area of automatic measurement will likely be an important undertaking so that more intensive data collection, e.g. from continuous Holter studies, resulting in hundreds if not thousands of readings, can be analyzed in a practical manner.

See also Wozniacka et al. (2006) and Yilmaz et al. (2007) for examples of the use of Holter monitoring in the assessment of drug cardiotoxicity in other circumstances.

14.2.3 Enhancing TQT Study Designs to Minimize False Positive Results

In Chapter 7 the results of a statistical study designed to describe the performance characteristics of the intersection-union-test (IUT) to evaluate QTc effects in the TQT study were discussed. The importance of the statistical research presented in Chapter 7 is that it demonstrates that a well-intentioned and rational approach to consider all time points in the TQT study can result in unusually high rates of false positive results. A positive TQT study result can increase the cost of further development (e.g., due to more intensive cardiac monitoring in later phases of development) or lead to abandonment of a new drug altogether. Further research into statistical approaches (e.g., modified testing strategies or modeling techniques) which do not yield high false positive results would seem to be a worthwhile endeavor.

14.2.4 Other Ion Channels in Addition to the KCNH2/hERG Channel Can Be Important

In Table 4.1 we presented three ionic currents involved in myocardial depolarization and repolarization: I_{Na}, I_{Ks}, and I_{Kr}. It was noted in Chapter 4 that these are a small subset of all of the ionic currents involved in these processes, and that our attention would focus on the repolarizing current I_{Kr}, i.e., the KCNH2/hERG current. This focus resulted from the observations that (to date) this is the repolarizing current most commonly blocked by small-molecule drugs that lead to QT interval prolongation via ion channel blockade, and that a wide array of drugs block this channel (see Jost et al., 2007, for a discussion of the I_{Ks} current). Although we noted in Chapter 4 that we do not discuss calcium ion channels in detail, at this point it is instructive to briefly consider their relevance with regard to assessing a drug compound's torsadogenic liability (see Doering and Zamponi, 2006, for further discussion of these channels).

Calcium ions flow into myocardial cells through calcium channels, and constitute a depolarizing ionic current. These ions play a role in excitation-contraction coupling in the heart. Their relevance here is as follows. The drug verapamil is a potent inhibitor of the KCNH2/hERG current, but it is not associated with clinical issues of QT interval prolongation. The reason for this is that verapamil also blocks the myocardial calcium channels, leading to reduced overall depolarizing current. By reducing both repolarizing and depolarizing ionic currents, the net effect is that verapamil does not impact the QT interval to any clinically significant degree.

The relevance of this observation for the development of new drugs is that, if a similarly acting compound were to be tested only for its ability to reduce the KCNH2/hERG current, its clear ability to do so might lead to the compound's development program being discontinued. Imagine a scenario where this compound may have proved to be an extremely useful therapeutic drug with a favorable benefit-risk balance. The development program's failure to identify the effect of the compound on both repolarizing and depolarizing ionic currents—and therefore to reveal that, despite blocking the KCNH2/hERG channel, the compound is not actually associated with torsadogenic liability—would deprive patients of the opportunity to benefit from the drug had it been approved.

Thus, in addition to failing to identify QT liabilities that do exist, identifying QT liabilities that likely do not exist can be problematic in drug development. (An analogous problem exists in efficacy evaluation: we do not want to say that a drug is efficacious when it truly is not, and we do not want to fail to identify drugs that truly are efficacious.)

14.2.5 KCNH2/hERG Trafficking Deficiencies Revisited

We noted in Section 4.7 that KCNH2/hERG channel trafficking deficiencies represent another mechanism for loss of function in hERG current (in both inherited LQTS and acquired QT prolongation). Hence, potential drug-induced KCNH2/hERG channel trafficking deficiencies need to be investigated in addition to testing for KCNH2/hERG channel blockade.

Another point of interest concerning trafficking deficiencies is that their influence on KCNH2/hERG current may operate over a different time scale from those due to KCNH2/hERG channel blockade: The onset of effects due to trafficking deficiencies may be slower. Van der Heyden et al. (2008) noted that long-term trafficking effects may not be identified in current drug development programs since, in contrast to routine screening for short-term effects of channel blockade, screening for long-term trafficking defects is not common. These authors also noted the existence of drugs with dual effects on KCNH2/hERG current: short-term effects via KCNH2/hERG channel blockade and longer-term effects via KCNH2/hERG channel trafficking deficiencies. As well as operating on different time scales, these two mechanisms of action may operate over different concentration scales. (For further discussion, see Hancox and Mitcheson, 2006, and Takemasa et al., 2008.)

14.2.6   Other Potential Indices

Section 4.6.1 discussed transmural dispersion of repolarization, and Section 4.6.2 identified other candidates for the preeminent designee(s) as indicators of torsadogenic liability. In addition to the references provided in those sections readers are referred to Extramiana et al. (2007) for discussions of T-wave morphology and to Hondeghem (2007, 2008) for discussions of TRIaD.

14.2.7   The Concentration-QT Relationship

Pharmacokinetic-pharmacodynamic (PK/PD) or exposure-response modeling techniques in evaluating torsadogenic potential were introduced in Section 7.16. A recent paper by Garnett et al. (2008) discussed the roles of concentration-QT relationships in more detail. The concentration-QT relationship can be helpful in several ways in regulatory decision making, including the planning and interpretation of TQT studies, quantification of a drug's benefit-risk balance, assessment of QT risk in subpopulations, making dose adjustments, determination of QTc prolongation for a given drug when a TQT study cannot be conducted, and writing informative labels. See also Bloomfield and Krishna (2008), Lin and Chan (2008), and Tsong et al. (2008).

14.3   THE PRESCRIPTION DRUG USER FEE ACT

The Prescription Drug User Fee Act (PDUFA) was passed in 1992. Under the terms of this act, sponsors pay a fee to the FDA every time an NDA is submitted. At the end of each five-year period since 1992 PDUFA has been reauthorized by a succession of differently named but related acts, and the acronyms PDUFA II, III, and IV are sometimes seen in the literature to denote these acts. The most recent reauthorization occurred in the FDAAA (PDUFA IV), which was signed by President Bush on September 27, 2007 and became operative on October 1, 2007.

The total of all fees paid under PDUFA has historically represented a sizable proportion of the FDA's funding. An FDA White Paper entitled "Prescription Drug User Fee Act (PDUFA): Adding Resources and Improving Performance in FDA Review of New Drug Applications" (FDA, 2005a, p. 1) noted the following:

> The Prescription Drug User Fee Act (PDUFA) program is the cornerstone of modern FDA drug review. User fees currently fund about half of new drug review costs. By providing needed funds, PDUFA ended slow and unpredictable review and approval of new drug applications, while keeping FDA's high standards.

PDUFA funds allowed FDA to accomplish a number of important goals. FDA hired more review and support staff to speed review. The number of full-time equivalent (FTE) staff devoted to the new drug review process has nearly doubled, growing from 1,277 FTE in 1992 to 2,503 FTE in 2004. FDA upgraded its data systems and gave industry guidance to help minimize unnecessary trials and generally improve drug development. FDA gave industry guidance on how to improve the quality of applications, with the goal of reducing misunderstandings and the need for sponsors to rework and resubmit applications. Finally, FDA improved procedures and standards to make reviews more rigorous, consistent, and predictable.

However, PDUFA has not been without its critics. The fact that PDUFA funds have comprised such a sizeable component of FDA's budget has prompted some observers to comment that conflict of interest is a potential outcome of such an arrangement: these funds have been used to pay reviewers' salaries. Additionally, and of particular relevance in this chapter, the Institute of Medicine (2007b) noted that the first two iterations of PDUFA (PDUFA in 1992 and PDUFA II in 1997) "specifically prohibited the use of fees for any postmarketing drug safety activities" (Institute of Medicine, 2007b, p. 16). In the 2002 reauthorization (PDUFA III), a small amount of fee revenues (about 5%) was permitted to be used for postmarketing drug safety activities, but the spending of these funds was heavily restricted. They could only be used in conjunction with drugs approved after 2002, and they could only be used for up to two years after a drug's approval, or up to three years for certain drugs that may have serious side effects. However, the provisions in the 2007 FDAAA (PDUFA IV) are set to change this state of affairs: this act is discussed in Section 14.12.

14.4 THREE RELATED FDA GUIDANCES ON RISK MANAGEMENT

The FDA released three related guidance documents in March 2005, each focusing on one aspect of risk management. These guidances addressed the following topics:

> ➢ Premarketing risk assessment (FDA, 2005a). This guidance addressed the generation, acquisition, analysis, and presentation of preapproval safety data. The FDA recommended that, from the outset of development, sponsors pay

careful attention to the overall design of safety evaluation to maximize the information gained from clinical trials.

➤ Good pharmacovigilance practices and pharmacoepidemiological assessment (FDA, 2005b).
➤ The development and use of risk minimization action plans (RiskMAPs) (FDA, 2005c).

The processes of risk assessment and risk minimization combine to form what the FDA terms risk management. Risk management is an iterative process consisting of several actions that should be conducted continuously throughout a drug's lifecycle, with the results of risk assessment informing a sponsor's decisions regarding risk minimization. The four-part process comprises the following:

➤ Assessing a product's benefit-risk balance.
➤ Developing and implementing tools to minimize the product's risks while preserving its benefits.
➤ Evaluating the effectiveness of these tools and reassessing the benefit-risk balance.
➤ Making any necessary adjustments to the risk minimization tools to further improve the benefit-risk balance.

The FDA therefore views risk management as "an iterative process encompassing the assessment of risks and benefits, the minimization of risks, and the maximization of benefits" (FDA, 2005c, p. 3).

14.5   THE FDA PREMARKETING RISK ASSESSMENT GUIDANCE

This guidance document (FDA, 2005a) discussed the generation, acquisition, analysis, and presentation of premarketing safety data. To maximize the information gained from clinical trials, the FDA recommends that, from the outset of development, sponsors pay careful attention to the overall design of safety evaluation. The agency is fully aware that "Even large clinical development programs cannot reasonably be expected to identify all risks associated with a product" (FDA, 2005a, p. 6), and it is therefore expected that "some risks will become apparent only after approval, when the product is used in tens of thousands or even millions of patients in the general population." Having said this, however, the FDA also acknowledges that the larger and more comprehensive the preapproval database, the more likely it is that serious adverse events (or safety signals) will be detected during preapproval drug development.

Several factors influence the determination of the appropriate size of a preapproval safety database for a new investigational drug:

> ➤ Its novelty (i.e., whether it represents a new treatment, or is similar to available treatments).
> ➤ The condition being treated and the intended population in which the treatment will be used.
> ➤ The intended duration of use.
> ➤ The availability of alternative therapies and the relative safety of those alternatives compared to that of the new product's safety profile.

As has been noted in previous chapters, assessment of both benefit and risk is needed for meaningful benefit-risk analysis. This observation has a direct impact on the quantity and quality of the safety database: generally, the fewer the drug's benefits, the less the uncertainty that may be acceptable with regard to its safety. Additionally, a larger safety database may be appropriate if a drug's nonclinical assessment or human pharmacology studies have identified signals of risk that warrant considerable clinical data to properly define the risk.

14.5.1 Issues to Be Addressed by Sponsors during New Drug Development

The FDA recommends that sponsors address the potential for serious adverse effects in various categories for all new small-molecule drugs, including the following:

> ➤ Drug-related QTc prolongation.
> ➤ Drug-related liver toxicity.
> ➤ Drug-related nephrotoxicity.
> ➤ Drug-related bone marrow toxicity.
> ➤ Drug-drug interactions.
> ➤ Polymorphic metabolism.

The meaning of the word address in this context varies with the circumstance. For example, consider the case of a drug that is intended to be applied topically. If it has been shown that the drug has no systemic bioavailability, systemic toxicities would not be of concern, and this issue could therefore be addressed in relatively less detail.

14.5.2 Analyzing Temporal Associations

We noted in Section 8.6.11 that temporal relationships between exposure to a drug and the occurrence of an adverse event can be very informative. As noted in the FDA's premarketing risk assessment guidance, when preparing individual participant safety reports, the temporal relationship between drug exposure and an adverse event is a critical consideration in the assessment of potential causality.

However, temporal parameters such as time-to-event and the duration of the event can be overlooked in aggregate inspections of safety data. As noted in this guidance (FDA, 2005a, p. 20), "Simple comparisons of adverse event frequencies between (or among) treatment groups, which are commonly included in product applications and reproduced in tabular format in labeling, generally do not take into account the time dependency of adverse events."

14.5.3   Narrative Summaries

Certain adverse events, e.g., those leading to discontinuation, death, and other serious adverse events, require narrative summaries to be written and submitted. These narratives should not simply repeat in sentence format the information that was adequately presented in the body of the clinical study report in numerical format. Rather, the narratives should permit an adequate understanding of the nature of each adverse event by providing "a complete synthesis of all available clinical data and an informed discussion of the case" (FDA, 2005a, p. 26). Useful components in a narrative include:

> ➢ The participant's age and sex.
> ➢ The participant's treatment group.
> ➢ Signs and symptoms related to the adverse event being discussed.
> ➢ An assessment of the relationship of exposure duration to the development of the adverse event.
> ➢ Concomitant medications, with start dates relative to the adverse event.
> ➢ Pertinent medical history, physical examination findings, and test results (e.g., laboratory data, ECG data, biopsy data).
> ➢ Discussion of the diagnosis as supported by available clinical data (for events without a definite diagnosis, a list of possibilities is useful).
> ➢ Outcomes and follow-up information.

14.6   THE FDA GOOD PHARMACOVIGILANCE PRACTICES AND PHARMACOEPIDEMIOLOGICAL ASSESSMENT GUIDANCE

Collection of postmarketing safety data and related risk assessment "are critical for evaluating and characterizing a product's risk profile and for making informed decisions on risk minimization" (FDA, 2005b, p. 3). Good pharmacovigilance practice is generally based on acquiring complete data from spontaneous adverse advent reports, since the quality of these reports is critical for appropriate evaluation of any relationship between the drug and the adverse event. As noted in this report, "FDA recommends that sponsors make a reasonable attempt to obtain complete information for case assessment during initial contacts and subsequent follow-up, especially for serious events, and encourages sponsors to use trained health care practitioners to query reporters" (FDA, 2005b, p. 4). When the report comes from a patient, obtaining permission to contact the patient's health care providers to obtain further medical information is an important consideration.

This guidance provided a discusion of the characteristics of a good case report, and developing a case series, presenting summary descriptive analysis of a case series, the use of data mining, pharmacoepidemiological studies, and registries. It also addresses the interpretation of safety signals, and the process of moving from a signal to a potential safety risk, and the development of a pharmacovigilance plan.

14.7 THE FDA DEVELOPMENT AND USE OF RISK MINIMIZATION ACTION PLANS GUIDANCE

A RiskMAP is defined as "a strategic safety program designed to meet specific goals and objectives in minimizing known risks of a product while preserving its benefits" (FDA, 2005c, p. 5). A RiskMAP targets safety-related goals and uses tools to achieve those goals. The FDA provided recommendations for using RiskMAPs, including the following:

> RiskMAPs should target the achievement of particular goals, i.e., health outcomes, related to known safety risks.
> Goals should be stated in such a way as to achieve maximum risk reduction.
> Goals should be translated into specific, pragmatic, and measurable objectives that result in processes or behaviors leading to achievement of a RiskMAP's goals.

Since evidence-based risk identification, risk assessment, and risk characterization should occur throughout a drug's lifecycle, a risk that warrants the consideration of a RiskMAP can occur during premarketing or postmarketing assessments. Several general considerations may determine whether the development of a RiskMAP is desirable:

> The nature and rate of known benefits and risks. Comparing the characteristics of the drug's benefits and risks may help clarify whether a RiskMAP could improve the benefit-risk balance.
> These characteristics might include:
  • The types, magnitude, and frequency of benefits and risks.
  • Patient populations likely to derive the most benefit and populations at the greatest risk.
> Improving the likelihood of benefit. A RiskMAP could improve the benefit-risk balance by increasing the benefit if factors are identified that can predict effectiveness.
> Decreasing the likelihood of risk. Identifiable serious adverse effects that can be minimized or avoided by preventive measures associated with the

prescription of drugs are the preferred candidates for RiskMAPs. In such cases, a RiskMAP could improve the benefit-risk balance by decreasing the risk.

14.7.1 Determining Appropriate Risk Minimization Approaches

The FDA believes that routine risk management measures are sufficient for most drugs. In a small number of cases, however, a RiskMAP should be considered. The FDA recommends that these plans "be used judiciously to minimize risks without encumbering drug availability or otherwise interfering with the delivery of product benefits to patients" (FDA, 2005c, p. 5).

14.7.2 Risk Minimization Action Plan Tools

Once the objectives of a RiskMAP have been identified, appropriate tools can be selected to achieve these objectives. The FDA guidance on RiskMAPs lists several categories of tools that are currently used in risk minimization plans. One of these categories is targeted education and outreach. Targeted education and outreach efforts are employed to educate key stakeholders, e.g., health care practitioners and patients, regarding preventing or lessening the risks of using a particular drug. Specific tools falling into this category include:

- ➢ Health care practitioner letters.
- ➢ Training programs for health care practitioners or patients.
- ➢ Prominent professional or public notifications.
- ➢ Continuing education for health care practitioners. One example of such continuing education would be product-focused programs developed by sponsors and/or accredited continuing education programs supported by the sponsor.

14.8   REPORTS ON THE STATUS OF POSTMARKETING STUDY COMMITMENTS

The Food and Drug Administration Modernization Act (FDAMA, also known as PDUFA II) was signed into law in November 1997, and Section 130 added Section 506B (Reports of Postmarketing Studies) to the federal Food, Drug, and Cosmetic Act. This section addressed the reporting of postmarketing studies, and provided for the FDA to be given additional authority to monitor the progress of postmarketing studies of both small-molecule drugs and biologicals that sponsors had agreed to conduct, or were required by the agency to be conducted. The regulations went into effect in April 2001, at which time the FDA issued a draft guidance relating to this rule. The FDA's final guidance, entitled *Reports on the Status of Postmarketing Study Commitments—Implementation of Section 130 of the Food and Drug*

Administration Modernization Act of 1997, was published in February 2006. This guidance described the content, format, and timing of the postmarketing study commitment reports required by Section 506B in more detail and also discussed the reporting of other postmarketing studies that are not subject to Section 506B. Addressing sponsors directly, this guidance noted the following (FDA, 2006, p. 2):

> If you are required by the FDA, or if you have entered into an agreement with the FDA, to conduct a postmarketing study concerning clinical safety, clinical efficacy, clinical pharmacology, or nonclinical toxicology, you are required to provide the Agency with an annual report on the status of the study until the FDA notifies you, in writing, that the Agency concurs with your determination that the study commitment has been fulfilled or that the study either is no longer feasible or would no longer provide useful information. This annual report must address the progress of the study or the reasons for your failure to conduct the study.

Section 506B also requires the FDA to make certain information available to the public about postmarketing study commitments and sponsors' progress in completing those studies. More specifically, under Section 506B(c), the FDA must develop and publish annually in the *Federal Register* a report on the status of postmarketing study commitments that sponsors have agreed to or are required to conduct and for which annual status reports have been submitted. Section 506B(b) indicates that any information necessary to identify sponsors as the applicant of a study and establish the status of a study and the reasons, if any, for any failure to carry out the study, is considered to be public information.

14.9 REPORTING ADVERSE EVENTS TO INVESTIGATIONAL REVIEW BOARDS

In April 2007 the FDA issued a draft guidance for clinical investigators, sponsors, and investigational review boards (IRBs) entitled *Adverse Event Reporting— Improving Human Subject Protection* (FDA, 2007). This guidance was intended to assist sponsors and investigators in interpreting requirements in the Code of Federal Regulations addressing the submission of reports of "unanticipated problems" to IRBs. The reason for the development and issuance of this guidance was considerable concern on the part of IRBs, in general, that many of the increasingly large number of individual adverse event reports being submitted to them were lacking in context and detail. Therefore, the large number of reports was felt to be inhibiting, rather than enhancing, the ability of IRBs to adequately protect human subjects.

The FDA regulates clinical trials of drugs and biologicals authorized under Section 505(i) of the Federal Food, Drug, and Cosmetic Act. Sponsors and investigators (the individuals who actually conduct a clinical investigation, i.e., those under whose direction and responsibility study drugs are administered or dispensed to study participants) have regulatory obligations during clinical trials conducted under an IND (21 CFR part 312). Obligations for sponsors include:

> ➢ Keeping each participating investigator informed of new observations discovered by or reported to the sponsor on the drug, particularly with respect to adverse effects and safe use.
> ➢ Notifying all participating investigators, in a written IND safety report, of any adverse experiences associated with the use of the drug that is both serious and unexpected, and any findings from tests in laboratory animals that suggest a significant risk for human participants. Additionally, sponsors are required to identify in these IND safety reports all previous safety reports concerning similar adverse experiences and to analyze the significance of the current adverse experience in the context of the previous reports.

Obligations for investigators include:

> ➢ Promptly reporting any adverse effect that may reasonably be regarded as being caused by, or probably caused by, the drug to the sponsor. If the adverse event is "alarming," the investigator must report the adverse effect immediately.
> ➢ Promptly reporting all unanticipated problems involving risks to human participants or others to the IRB.

However, fulfillment of these obligations requires determination of precisely which occurrences represent unanticipated problems. Because this determination may be difficult, and because investigators (laudably) want to fulfill both the letter and the spirit of these requirements, they are sending a tremendous number of reports to IRBs. However, as noted a few moments ago, many of these reports lack sufficient context and detail, thereby impeding IRBs' function as effective monitors of safety. Specific problems include:

> ➢ Sponsors may not explain to investigators why an event constitutes an unanticipated problem in a given clinical trial and how the event relates to that particular study.
> ➢ Events that were anticipated—events described in the related Investigator's Brochure, the study protocol, and the study's informed consent form—are often reported, adding to the number of reports that IRBs must go through.
> ➢ Some events are part of the underlying process of the disease being studied, and/or they may occur at reasonably large background rates in the participant population. The IRBs have found that, in reports of such events, individual reports of their occurrence in a clinical trial are almost never informative. Before such events can be determined to be unanticipated, and their

significance (or otherwise) can therefore be assessed, a comparison of the incidence of the event in treated participants and untreated participants/patients is needed.

In general, the FDA's position is that it is difficult to determine from an individual adverse event report whether or not the event represents an unanticipated problem, even if the event is not addressed in the investigator's brochure, study protocol, or informed consent form, and therefore may initially (and reasonably) be thought to be an unanticipated problem. The assessment of an adverse event in the context of other such events (if they exist) provides some assurance that any determination made will have a certain degree of validity. Similarly, in the context of reporting to IRBs, individual adverse event reports generally require an evaluation of their relevance and significance to the study, including an evaluation of other adverse events, before they can be considered to be an unanticipated problem.

The FDA therefore believes that reports that lack such assessment should not be submitted to IRBs, since the IRB will be unable to assess the significance of the report. Reports of unanticipated problems that are submitted to IRBs should provide information that is of some relevance to the IRB's responsibility to ensure the protection of participants (e.g., new information that might affect the IRB's view of the study or that suggests a beneficial change to the study protocol or consent form). These reports should explain clearly why the event described represents a problem for the study, and why it is unanticipated. Sponsors are required to notify investigators of serious and unexpected adverse experiences, and must keep investigators informed of new observations discovered by or reported to the sponsor, particularly with respect to adverse effects and safe use.

This guidance therefore clarifies the FDA's position that only the following adverse experiences (or events) should be reported to the IRB as unanticipated problems:

- ➤ Any adverse experience that, even without detailed analysis, represents a serious unexpected adverse event that is rare in the absence of drug exposure (e.g., agranulocytosis, hepatic necrosis, Stevens-Johnson syndrome).
- ➤ A series of adverse events that, on analysis, is both unanticipated and a problem for the study. There would be a determination that the series of adverse events represents a sign that the adverse events were not just isolated occurrences and were significant to the rights and welfare of participants. The FDA recommends that a summary and analyses supporting the conclusion accompany the report.
- ➤ An adverse event that is described or addressed in the investigator's brochure, protocol, or informed consent documents, or expected to occur in study participants at an anticipated rate (e.g., expected progression of disease, occurrence of events consistent with the background rate in the participant population), but that occurs at a greater frequency or greater severity than expected. The FDA recommends that a discussion of the divergence from expected rates of occurrence accompany the report.

> Any other adverse event that would cause the sponsor to modify the investigator's brochure, study protocol, or informed consent documents, or would prompt other action by the IRB to ensure the protection of participants. The FDA recommends that an explanation of the conclusion accompany the report.

Sponsors typically have considerably more experience and expertise with the study drug than individual investigators, and are therefore in a better position to process and analyze the significance of adverse event information from multiple sites and determine whether an adverse event is an unanticipated problem or not. It is therefore beneficial, from the IRB's perspective, to receive thorough analyses from sponsors rather than less detailed (and more speculative) reports from investigators. However, investigators are also obligated to provide such reports. Fortunately, this guidance provides a solution that is beneficial to all concerned. To satisfy their responsibility to inform their IRBs of unexpected problems, investigators may rely on the sponsor's assessment and provide their IRB with a report of the unanticipated problem prepared by the sponsor. Further, if an explicit agreement between the sponsor, investigators, and IRBs is made up front to this effect, investigators will be regarded as having fulfilled their reporting responsibilities when the sponsor provides a report to the IRB and sends a copy to the investigators.

In this manner, sponsors, investigators, IRBs, and, most importantly, patients are well served since the IRBs obtain the most useful information possible.

14.10   FDA's COMMUNICATION TO THE PUBLIC

In March 2007, the FDA issued a guidance entitled *Drug Safety Information—FDA's Communication to the Public* (see http://www.fda.gov/cder/guidance/7477fnl.pdf, accessed May 30, 2008). This document provided guidance "on how the FDA is developing and disseminating information to the public regarding important drug safety issues, including emerging drug safety information" (p. 1). The document regards an important drug safety issue as "one that has the potential to alter the benefit/risk analysis for a drug in such a way as to affect decisions about prescribing or taking the drug," and regards emerging drug safety information as "information about an important drug safety issue that has not yet been fully analyzed or confirmed" (p. 1).

The broad range of methods used by the FDA to communicate drug safety information to the public (including both prescribing physicians and patients) includes the following:

> Professional labeling for prescription drugs.
> Patient-directed labeling for prescription drugs (patient package inserts and medication guides).
> Over-the-counter (OTC) "drug facts" labeling.

> ➢ Public health advisories.
> ➢ Patient information sheets.
> ➢ Healthcare professional information sheets.
> ➢ Alerts on patient information and healthcare professional sheets.

The FDA also noted that it is "assessing other communication tools, including broadcasts and conference calls to disseminate drug safety information."

Another development related to communicating with the public is the formation of the FDA's Risk Communication Advisory Committee. The FDA announced the establishment of the advisory committee on June 5, 2007, and announced the members selected on November 5, 2007. In its press release, the FDA noted the following (see http://www.fda.gov/bbs/topics/NEWS/2007/NEW01739.html, accessed March 1, 2008):

> The advisory committee's 15 voting members include independent experts and public members. Experts were chosen from the fields of risk communication, risk perception, decision analysis, communication, [and others]. Public members include those who can provide the perspective of users of FDA-regulated products, such as consumers, patients, caregivers and health care providers. For some meetings, one or more industry representatives may be invited to participate in a nonvoting capacity.

Formation of this Advisory Committee resulted from a recommendation made in the Institute of Medicine report discussed in the next section.

14.11   THE INSTITUTE OF MEDICINE'S REPORT *THE FUTURE OF DRUG SAFETY*

In September 2006, the Institute of Medicine's Committee on the Assessment of the U.S. Drug Safety System released a report, commissioned by FDA, entitled *The Future of Drug Safety: Promoting and Protecting the Health of the Public.* This report was then published in book format by the National Academies Press in 2007, and hence citations to the contents of this report are presented here as "Institute of Medicine, (2007b)," along with the respective page numbers from the book. This report addresses the FDA's function in a broad manner, commenting on its structure, operations, and how it might best be funded by Congress in order to carry out its mandates.

While this report is not a regulatory document *per se,* its contents are summarized here since the report made explicit recommendations for modifications to the FDA's regulatory activities. Following this, the next three sections discuss the FDAAA (October 2007) and two documents released by FDA in March and May of 2008, respectively. Each of these documents is relevant to current FDA initiatives addressing these recommendations.

The intent of the broad set of recommendations in *The Future of Drug Safety* was to ensure that consideration of safety extends from before drug approval throughout the entire time the drug is marketed and used. The reported noted that "The approval decision does represent a singular moment of clarity about the risks and benefits associated with a drug—preapproval clinical trials do not obviate continued formal evaluations after approval" (Institute of Medicine, 2007b, p. 27). It also noted the following (p. 19):

> No one in FDA, industry, or academic research enterprise would disagree with the importance of implementing a lifecycle approach to the assessment of drug risks and benefits. Nevertheless, a great deal of separation persists between premarket and postmarket activities and functions. The separation, both structural and cultural, is reinforced by user-fee funding that is predominantly devoted to premarket activities and funding from appropriations that has not kept up with need in vital areas of the agency's work, by regulatory authority that is stronger and clearer preapproval, and by data requirements that are more structured and intensive for approval than for the postmarketing period.

It was recommended that the FDA should:

> ➢ Appoint a staff member from the Office of Surveillance and Epidemiology to each New Drug Application review team, and assign authority for postapproval regulatory actions related to safety jointly to the Office for New Drugs and the Office of Surveillance and Epidemiology.
> ➢ Ensure the performance of timely and scientifically-valid evaluations of RiskMAPs.
> ➢ Develop a systematic approach to benefit-risk analysis for use throughout the FDA in both preapproval and postapproval settings, and should continually improve this approach once developed and implemented.
> ➢ Build internal epidemiological and informatics capacity to improve the postmarketing assessment of drugs.
> ➢ Form review teams to regularly and systematically analyze all postmarketing study results and make their assessment of the significance of the results, with regard to their integration of risk and benefit information, available to the public.

It was further recommended that Congress should:

> ➢ Ensure that the FDA has the ability to require such postmarketing risk assessment and risk management programs as needed to monitor and ensure safe use of drugs.
> ➢ Enact legislation establishing a new FDA advisory committee on communication with patients and consumers. The committee would be

composed of members who represent consumer and patient perspectives and organizations (recall the discussions in the previous section).
➢ Approve, at the Administration's request, substantially increased resources in both funds and personnel for the FDA in order to support improvements in drug safety and efficacy activities over a drug's lifecycle.

Immediately following the last recommendation listed here, the report continued as follows (Institute of Medicine, 2007b, p. 198):

> The committee favors appropriations from general revenues, rather than user fees, to support the full spectrum of new drug safety responsibilities proposed in this report. This preference is based on the expectation that CDER will continue to review and approve drugs in a timely manner and that increasing attention to drug safety will not occur at the expense of efficacy reviews but rather it will complement efficacy review for a lifecycle approach to drugs. Congressional appropriations from general tax revenues are a mechanism by which the public can directly, fairly, and effectively invest in the FDA's postmarket drug safety activities.

A paradoxical state of affairs has existed in the past: the best information about a drug's safety and effectiveness is gathered once it has been approved and is being used by many patients, yet regulatory governance of the collection and dissemination of postmarketing information has been considerably less than the regulatory governance of premarketing nonclinical and clinical research. Integrated and equally stringent regulatory governance throughout a drug's lifecycle is a worthwhile goal. The Institute of Medicine's report noted that FDA's critical mission, to protect and advance the public's health, requires that it be given adequate resources (financial and personnel) and authority to enforce defined penalties and sanctions in the domain of postmarketing evaluation of a drug's safety.

As noted earlier, the following three sections discuss events relevant to current FDA initiatives addressing these recommendations.

14.12   THE FOOD AND DRUG ADMINISTRATION AMENDMENTS ACT OF **2007**

As noted in Section 14.3, the FDAAA (PDUFA IV) became operative on October 1st 2007. Schultz (2007) noted that the key drug safety provisions in this act are:

➢ Power to require postmarketing studies, order changes in a drug's label, and restrict distribution of a drug.
➢ New resources of $225 million over five years for drug safety activities ($25 million for financial year 2008, rising incrementally by $10 million per year to reach $65 million for financial year 2012).

> Modernization of the AERS and access to large governmental and private databases on adverse drug reactions.
> Elevation of the drug safety group's organizational status.

14.12.1   Legal Issues Surrounding Drug Labeling

A drug's label includes warnings and other information critical to the safe use of the drug. In the first three iterations of the PDUFA, the FDA never actually had the power to order companies to make labeling changes for a drug that was already on the market. Now, after a 30-day period of negotiation, the FDAAA says that the agency may order such a change. However, there may be legal repercussions from various challenges to this.

In addition to discussing the Supreme Court and its past and potential future rulings on medical device issues, Korobkin (2007) addressed state and federal involvement in pharmaceutical issues. The FDA's current position (at the time of writing) on labeling rules for prescription drugs is that its approval of label language preempts private lawsuits alleging that a manufacturer did not provide an adequate warning of a drug's risks. Currently, there is no federal law that expressly provides that FDA requirements for drugs should preempt state law. Therefore, "the survival of the FDA's claim of preemption depends largely on whether courts will defer to the agency's view that state-court verdicts undermine its mission and are therefore implicitly preempted because the Constitution provides for the supremacy of federal law over conflicting state law" (Korobkin, 2007, p. 1681). Political commentary along party lines and litigation followed this preemption provision in the drug-labeling regulations. Korobkin noted that the Supreme Court is likely to agree to consider this issue in the next several years. If so, the Supreme Court's decision could have considerable ramifications for state versus federal control of both drugs and medical devices. As Korobkin (2007, p. 1681) further commented:

> The outcome could have an effect on the willingness of pharmaceutical companies to invest in, and on the prices they charge for, new classes of products with unknown medical risks and thus more uncertain legal ones. The balance between two important goals—the safety and the availability of new treatments—is at stake.

Glantz and Annas (2008) noted that the Supreme Court is now scheduled to consider this issue in late 2008 (Wyeth v. Levine, cert. granted, 2008: Glantz and Annas, 2008, p. 1885).

14.13   THE FDA'S DRUG SAFETY FIVE-YEAR PLAN

In March 2008 the FDA released a draft of the *Prescription Drug User Fee Act (PDUFA) IV Drug Safety Five-year Plan* (see http://www.fda.gov/cder/pdufa/ PDUFA_IV_5yr_plan_draft.pdf, accessed May 30, 2008). The purpose of this plan is "to communicate FDA's strategy for meeting the commitments for enhancing and modernizing the drug safety system" within the context of FDAAA (p.1). The FDA intends to use this plan to:

> ➤ Communicate their strategies for using the drug safety resources provided by the FDAAA.
> ➤ Communicate their current activity and establish measures to report progress.
> ➤ Provide FDA leadership and management with a foundation for understanding planned FDAAA drug safety activities.

Under the FDAAA program, $29.29 million (plus an inflation factor) will be allocated annually to enhance the Agency's drug safety capabilities. With these funds, FDA will be able to:

> ➤ Increase the number of employees dedicated to safety evaluation of marketed medications.
> ➤ Add resources for adopting new scientific approaches to drug safety, improving the utility of existing tools for detection and prevention of adverse events, and incorporating the new approaches into the Agency's drug safety program.

In addition to these funds, Congress authorized FDA to collect additional user fees to broaden the focus of drug safety. As noted in the previous section, these amounts are set at $25 million for financial year 2008, rising incrementally by $10 million per year to reach $65 million for financial year 2012. The report noted that "We believe that Congress intended these additional resources to increase the Agency's capacity for handling new authorities and requirements of FDAAA" (p. 2), including efforts associated with the implementation of:

> ➤ Risk evaluation and mitigation strategies (REMS).
> ➤ Postmarketing study/trial requirements.
> ➤ Safety labeling changes.
> ➤ Active postmarketing risk identification (see Section 14.14.2 for FDA's view of active postmarketing surveillance).

With this funding, FDA will support and strengthen its postmarketing activities by increasing staff levels of:

> ➤ Safety evaluators responsible for reviewing adverse events reported for, and evaluating the safety of, marketed drugs.
> ➤ Epidemiologists responsible for reviewing protocols and study reports and conducting nonexperimental pharmacoepidemiological studies.
> ➤ Risk management experts, including risk management analysts, program evaluators, and behavioral and social science experts. These personnel will be responsible for reviewing proposed and implemented RiskMAPs or REMS, and reviewing and developing risk management communication tools.
> ➤ Medication experts devoted to medication error analysis and prevention.
> ➤ Regulatory project managers responsible for providing regulatory input relevant to the management, tracking, and facilitation of projects related to drug safety, and the improvement of communication.

The FDAAA recognized and emphasized the FDA's vital role in ensuring the safe and appropriate use of marketed drugs. This act provided the FDA with substantial new resources for medical product safety, as well as "a variety of regulatory tools and authorities" to ensure such use (p. 2). The plan continued as follows (p. 2):

> The Congress, consistent with many recommendations made over the past two years by the Institute of Medicine, the GAO [US General Accountability Office: see http://www.gao.gov], and a multitude of others, directs FDA to shift its regulatory paradigm to recognize that ensuring that marketed drugs are used as safely and effectively as possible is equally as important as getting new safe and effective drugs to market quickly and efficiently. With the goal of maintaining a systematic and scientific approach to the evaluation of benefit/risk throughout the product lifecycle, FDA must build the scientific and administrative capacity needed to become active and collaborative players in the U.S. healthcare delivery system.

The paradigm shift cited in this quote is a critical one in the context of this book's discussions: it makes clear that an integrated evaluation of drug safety, operationalized in terms of benefit-risk balance assessments, must be conducted throughout lifecycle drug development, and that equal weight must be given to preapproval and postapproval safety investigations.

14.14   THE FDA'S *SENTINEL INITIATIVE* **AND THE SCIENCE OF SAFETY**

In May 2008 the FDA released a report entitled *The Sentinel Initiative: A National Strategy for Monitoring Medical Product Safety* (see http://www.fda.gov/oc/ initiatives/advance/reports/report0508.pdf, accessed May 30, 2008). This report commenced with a message from FDA Commissioner Andrew von Eschenbach, MD, the first part of which reads as follows (FDA, 2008, p. 1):

> Imagine a national electronic safety system capable of tracking the performance of a drug or medical product, beginning with the earliest stages of clinical research through its effects on millions of Americans who use it to treat or to recover from an illness or condition.
>
> The U.S. Food and Drug Administration of the 21st century needs such an electronic system to serve as *sentinel* over the safety of medical products and help FDA fulfill its responsibility to protect the health and well being of the American people. Learning all we can about the risks and benefits of medical products is essential. Accurate and reliable information must be obtained before products are approved and afterwards when they are being used by large and diverse populations.
>
> The FDA works hard to learn all we can about the risks and benefits of medical products, beginning before they are approved and continuing after they reach the market. Nevertheless, uncertainties about the safety of medical products regulated by the FDA will always remain. Once a product goes on the market, additional information about the possible risks of its use can almost always be gained. Postmarket safety monitoring is a critical part of our job, and we analyze this information to help guide the best uses of medical products.

The goal of the sentinel initiative is to create the sentinel system, "a national, integrated, electronic system for monitoring medical product safety" (p. 11). A key aspect of the sentinel initiative is the application of information technologies to the way health-related information is collected, managed, and shared. Technologies such as electronic health records (EHRs), e-prescribing, and electronic decision support tools will make the FDA's risk management systems more efficient, improve their ability to protect the public, and, potentially, to reduce healthcare costs. The FDA's *Critical Path Initiative* (e.g., see http://www.fda.gov/oc/initiatives/criticalpath/ initiative.html, accessed May 30, 2008) has been instrumental in movement toward an entirely electronic environment for information management. As the sentinel initiative report notes, FDA will soon be able "to receive, analyze, and disseminate important health information wholly electronically" (p. 2).

We discussed the Institute of Medicine's 2000 report *To Err Is Human* and their 2001 report *Crossing the Quality Chasm* in the previous chapter (Sections 13.3 to 13.5). As the sentinel initiative report noted, those reports "make clear that a modernized medical product safety system must establish robust links with quality and safety managers and researchers within the broad health care system to enable exchange and feedback of information" (p. 3).

14.14.1 The Science of Safety

The increased focus on safety and quality discussed in the previous section are in part "a result of an emerging science of safety, which combines a growing understanding of disease and its origins with new methods of safety signal detection" (FDA, 2008, p. 3). The science of safety is an integrative science. As the sentinel initiative report noted, investigations at the molecular biological level are permitting a greater understanding of the origins and nature of diseases and conditions of clinical interest, and of adverse drug reactions to—and therapeutic benefit from—pharmacological therapy. Second, new methods of signal detection, data mining, and data analysis are enabling researchers to identify and then to generate and test hypotheses about safety problems in the populations using medical products. Third, precision medicine is generating information about "the unique genetic and biologic features of each person that some day will help determine how he or she responds to treatment" (FDA, 2008, p. 3). The report continued (p. 5):

> Using these tools, FDA has increasingly adopted a life-cycle approach to product development and evaluation. This kind of approach should be used for all medical products so that safety signals generated at any point in the process can be evaluated along with relevant benefit-risk data to inform treatment choices and regulatory decision making.

With regard to benefit-risk data, the FDA regards benefit-risk analysis to be "one of the important facets of the science of safety that urgently requires additional development" (FDA, 2008, p. 5).

14.14.2 Active Surveillance

To date, most postmarketing surveillance has been passive in nature. The FDA is keen to supplement this monitoring with active surveillance activities. These include (FDA, 2008, pp. 3–4):

➤ Linking, in a secure fashion, existing electronic databases run by private health plans, insurance plans, government agencies, and industry.
➤ Querying electronic health records, claims databases, and other such repositories to pick up early warnings of adverse events.
➤ Studying deidentified data on millions of people in something much closer to real time.

Active surveillance systems incorporating the appropriate security and privacy safeguards will facilitate FDA's identification of priority safety questions and the development of mechanisms to protect patients in a more efficient and timely manner.

14.15 DECISION MAKING RELATED TO BENEFIT-RISK ASSESSMENTS

Benefit-risk assessments (or, perhaps more correctly, benefit-risk estimations—recall the discussions in Section 1.6) are informed throughout lifecycle drug development by numerical representations of estimations of safety and efficacy/effectiveness. However, these benefit-risk estimations are not themselves the final step in the process: rather, they provide the most rational foundation we have for making decisions. These decisions include sponsors' go/no-go decisions during drug development, regulatory marketing decisions, and regulatory postmarketing decisions to modify a drug's labeling or availability.

During its clinical development program, new data concerning the benefits and risks of a drug emerge. In early stages of development, estimates of the benefits (e.g., efficacy in terms of a clinically relevant endpoint) and risks (e.g., a safety profile containing multiple adverse effects) are associated with a great deal of uncertainty owing to the relatively small sample sizes of early phase studies. This inherent uncertainty regarding the drug's profile can complicate the decision making process of sponsors who must make a number of decisions regarding further development choices among multiple drug candidates within their portfolios. These decisions often are made in a broader context of the competitive marketplace by considering the emerging product profiles of other drugs in development. With a number of competing products on the market, the product with the greatest advantage would be the one with the most favorable benefit-risk profile, as evidenced by its labeling. Those drugs that have been found to have torsadogenic liability (e.g., in a TQT study) may well have this information appear in their approved labeling. This potential outcome may be successfully managed during the complex decision making process that goes on through many years of clinical development.

Many pharmaceutical companies use a quantitative method called decision analysis to prioritize the products in their portfolios. Decision analysis enables one to quantify various aspects of a decision so that the consequences of various decision alternatives are more readily apparent (e.g., see Clemen, 1996). Comparisons of alternatives are made possible by construction of a decision model, which identifies the various decisions to be made (e.g., initiate a therapeutic confirmatory trial, conduct an additional therapeutic exploratory trial, or abandon development) and the consequences of each decision. In the context of decision analysis, a consequence called a utility can be quantified. For sponsors, the utility of a given course of action is typically expressed in financial terms. That is, a sponsor would like to maximize their utility (e.g., by making a profit once a product is marketed). A decision model can become quite complex by including several decisions to be made, uncertain events which are out of the decision maker's control (e.g., success or not of a therapeutic exploratory study), and accounting for uncertainty (both in terms of outcomes of uncertain events and financial components of a model).

A simple example may be helpful to illustrate these concepts. Imagine that a sponsor is developing three compounds, all for the same chronic condition. One compound is suspected of having some effect on the QTc interval, but early studies suggest dramatic benefit in terms of efficacy as long as it is taken three times daily. A second compound is not thought to have adverse cardiac effects, but its efficacy is much less impressive than the first compound and it must still be taken three times per day. The cardiac effects of the third compound are unknown and it is the least potent of the three compounds under consideration, but due to its pharmacokinetic properties it can be used once per day with modest, yet minimally clinically relevant, benefits. If the company could choose only one of these drugs to invest in, decision analysis could shed light on the importance of a number of the factors in the decision process. The company would estimate the value of each drug by considering the following:

> How likely is the drug to survive each successive stage of clinical development (early therapeutic trials, a TQT study, and therapeutic confirmatory trials)?
> What is the cost of development of the drug?
> How likely is the drug to be approved, given its successful development?
> Once approved, how much revenue will the drug generate?

The three imaginary compounds in this scenario have different characteristics according to these factors, which clearly influence the decision to be made. A modestly effective drug may be less likely to be successful in development than a more effective drug. A drug with a safety liability may be less attractive in the marketplace than a drug without a safety liability at the time of marketing approval. A drug with early signs of cardiac effects will be more expensive to develop than one without such signals.

The outputs of a decision analysis are semiquantitative, providing a decision maker with additional insights about which characteristics have the most impact on the value of a potential new drug. The resulting value information can then be used to prioritize the most valuable drugs in the portfolio. Additionally, and perhaps more importantly, decision analysis enables a decision maker to choose alternative strategies to mitigate those factors which seemingly make a drug less valuable. If a drug is found to be positive for QTc prolongation but otherwise has an exceptional profile, a company may well benefit from its continued clinical development in conjunction with the development of risk mitigation programs which would limit its unwanted effects on the public health. On the other hand, a drug that is positive for QTc prolongation and additionally has a less-than-desirable overall profile may well be abandoned because such an analysis would reveal that the drug would not be useful in light of its other characteristics. From the public health perspective, this would be a favorable outcome, provided the result was not a false positive. The difficulty of making decisions in the presence of great uncertainty, especially when the consequences are potentially significant (e.g.., drug abandonment), highlights again the importance of designing studies to minimize the chances of a false positive result.

Decision making must continue throughout a marketed drug's entire life on the market. It is appropriate to reevaluate previous decisions on the basis of new information, and reaching a different decision than was reached in the past is not a statement that the previous decision was wrong, but rather that additional information suggests a different decision: We can only make decisions with the information available at the time of the decision. Decision making is predicated on benefit-risk estimates that require calculation: as Senn (2007, p. 399) observed, "in order to prescribe medicines rationally, calculation and yet more calculation is needed."

14.16 PHARMACOGENETICS, PHARMACOGENOMICS, AND PRECISION MEDICINE

Pharmacogenetics studies the contribution of genetic variation to variation in response to pharmacotherapy. Interest lies with both the desired therapeutic effects and the range and severity of adverse drug reactions. While other factors (e.g., existing disease, concomitant medication use, and use of tobacco and alcohol) can influence individual differences in response to a given drug, the predominant factor is genetic variation. Genetic variation in the structure of the target receptor and nontarget receptors plays a role. So too does genetic influence on pharmacokinetic processes. This influence may lead to enhanced drug clearance, impaired drug clearance, or inactivation of the drug, and the respective pharmacodynamic consequences: less efficacy, more efficacy, and no efficacy. Genetic variation and the resultant individual differences in drug responses therefore lead to outcomes that permit the following classification system for a given drug:

- Optimal responders: individuals who show the desired therapeutic response to the drug and do not have an adverse drug reaction.
- Suboptimal responders: individuals who show less than the desired level of therapeutic response.
- Supraoptimal responders: individuals who show a greater therapeutic response than desired (e.g., becoming hypotensive rather than normotensive following the administration of an antihypertensive drug).

> ➢ Adverse responders: individuals who show relatively serious adverse drug reactions.

Primrose and Twyman (2006, pp. 504–505) provided a telling illustration of the ramifications of genetic influences on metabolism. Most patients require 75–150 milligrams per day (mg/day) of the drug nortriptyline, a tricyclic antidepressant, in order to reach a steady-state plasma concentration of 50–150 micrograms per liter. In contrast, poor metabolizers need only 10–20 mg/day, while ultrarapid metabolizers need 300–500 mg/day to achieve the same plasma concentration. The ultrarapid metabolism is caused by amplification of the CYP2D6 locus. The cytochrome P450 group of enzymes mediate most drug functional group metabolic modifications, and these enzymes are therefore very important in the study of drug responses. Particularly important enzymes include CYP1A2, CYP3A, CYP2C9, CYP2C19, CYP2D6, and CYP2E1 (Wijnen et al., 2007). As an example of genetic variance here, over 70 allelic variants of the CYP2D6 locus have been described: this polymorphism is of particular importance since this locus is implicated in the metabolism of over 100 drugs (Primrose and Twyman, 2006).

A direct molecular genetic link between genetic variation and individual variation in drug response is thus provided by the facts that proteins are biological products of an individual's genetic information, proteins commonly function as drug receptors (target and nontarget), and proteins commonly function as metabolic enzymes. (See Turner, 2007, pp. 228–234, for additional discussion of pharmacoproteomics.)

The field of pharmacogenomics involves the use of genomic technologies in predicting and assessing differential responses to drugs and hence the possibility of pharmacological therapy targeted for particular individuals, and not for others, based on this knowledge. The terms pharmacogenetics and pharmacogenomics are not synonymous. Meyer (2002, p. 3) noted that "The term pharmacogenomics reflects the evolution of pharmacogenetics into the study of the entire spectrum of genes that determine drug response, including the assessment of the diversity of the human genome and its clinical consequences" (see also the article entitled *Pharmacogenetics goes Genomic* by Goldstein et al., 2003). Monkhouse (2006, pp. 26–27) commented as follows:

> Pharmacogenomic studies promise to revolutionize medicine by providing clinicians with prospective knowledge regarding the likelihood of an individual patient's response to a particular medication and, ultimately, the identification of patients who might benefit from targeted dosing of the drug or alternate drug therapy.

As was the case in Chapter 10 with regard to the terms pharmacovigilance, pharmacoepidemiology, and postmarketing surveillance, the nomenclature used by other authors cited here is respected.

14.16.1 Precision Medicine

The term precision medicine is deliberately used here instead of other common general terms such as individualized medicine and personalized medicine (the term personalized medicine is used shortly as employed in a specific manner by another author). Clinicians, as many will argue both reasonably and forcefully, have always practiced individualized medicine to the limit of knowledge at that point in time. Clinical care of a patient has always involved, and will always involve, using all available evidence concerning an individual patient's unique set of circumstances and knowledge of all available treatment options to tailor a course of individualized treatment accordingly. The major difference in the context of the present discussions is the availability and incorporation of information regarding the biological makeup of individual patients in their care, information not previously available.

Kaitin (2008) described a pharmacotherapeutic continuum consisting of generalized medicine, stratified medicine, and personalized medicine. Generalized medicine includes the use of most of today's drugs and vaccines, which are prescribed without concern for individual genetic makeup. Stratified medicine refers to the prescription of certain drugs in which genomic technology plays a part: such drugs include herceptin, gleevac, and camptosar. Genomic technology permits the prediction of individuals who will and will not likely benefit from treatment with a given drug, and accordingly stratification of individuals is thereby made possible. Personalized medicine is exemplified by a cancer vaccine whose manufacture incorporates the use of an individual's biological material in preparing a treatment uniquely tailored to that individual alone (Kaitin, 2008).

Ingelman-Sundberg (2008) discussed the employment of pharmacogenomic biomarkers in the prediction of severe adverse drug reactions. As the author noted (p. 637):

> The search for pharmacogenomic biomarkers that could be used to identify patients at increased risk for drug-related toxic effects has often focused on variation within genes encoding drug-metabolizing enzymes. Altered enzymatic activity can lead to elevated levels of the substrate drug, or alternatively, increased amounts of a reactive metabolite, either of which could have toxic effects.

Ingelman-Sundberg's editorial focused largely on abacavir, an antiretroviral treatment used against infection with HIV, the human immunodeficiency virus, since an original article in the same copy of the journal reported a related prospective randomized study (Mallal et al., 2008). However, many general aspects of biomarker use are well exemplified by both the editorial and the article. In white populations, approximately 6% of individuals carry the HLA-B*5701 allele, a genetic variant that is strongly associated with hypersensitivity to abacavir (for unknown reasons, the association between HLA-B alleles and hypersensitivity reactions is less clear in black populations). Screening individuals who are being considered by their physicians for abacavir therapy for the presence of the HLA-B*5701 allele has proved to be a successful strategy in reducing hypersensitive reactions to the drug (see Mallal et al., 2008; Ingelman-Sundberg, 2008).

Pharmacogenomic biomarkers are also proving of interest with regard to the drug warfarin, "the most widely used oral anticoagulant in the world for patients with venous thrombosis, pulmonary embolism, chronic atrial fibrillation, and prosthetic heart valves" (Krynetskiy and McDonnell, 2007, p. 427). Warfarin drug response is a polygenic pharmacogenetic trait. Krynetskiy and McDonnell (2007) reported finding an association between individual variation in the anticoagulant effect of warfarin and genetic polymorphisms in six genes, the two strongest predictors of which were VKORC1 and CYP2C9 (the latter gene encodes a metabolic enzyme in the cytochrome P450 family).

14.17   BIOMARKERS AND CLINICAL ENDPOINTS

The topic of biomarkers and their use in pharmacotherapy and in drug development is a complex and fascinating one that is currently receiving a lot of attention. Kaitin's (2008) pharmacotherapeutic continuum was described in the previous section, and it was noted that the majority of today's drugs and vaccines fall within the generalized medicine category. The predominant historical pharmaceutical model is one in which a drug is developed with the intention of its being useful to everyone with the disease or condition of interest, a model that leads to the blockbuster concept that has driven drug development so powerfully for many reasons, including financial.

Pharmaceutical companies are for-profit organizations, and if they are not financially viable, they will not be able to develop any future drugs that would benefit patients. An alternative model, one in which a drug is developed for use in a selected stratification of a disease population and not for use in another (i.e., it is not suitable for the entire population with the disease), may therefore initially seem financially counterintuitive: why develop a drug that is only suitable for a limited patient population when this strategy leads to fewer sales and therefore makes it harder for the sponsor to recoup development costs? This, however, may not be the case.

Ingelman-Sundberg (2008) noted that the rate of prescription of abacavir in the United Kingdom actually increased following the introduction of prospective HLA-B*5701 genotyping. This observation may herald a new paradigm. The integration of diagnostic tools and pharmacotherapy has historically presented a paradoxical challenge to sponsors developing these items. Pharmaceutical companies do not want to develop a drug that would work very well for some identified patients if there is no currently available diagnostic test to identify those patients, and diagnostic test manufacturers do not want to produce a test that identifies individuals who would benefit from a particular targeted drug if that drug does not yet exist. Thus, each side would like to be just slightly behind the other in respective development programs: they would like to know that the other side's product will become available for certain, and then have theirs ready as soon as possible after this occurrence. A model that encourages one manufacturer to be just slightly behind another, however, is not the typical business model.

A solution to this paradox is to fully integrate diagnostic development with drug development. Ingelman-Sundberg (2008, p. 639) commented that the use of validated biomarkers "might result in increased, rather than decreased, use of medication and, in my opinion, the development of pharmacogenetic biomarkers may in many cases constitute an integral part of drug development." Kaitin (2008) presented various ways that stratified and personalized medicine will profoundly alter research and development and business strategies. Two of these are increased reliance on biomarkers and increasing partnerships between pharmaceutical companies and diagnostic companies. Having both activities proceed side-by-side in the same company is also a possible outcome here. As well as the (real and important) financial considerations here, this strategy could be extremely beneficial to the most important person in all of our discussions: the patient who benefits from appropriate pharmacotherapy.

Wood (2006) proposed one potential avenue when a biomarker has proved helpful but evidence of therapeutic benefit via the assessment of actual clinical outcomes is needed. In the case of chronic diseases, taking the time needed to demonstrate a clinically meaningful benefit in preapproval clinical trials would typically be considered impractical, and so drugs have previously been approved on the basis of surrogate biomarkers. One strategy would be to provide initial marketing approval on the basis of biomarker results but limit the period of exclusivity for the drug. During this period the sponsor would be required to demonstrate a clinically meaningful therapeutic benefit, such as a meaningful improvement in function or a reduction in morbidity or mortality. Then, "The timely provision of such data would result in an extension of the period of exclusivity" (Wood, 2006). (See also Biomarkers Definitions Working Group, 2001.)

14.18   DRUG DEVELOPMENT AND DRUG THERAPY: BENEFIT-RISK ASSESSMENTS

As Turner (2007, p. 14) noted, the ultimate goal of new drug development is to produce a biologically active drug that is acceptably safe, well tolerated, and useful in the treatment or prevention of biological states of clinical concern. These drugs can then be used to improve patients' health, well-being, and quality of life by changing their biology for the better. All of the activities discussed in this book—from *in silico* modeling to active postmarketing surveillance—are conducted with patients in mind (recall our comment in Section 8.2.2 that clinical research might be defined concisely as any research undertaken with the intent of improving patient care).

However, since no drug is immune from the possibility of side effects, there is some degree of risk inherent in all drug therapy. Such risk, addressed in the context of benefit-risk balance, has to be considered at the public health level (the remit of regulatory agencies) and at the individual patient level by prescribing physicians and their patients.

14.18.1   Regulatory Benefit-risk Decision Making

Sometimes, regulatory decisions are neither straightforward nor easy. A question of current interest is: how are regulatory agencies to address the case of drugs that may be extremely beneficial to a very large number of patients but, very unfortunately, may cause some degree of harm to a small number of other patients if prescribed? It is our perspective that regulatory decisions must be made from the standpoint that the greatest therapeutic benefit should be made available to the greatest number of people, while, at the same time, physicians and patients should be made fully aware of the risks as well as the benefits of all marketed drugs. This approach allows prescribing physicians an array of treatment options from which to choose the drug they consider best suited for an individual patient, and, where appropriate, to consider other treatment modalities that are in an individual patient's best interests. This viewpoint is not unique: many authors have expressed these sentiments, as demonstrated by the following selection of quotes.

Inman founded two national systems for adverse drug monitoring in the United Kingdom. In the second edition of the classic textbook, *Monitoring for Drug Safety*, Inman and Weber (1986, p. 39) wrote:

> Risk-benefit judgments are complex...Irresponsible reporting by the lay press frequently leads to political pressure to restrict or ban drugs...The continued use of many valuable drugs must depend on the ability of the monitoring and regulatory agency to withstand criticism. Their policy on the whole is to warn about dangers rather than ban drugs because of them.

In a later chapter in the same book, Herxheimer (1986, p. 699) wrote:

> If we want to benefit from medicine, we must accept some risks. We first need to consider the risks when deciding whether or not to use the medicine. When we have decided to take the medicine, because the likely benefit sufficiently outweighs the risks, we have to understand how to minimize these risks. The user thus needs two quite separate kinds of information about possible harm: first, a realistic assessment of benefits and risks when the drug is properly used; second, what precautions and circumspections "proper use" requires.

The FDA's document "Guidance for Industry: Development and Use of Risk Minimization Action Plans" (2005d, p. 5) stated that:

> FDA recommends that RiskMAPs be used judiciously to minimize risks without encumbering drug availability or otherwise interfering with the delivery of product benefits to patients.

Shah (2005a, p. 290) commented as follows in the context of proarrhythmic cardiac safety:

> With respect to drug-induced TdP, there is also a more philosophical question of the definition of "clinical risk" and the level of risk that is unacceptable or tolerable. It seems inappropriate to categorize together a drug with an incidence of TdP of 1 in 500,000 patients with another with an incidence of 1 in 3000. As with other potentially fatal adverse drug reactions such as myelotoxicity, gastrointestinal hemorrhage, hepatotoxicity, or rhabdomyolysis, a level of risk may have to be tolerated. Whereas an incidence of a potentially fatal event at the rate of 1 in 3000 may be unacceptable, an incidence of 1 in 500,000 may be considered acceptable with a whole range in between. This perceived risk has to be seen in the context of benefit and available alternatives. The risk of not treating a disease is also an important component in risk assessment.

In their report *The Future of Drug Safety,* the Institute of Medicine (2007b, pp. 146–147) commented that:

> The role of the regulator is not to impede the development of innovative medicines, but to ensure that needed drugs are available to patients and that risk-benefit information is accurate and widely available.

The final quote here comes from a chapter by Gardner and Schultz (2007, p. 484) that discussed the postmarketing surveillance of medical devices, but the sentiments expressed are equally relevant to drugs:

> In acting on the information provided by our postmarket surveillance systems, we must be aware of the potential negative consequences of what we do. For example, if we were to remove from the market the only product available to treat a critical condition because we discovered that it could produce a relatively rare adverse event, this could do more harm to patients than allowing it to remain on the market and working to correct

the problem through other means, such as labeling changes, training programs, or safety messages. And if our actions were to result in patients foregoing needed treatment, or opting for riskier alternatives, this too would compromise public health.

In the scenario of a drug that is useful to many patients but potentially harmful to a few, it seems to us that removing the drug from the market is not the most beneficial action that a regulatory agency can take. Rather, alerting and educating physicians about the "precautions and circumspections" (Herxheimer, 1986, p. 699) that appropriate prescription and use of the drug requires is much more fruitful from the perspective of public health, the perspective that a regulatory agency is charged to take. This allows the many patients who benefit from the drug to continue to do so, and affords maximum protection to those individuals who, in the judgment of their physicians, might be at risk were they to be prescribed the drug. For these latter patients, their physicians may recommend to them that the risks of prescribing the drug outweigh the likely benefits, and therefore these physicians and patients would work together on a case-by-case basis to consider alternative treatment options.

14.18.2   Physician and Patient Benefit-risk Decision Making

As just noted, physicians, in conjunction with their patients, have to make benefit-risk evaluations and decisions at the level of the individual patient. However, there is often an inherent challenge when trying to apply the information obtained during clinical trials to an individual patient's care: The benefits and risks are both quantified for a population, not for an individual patient. For example, a relative risk of 0.86 for death or myocardial infarction in a therapeutic confirmatory trial of a new cardiovascular agent indicates that these events are less likely among participants treated with the new drug than the control. This result would suggest a benefit at the population (public health) level, but its interpretation may be viewed quite differently for a patient considering using this drug. For an individual, the benefit is a "yes or no" proposition. Likewise, patients and their physicians must consider the risks of a therapy, again quantified for a specific population, when weighing individual treatment decisions.

14.19   LOSING GOOD DRUGS FOR BAD REASONS

The following quote from Senn (2007, p. 384) concerning drug safety extends a quote cited in Section 8.2.3 by adding the final sentence:

> The subject is extremely important. Safety issues can cause drugs to be abandoned and companies to fail. If there are problems with a drug, then the sooner they are discovered the better. But it is also the case that some drugs have been lost

through witch-hunts, and occasionally such persecutions have been justified by fraudulent research.

In addition to emphasizing awareness of the benefits of pharmacovigilance, the WHO (2002, p. 17) observed the following:

> A more difficult question is whether pharmacovigilance has resulted in inappropriate removal from the market of potentially useful medicines as the result of misplaced fears or false signals.

Concern has also been expressed by many individuals involved with drug development that the increasingly conservative approach to safety in early drug development is leading to the abandonment of compounds by sponsors at the first hint of safety concerns that may have become useful drugs with positive benefit-risk balances. DePonti (2008, p. 57) noted that "as many as 60% of new molecular entities developed as potential therapeutic agents, when assayed for hERG blocking liability, test positive and are thus abandoned early in development, although their true torsadogenic potential is unknown."

14.20   REFLECTIONS ON CENTRAL THEMES IN THE BOOK

Several themes have recurred throughout the book. One of these themes is that a lifecycle approach is beneficial throughout all aspects of drug development. The term lifecycle drug development was used in the first section of the book, and the stages of drug discovery and design, nonclinical development, preapproval clinical development, and postmarketing surveillance were discussed in the second section. These stages have been used as an architectural framework for subsequent discussions, and the importance of viewing each of the stages as an integral part of the continuum of lifecycle drug development has resonated throughout the book.

   Another recurring theme is that interaction between government, industry, and academia can be very beneficial in the drug safety domain. As Lo Re and Strom (2007, p. 818) commented:

> Greater partnership between academia and the FDA could facilitate the prioritization of important issues on drug safety, allow more research questions on drug safety to be answered in a timely fashion, promote the development of networks for answering these questions, and help generate additional research ideas, ultimately providing enormous benefit to the public health.

In this regard, it might usefully be noted that Strom's (2005a) edited volume entitled *Pharmacoepidemiology* contains chapters that present academic, industry, and regulatory agency perspectives on pharmacoepidemiology.

A third central theme has been that an integrative approach is beneficial throughout all aspects of drug safety. This book has taken an integrated approach in all of its discussions. The lifecycle approach to drug development is itself an integrated approach, and, as already noted, we have discussed drug safety issues in all phases of lifecycle drug development. We have also emphasized that the progression through these stages is not always linear: concern regarding a safety signal identified in a later stage may be beneficially informed by data (either existing or to be collected) from an earlier stage. In the spirit of integration, the book has brought together research in three areas of cardiac safety that are typically addressed separately: proarrhythmic, generalized, and behavioral cardiac safety. While the third of these was discussed in less detail than the first two, its inclusion is still informative: As noted in Section 14.13, strengthening medication error analysis and prevention is part of the FDA's Drug Safety Five-year Plan.

A fourth theme is the pervasiveness of benefit-risk assessments. These occur at every stage of lifecycle drug development, and they occur at both the regulatory (public health) level and at the level of providing treatment to individual patients. Given the central importance of benefit-risk analysis in the science of safety, we noted in Section 14.14.1 that the FDA regards this process as one that "urgently requires additional development" (Sentinel Initiative Report, 2008, p. 5).

While this book has not addressed the assessment of benefit, we have noted that, by definition, benefit-risk assessment necessitates assessment of both the benefits and the risks associated with a drug. It should be noted here that each of these poses difficulties. Of interest in the context of the assessment of effectiveness is the Comparative Effectiveness Research Act of 2008 (see http://finance.senate.gov/ press/Bpress/2008press/prb030408.pdf, accessed May 30, 2008). As this news release (March 4, 2008) observed:

> The Comparative Effectiveness Research Act of 2008 establishes a private, nonprofit corporation [Institute] to generate evidence on what works in health care through comparative effectiveness research. Comparative effectiveness research compares treatment outcomes, or the "clinical effectiveness," of alternative therapies for the same condition. Better evidence on what works will lead to better health care choices and thus improved quality of care, improved efficiency, and ultimately to potential for cost savings...A crucial goal of the Institute will be to develop the field of comparative effectiveness research. To accomplish this, the bill calls for the establishment of an expert methodology committee to develop methodological standards to be used in the conduct of comparative effectiveness research.

Further discussions of comparative effectiveness can be found in Ray (2008) and Strom (2007).

14.21   THE FDA'S CRITICAL PATH INITIATIVE: THE RIGHT PATH

While the FDA's Critical Path Initiative has not been mentioned explicitly as often as the central themes discussed in the previous section, it is relevant to all of our discussions. The Critical Path Initiative reflects the FDA's work "to stimulate and facilitate a national effort to modernize the scientific process through which a potential human drug, biological product, or medical device is transformed from a discovery or "proof of concept" into a medical product" (http://www.fda.gov/oc/initiatives/criticalpath/, accessed May 30, 2008). The initiative was launched in March 2004 and followed in March 2006 by the Critical Path Opportunities List, which "describes the areas of greatest opportunity for improvement in the product development sciences" (http://www.fda.gov/oc/initiatives/criticalpath/initiative.html, accessed May 30, 2008). These areas are being addressed by the establishment of greater collaboration between regulators, academics, physicians, and scientists from industry, an occurrence discussed in the previous section.

Two points are noteworthy here. First, the phrases "scientific process" and "product development sciences" in the quotes in the previous paragraph exemplify that our interest lies with the application of science—e.g., computer simulation science, biological science, statistical science, clinical science—in developing drugs with favorable benefit-risk balances. Second, in the context of this book, two of the items that we have encountered are closely related to the Critical Path Initiative.

One is the Cardiac Safety Research Consortium, discussed in Section 7.20. As noted there, the mission of the CSRC is to advance scientific knowledge on cardiac safety for new and existing medical products by building a collaborative environment based upon the principles of the Critical Path Initiative and other public health priorities. As noted on the CSRS's web site (see http://www.cardiac-safety.org/about-us, accessed May 30, 2008):

> A central tenet to *Critical Path Initiative* is a focus on the evaluative science of the approval process, including both efficacy and safety measures...[The CSRC] is a first step in bringing together key constituencies to focus on cardiac safety issues during the new medical product development process. By utilizing the principals of the *Critical Path Initiative*, the CSRC will focus on improving the evaluative sciences specifically in relation to cardiac safety.

A second item is the Sentinel Initiative, discussed earlier in this chapter in Section 14.14. As noted in the Sentinel Initiative Report (2008, p. 1):

> FDA's focus on safety and the promise of collaborating with other experts are critical to creating a successful safety system. The Sentinel Initiative's value to other ongoing medical product

performance activities, such as FDA's Critical Path Initiative, makes it an invaluable asses in helping the FDA make the best possible regulatory decisions with the goal of protecting and promoting public health.

This report provides an overview of the projects already under way and outlines the Agency's vision and proposed next steps in the creation of a public-private partnership that could design and implement a national strategy for monitoring medical product safety.

The Critical Path will positively impact drug safety activities for many years to come.

14.22   EUROPEAN DRUG SAFETY ACTIVITIES

We noted in Section 14.1 that discussions in this chapter focus primarily on the FDA, simply because we are more familiar with their activities. However, it is appropriate here to address European regulatory activities in the domain of drug safety, and to provide some web sites that facilitate your further reading (the EMEA's website is http://www.emea.europa.eu/; recall also the discussions in Section 1.4.2).

In December 2005, the EMEA released a document entitled *Implementation of the Action Plan to Further Progress the European Risk Management Strategy: Rolling Two-year Work Programme (Mid 2005—Mid 2007)* (Doc. Ref: EMEA/ 372687/2005: see http://www.emea.europa.eu/pdfs/human/phv/37268705en.pdf, accessed May 30, 2008). The European Risk Management Strategy (ERMS) is focused upon achieving high standards of public health protection for all medicines available on the EU market. This action plan addressed the three priority initiatives to be taken during the second implementation phase of the ERMS, one of which was a further strengthening of the EU Pharmacovigilance System. Activities in the field of risk detection were undertaken to establish a framework that facilitates the earliest possible detection of important safety signals. These included:

> ➤ Speeding-up the implementation of electronic reporting to EudraVigilance in accordance with ICH standards, at the National Competent Authorities (NCAs) and the pharmaceutical industry levels.
> ➤ Further developing the EudraVigilance database by introducing additional functionalities, especially in the field of signal detection and data mining.
> ➤ Developing a network of academic centers to be involved in intensive drug monitoring.

A report on the activities undertaken during this two-year plan was released in July 2007 (Doc. Ref: 168954/2007: see http://www.emea.europa.eu/pdfs/human/phv/

16895407en.pdf, accessed May 30, 2008). This report noted that "Overall, very good progress has been achieved on the implementation of the ERMS." Readers are encouraged to read these releases. Information about the CHMP Pharmacovigilance Working Party's activities in 2008 can be found at http://www.emea.europa.eu/pdfs/ human/phvwp/phvwpworkprogramme.pdf (accessed May 30, 2008).

Another document of interest is the *European Medicines Agency Road Map to 2010: Preparing the Ground for the Future* (see http://www.emea.europa.eu/ pdfs/general/direct/directory/3416303enF.pdf, accessed May 30, 2008). As this document noted (p. 2):

> The key aspects of the Agency's vision for the coming years are to allow rapid access to safe and effective medicines, provide for adequately informed patients and users of medicines, encourage and facilitate innovation and research in the EU, tackle emerging public health challenges, prepare for developments in the pharmaceutical field, and reinforce the partnership between the EMEA and the NCAs to establish a network of excellence at EU level.

Other web sites of interest include the following:

➢ European Network of Centres for Pharmacoepidemiology and Pharmaco-vigilance: see http://www.emea.europa.eu/pdfs/human/phv/60110707en.pdf (accessed May 30, 2008).
➢ Guidelines on the use of statistical signal detection methods in the EudraVigilance Data Analysis System: see http://www.emea.europa.eu/pdfs/ human/phvwp/10646406en.pdf (accessed May 30, 2008).
➢ Further progress on the European Risk Management Strategy: see http: //www.emea.europa.eu/pdfs/human/phv/28008907en.pdf (accessed May 30, 2008). As noted in this document, regulatory cooperation between the European Commission and the EMEA and both the FDA and the Japanese Ministry of Health, Labour, and Welfare is envisioned.
➢ Guideline on Strategies to Identify and Mitigate Risks for First-in-Human Clinical Trials with Investigational Medicinal Products: see http:// www.emea.europa.eu/pdfs/human/swp/2836707enfin.pdf (accessed May 30, 2008). Recall the discussion of the first-in-human clinical trial of compound TGN1412 in Section 7.1.
➢ EudraVigilance Expert Working Group—Volume 9A Implementation Questions and Answers: see http://www.emea.europa.eu/pdfs/human/phv/ 11197208en.pdf (accessed May 30, 2008).
➢ EudraVigilance Human Version 7.1—Processing of Safety Messages and Individual Case Safety Reports (ICSRs): see http://www.emea.europa.eu/ pdfs/human/swp/2836707enfin.pdf (accessed May 30, 2008).

As noted in Section 14.1, while the precise operational implementation of activities may differ between regulatory agencies, many issues of concern to the FDA can be generalized to other agencies' deliberations in the drug safety arena.

14.23   CONCLUDING COMMENTS

Turner (2007, p. 239) commented that new drug development is a very complicated and difficult undertaking, requiring "attention to be paid to ethical, intellectual, scientific, biological, clinical, organizational, regulatory, financial, legal, congressional, social, and political considerations." Despite these challenges, it is important to remind ourselves why we do the work we do: Pharmaceutical therapy makes an enormous difference to the health, well-being, and quality of life of patients across the globe. Ethical, scientific, biological, regulatory, and clinical considerations are central to the development of drugs with favorable benefit-risk balances, but the reality of modern life requires that other considerations listed are addressed too.

We noted in Section 14.20.3 that integration has been a central theme in our discussions, a theme captured in the book's title, *Integrated Cardiac Safety*. Many professionals bring diverse sets of skills to the domain of drug safety. The more integrated the efforts of everyone concerned, the better all patients will be served.

14.24   FURTHER READING

Many of the sources cited in the book's text—and hence listed in the formal reference section—are book chapters, review articles, and regulatory guidances intended to be read in concert with the text to enhance your fundamental knowledge of issues within the realm of integrated cardiac safety. Moreover, further reading lists at the end of previous chapters have provided additional material specific to the topics discussed within individual chapters. At this point, an integrated list of further readings is provided. Most of them are articles published shortly before this book's publication. They address issues within proarrhythmic, generalized, and behavioral cardiac safety, and issues in the broader field of overall drug safety. It is our hope that your study to date will have provided you with the understanding, knowledge, and desire to obtain maximum benefit from these readings.

Aagaard, L., Stenver, D.I., and Hansen, E.H., 2008, Structures and processes in spontaneous ADR reporting systems: A comparative study of Australia and Denmark, *Pharmacy World and Science*, March 19 [E-publication ahead of print].

Abbott, G.W., Xu, X., and Roepke, T.K., 2007, Impact of ancillary subunits on ventricular repolarization, *Journal of Electrocardiology*, 40(6 Suppl.):S42–S46.

Aerssens, J. and Paulussen, A.D., 2005, Pharmacogenomics and acquired long QT syndrome, *Pharmacogenomics*, 6:259–270.

Agin, M.A., Aronstein, W.S., Ferber, G., et al., 2008, QT/QTc prolongation in placebo-treated subjects: A PhRMA collaborative data analysis, *Journal of Biopharmaceutical Statistics*, 18:408–426.

Ahmad, K. and Dorian, P., 2007, Drug-induced QT prolongation and proarrhythmia: An inevitable link? *Europace*, 9(Suppl. 4):iv16–iv22.

Alonso-Ron, C., de la Pena, P., Miranda, P., Dominguez, P., and Barros, F., 2008, Thermodynamic and kinetic properties of amino-terminal and S4-S5 loop hERG channel mutants under steady-state conditions, *Biophysical Journal*, 94:3893–3911.

Altar, C.A., The Biomarkers Consortium: On the critical path of drug discovery, *Clinical Pharmacology and Therapeutics*, 83:361–364.

Altar, C.A., Amakye, D., Bounos, D., et al., 2008, A prototypical process for creating evidentiary standards for biomarkers and diagnostics, *Clinical Pharmacology and Therapeutics*, 83:368–371.

Anghelescu, A.V., Delisle, R.K., Lowrie, J.F., et al., 2008, Technique for generating three-dimensional alignments of multiple ligands from one-dimensional alignments, *Journal of Chemical Information and Modeling*, April 16 [E-publication ahead of print].

Antzelevitch, C., 2007, Ionic, molecular, and cellular bases of QT-interval prolongation and torsade de pointes, *Europace*, 9(Suppl. 4):iv4–v-15.

Aronov, A.M., 2008, Tuning out of hERG, *Current Opinion in Drug Discovery and Development*, 11:128–140.

Astrom-Lilja, C., Odeberg, J.M., Ekman, E., and Hagg, S., 2008, Drug-induced torsades de pointes: A review of the Swedish pharmacovigilance database, *Pharmacoepidemiology and Drug Safety*, May 1 [E-publication ahead of print].

Au, W.Y. and Kwong, Y.L., 2008, Arsenic trioxide: Safety issues and their management, *Acta Pharmacologica Sinica*, 29:296–304.

Avorn, J. and Shrank, W.H., 2008, Adverse drug reactions in elderly people: A substantial cause of preventable illness, *British Medical Journal*, 336:956–957.

Badilini, F., Maison-Blanche, P., Childers, R., and Coumel, P., 1999, QT interval analysis on ambulatory electrocardiogram recordings: A selective beat averaging approach, *Medical and Biological Engineering and Computing*, 37:71–79.

Baker, S.G. and Kramer, B.S., 2003, A perfect correlate does not a biomarker make, *BMC Medical Research Methodology*, 3:16.

Baldrick, P., 2008, Safety evaluation to support First-in-Man investigations I: Kinetic and safety pharmacology studies, *Regulatory Toxicology and Pharmacology*, May 21 [E-publication ahead of print].

Baldrick, P., 2008, Safety evaluation to support First-in-Man investigations II: Toxicology studies, *Regulatory Toxicology and Pharmacology*, May 21 [E-publication ahead of print].

Bass, A.S., Siegl, P.K.S., Gintant, G.A., Murpy, D.J., and Porsolt, R., 2008, Current practices in safety pharmacology. In Gad, S.C. (Ed.), *Preclinical development handbook: Toxicology,* Hoboken, NJ: John Wiley & Sons, 611–694.

Bass, A., Valentin, J.P., Fossa, A.A., and Volders, P.G., 2007, Points to consider emerging from a mini-workshop on cardiac safety: Assessing torsades de pointes liability, *Journal of Pharmacological and Toxicological Methods*, 56:91–94.

Beasley, C.M., Jr., Mitchell, M.I., Dmitrienko, A.A., et al., 2005, The combined use of ibutilide as an active control with intensive electrophysiological sampling and signal averaging as a sensitive method to assess the effects of tadalafil on the human QT interval, *Journal of the American College of Cardiology*, 46:678–687.

Becucci, L., Carbone, M.V., Biagiotti, T., et al., 2008, Incorporation of the hERG potassium channel in a mercury supported lipid bilayer, *Journal of Physical Chemistry*, 112:1315–1319.

Beghetti, M., Hoeper, M.M., Kiely, D.G., et al., 2008, Safety experience with bosentan in 146 children 2–11 years with pulmonary arterial hypertension: Results from the European post-marketing surveillance program, *Pediatric Research*, April 9 [E-publication ahead of print].

Bertera, F.M., Mayer, M.A., Opezzo, J.A., Taira, C.A., and Hocht, C., 2008, Comparison of different pharmacodynamic models for PK-PD modeling of verapamil in renovascular hypertension, *Journal of Pharmacological and Toxicological Methods*, March 19 [E-publication ahead of print].

Betteridge, D.J., DeFronzo, R.A., and Chilton, R.J., 2008, PROactive: Time for a critical appraisal, *European Heart Journal*, 29:969–983.

Bittner, H.B., Lemke, J., Lange, M., Rastan, A., and Mohr, F.W., 2008, The impact of aprotinin on blood loss and blood transfusion in off-pump coronary artery bypass grafting, *Annals of Thoracic Surgery*, 85:1662–1668.

Bloomfield, D., Kost, J., Ghosh, K., et al., 2008, The effect of moxifloxacin on QTc and implications for the design of thorough QT studies, *Clinical Pharmacology and Therapeutics*, March 26th [E-publication ahead of print].

Bonney, G.K., Craven, R.A., Prasad, R., et al., 2008, Circulating markers of biliary malignancy: Opportunities in proteomics? *Lancet Oncology*, 9:149–158.

Braunwald, E., 2008, Biomarkers in heart failure, *New England Journal of Medicine*, 358:2148–2159.

Broeyer, F.J., Osanto, S., Ritsema van Eck, H.J., et al., 2008, Evaluation of biomarkers for cardiotoxicity of anthracycline-based chemotherapy, *Journal of Cancer Research and Clinical Oncology*, March 15 [E-publication ahead of print].

Brugts, J.J., Danser, A.J., de Maat, M.P., et al., 2008, Pharmacogenetics of ACE inhibition in stable coronary artery disease: Steps towards tailored drug therapy, *Current Opinion in Cardiology*, 23:296–301.

Bryant, J., Picot, J., Baxter, L., et al., 2007, Use of cardiac markers to assess the toxic effects of anthracyclines given to children with cancer: A systematic review, *European Journal of Cancer*, 43:1959–1966.

Budnitz, D.S., Pollock, D.A., Weidenbach, K.N., et al., 2006, National surveillance of emergency department visits for outpatient adverse drug reactions, *Journal of the American Medical Association*, 296:1858–1866.

Campbell, S.C., Criner, G.J., Levine, B.E., et al., 2007, Cardiac safety of formoterol 12 microg twice daily in patients with chronic obstructive pulmonary disease, *Pulmonary Pharmacology and Therapeutics*, 20:571–579.

Carini, C., 2007, Biomarkers: A valuable tool in clinical research and medical practice, *IDrugs*, 10:395–398.

Carpenter, D., Zucker, E.J., and Avorn, J., 2008, Drug-review deadlines and safety problems, *New England Journal of Medicine*, 358:1354–1361.

Chaves, S.S., Haber, P., Walton, K., et al., 2008, Safety of varicella vaccine after licensure in the United States: Experience from reports to the vaccine adverse event reporting system, 1995–2005, *Journal of Infectious Diseases*, 197(Suppl. 2):S170–S177.

Chekmarev, D.S., Kholodovych, V., and Balakin, K.V., 2008, Shape signatures: New descriptors for predicting cardiotoxicity *in silico*, *Chemical Research in Toxicology*, May 8 [E-publication ahead of print].

Cheng, B., Chow, S-C., Burt, D., and Cosmatos, D., 2008, Statistical assessment of QT/QTc prolongation based on maximum of correlated normal random variables, *Journal of Biopharmaceutical Statistics*, 18:494–501.

Chow, S-C., Cheng, B., and Cosmatos, D., 2008, On power and sample size calculation for QT studies with recording replicates at given time point, *Journal of Biopharmaceutical Statistics*, 18:483-493.

Chu, T.F., Rupnick, M.A., Kerkela, R., et al., 2007, Cardiotoxicity associated with tyrosine kinase inhibitor sunitinib, *Lancet*, 370:2011–2019.

Chuang-Stein, C., Entsuah, R., and Pritchett, Y., 2008, Measures for conducting comparative benefit:risk assessment, *Drug Information Journal*, 42:223–233.

Christ, T., Wettwer, E., Wuest, M., et al., 2008, Electrophysiological profile of propiverine—Relationship to cardiac risk, *Naunyn-Schmiedebergs Archives of Pharmacology*, 376:431–440.

Clarke, C.J. and Haselden, J.N., 2008, Metabolic profiling as a tool for understanding mechanisms of toxicity, *Toxicologic Pathology*, 36:140–147.

Cohen, A.L., Budnitz, D.S., Weidenbach, K.N., et al., 2008, National surveillance of emergency department visits for outpatient adverse drug events in children and adolescents, *Journal of Pediatrics*, 152:416–421.

Coi, A., Massarelli, I., Testai, L., Calderone, V., and Bianucci, A.M., 2008, Identification of "toxicophoric" features for predicting drug-induced QT interval prolongation, *European Journal of Medicinal Chemistry*, January 5 [E-publication ahead of print].

Coker, S.J., 2008, Drugs for men and women—How important is gender as a risk factor for TdP? *Pharmacology and Therapeutics*, April 7 [E-publication ahead of print].

Cooper, A.J., Lettis, S., Chapman, C.L., et al., 2008, Developing tools for the safety specification in risk management plans: Lessons learned from a pilot project, *Pharmacoepidemiology and Drug Safety*, 17:445–454.

Couderc, J.P., McNitt, S., Hyrien, O., et al., 2008, Improving the detection of subtle I_{Kr}-inhibition: Assessing electrocardiographic abnormalities of repolarization induced by moxifloxacin, *Drug Safety*, 31:249–260.

Crespo, A. and Fernandez, A., 2008, Induced disorder in protein-ligand complexes as a drug-design strategy, *Molecular Pharmaceutics*, February 16 [E-publication ahead of print].

Crumb, W.J., Jr., Ekins, S., Sarazan, R.D., et al., 2006, Effects of antipsychotic drugs on I_{to}, I_{Na}, I_{sus}, I_{K1}, and hERG: QT prolongation, structure activity relationship, and network analysis, *Pharmaceutical Research*, 23:1133–1143.

Curigliano, G., Spitaleri, G., Fingert, H.J., et al., 2008, Drug-induced QTc interval prolongation: A proposal towards an efficient and safe anticancer drug development, *European Journal of Cancer*, 44:494–500.

Dahabreh, I.J., 2008, Meta-analysis of rare events: An update and sensitivity analysis of cardiovascular events in randomized trials of rosiglitazone, *Clinical Trials*, 5:116–120.

Dale, T.J., Townsend, C., Hollands, E.C., and Trezise, D.J., 2007, Population patch clamp electrophysiology: A breakthrough technology for ion channel screening, *Molecular Biosystems*, 3:714–722.

Darpo, B., 2007, Detection and reporting of drug-induced proarrhythmias: Room for improvement, *Europace*, 9(S4):iv23–iv36.

Darpo, B. and Sager, P., 2008, Design of the "Thorough QT Study," *Clinical Pharmacology and Therapeutics*, 83:529 (Author reply, 530).

Darpo, B., Agin, M., Kazierad, D.J., et al., 2006, Man versus machine: Is there an optimal method for QT measurements in thorough QT studies? *Journal of Clinical Pharmacology*, 46:598–612.

Darpo, B., Nebout, T., and Sager, P., 2006, Clinical evaluation of QT/QTc prolongation and proarrhythmic potential for nonantiarrhythmic drugs: The International Conference on Harmonization of Technical Requirements for Registration of Pharmaceuticals for Human Use E14 guideline, *Journal of Clinical Pharmacology*, 46:498–507.

Davis, J.D., Hackman, F., Layton, G., et al., 2008, Effect of single doses of maraviroc on the QT/QTc interval in healthy subjects, *British Journal of Clinical Pharmacology*, 65(Suppl. 1): 68–75.

Dearden, J.C., 2007, *In silico* prediction of ADMET properties: How far have we come? *Expert Opinion on Drug Metabolism and Toxicology,* 3:635–639.

Delbanco, T. and Bell, S.K., 2007, Perspective: Guilty, afraid, and alone—Struggling with medical error, *New England Journal of Medicine*, 357:1682–16383.

de Leon, J., 2006, AmpliChip CYP450 test: Personalized medicine has arrived in psychiatry, *Expert Reviews in Molecular Diagnostics*, 6:277–286.

de Leon, J., Armstrong, S.C., and Cozza, K.L., 2006, Clinical guidelines for psychiatrists for the use of pharmacogenetic testing for CYP450 2D6 and CYP450 2C19, *Psychosomatics*, 47:75–85.

Demetri, G.D., 2007, Structural reengineering of imatinib to decrease cardiac risk in cancer therapy, *Journal of Clinical Investigation*, 117:3650–3653.

Dennis, A., Wang, L., Wan, X., and Ficker, E., 2007, hERG channel trafficking: Novel targets in drug-induced long QT syndrome, *Biochemical Society Transactions*, 35:1060–1063.

Desai, M., Stockbridge, N., and Temple, R., 2006, Blood pressure as an example of a biomarker that functions as a surrogate, *AAPS Journal*, 8:E146–E152.

Devchand, P.R., 2008, Glitazones and the cardiovascular system, *Current Opinion in Endocrinology, Diabetes, and Obesity*, 15:188–192.

Diamond, G.A. and Kaul, S., 2004, Prior convictions: Bayesian approaches to the analysis and interpretation of clinical megatrials, *Journal of the American College of Cardiology*, 43:1929–1939.

Dieterle, F. and Marrer, E., 2008, New technologies around biomarkers and their interplay with drug development, *Analytical and Bioanalytical Chemistry*, 390: 141–154.

Du, W., Guo, J.J., Jing, Y., Li, X., and Kelton, C.M., 2008, Drug safety surveillance in China and other countries: A review and comparison, *Value in Health*, 11 (Suppl. 1): S130–S136.

DuMouchel, W., Fram, D., Yang, X., et al., 2008, Antipsychotics, glycemic disorders, and life-threatening diabetic events: A Bayesian data-mining analysis of the FDA adverse event reporting system (1968–2004), *Annals of Clinical Psychiatry*, 20:21–31.

Dunlop, J., Bowlby, M., Peri, R., Vasilyev, D., and Arias, R., 2008, High-throughput electrophysiology: An emerging paradigm for ion-channel screening and physiology, *Nature Reviews Drug Discovery*, 7:358–368.

Dustan Sarazan, R., Crumb, W.J., Jr., Beasley, C.M., Jr., et al., 2004, Absence of clinically important hERG channel blockade by three compounds that inhibit phosphodiesterase 5: Sildenafil, tadalafil, and vardenafil, *European Journal of Pharmacology*, 502:163–167.

Eaton, M.L., Muirhead, R.J., Mancuso, J.Y., and Kolluri, M.L., 2006, A confidence interval for the maximal mean QT interval change caused by drug effect, *Drug Information Journal*, 40:267–271.

Eichelbaum, M., Ingelman-Sundberg, M., and Evans, W.E., 2006, Pharmacogenomics and individualized drug therapy, *Annual Reviews of Medicine*, 57:119–137.

Etwel, F.A., Rieder, M.J., Bend, J.R., and Koren, G., 2008, A surveillance method for the early identification of idiosyncratic adverse drug reactions, *Drug Safety*, 31:169–-180.

Evans, B.J. and Flockhart, D.A., 2006, The unfinished business of U.S. drug safety regulation, *Food Drug Law Journal*, 61:45–63.

Extramiana, F., Maison-Blanche, P., Cabanis, M.J., et al., 2005, Clinical assessment of drug-induced QT prolongation in association with heart rate change, *Clinical Pharmacology and Therapeutics*, 77:247–258.

Extramiana, F., Maison-Blanche, P., Tavernier, R., et al., 2002, Cardiac effects of chronic oral beta-blockade: Lack of agreement between heart rate and QT interval changes, *Annals of Noninvasive Electrocardiology*, 7:379–388.

Extramiana, F., Maison-Blanche, P., Badilini, F., Beaufils, P., and Leenhardt, A., 2005, Individual QT-RR relationship: Average stability over time does not rule out an individual residual variability: Implication for the assessment of drug effect on the QT interval, *Annals of Noninvasive Electrocardiology*, 10:169–178.

Extramiana, F., Maison-Blanche, P., Haggui, A., et al., 2006, Control of rapid heart rate changes for electrocardiographic analysis: Implications for thorough QT studies, *Clinical Cardiology*, 29:534–539.

Extramiana, F., Maury, P., Maison-Blanche, P., et al., 2008, Electrocardiographic biomarkers of ventricular repolarisation in a single family of short QT syndrome and the role of the Bazett correction formula, *American Journal of Cardiology*, 101:855–860.

Fanikos, J., Cina, J.L., Baroletti, S., et al., 2007, Adverse drug events in hospitalized cardiac patients, *American Journal of Cardiology*, 100:1465–1469.

Feldman, A.M., Kock, W.J., and Force, T.L., 2007, Developing strategies to link basic cardiovascular sciences with clinical drug development: Another opportunity for translational sciences, *Clinical Pharmacology and Therapeutics*, 81:887–892.

Fergusson, D.A., Hebert, P.C., Mazer, C.D., et al., for the BART Investigators, 2008, A comparison of aprotinin and lysine analogues in high-risk cardiac surgery, *New England Journal of Medicine*, 358:2319–2131.

Fernandez, A., Sanguino, A., Peng, Z., et al., 2007, An anticancer C-Kit kinase inhibitor is re-engineered to make it more active and less cardiotoxic, *Journal of Clinical Investigation*, 117:4044–4054.

Ferranti, J., Horvath, M.M., Cozart, H., Whitehurst, J., and Eckstrand, J., 2008, Reevaluating the safety profile of pediatrics: A comparison of computerized adverse drug event surveillance and voluntary reporting in the pediatric environment, *Pediatrics*, 121:1201–1207.

Fielden, M.R. and Kolaja, K.L., 2008, The role of early *in vivo* toxicity testing in drug discovery toxicology, *Expert Opinion on Drug Safety*, 7:107–110.

Force, T., Krause, D.S., and Van Etten, R.A., 2007, Molecular mechanisms of cardiotoxicity of tyrosine kinase inhibition, *Nature Reviews Cancer*, 7:332–344.

Fossa, A.A., 2008, Assessing QT prolongation in conscious dogs: Validation of a beat-to-beat method, *Pharmacology and Therapeutics*, 118:231–238.

Fossa, A.A., Gorczyca, W., Wisialowski, T., et al., 2007, Electrical alternans and hemodynamics in anesthetized guinea pigs can discriminate the cardiac safety of antidepressants, *Journal of Pharmacological and Toxicological Methods*, 55: 78–85.

Fossa, A.A., Wisialowski, T., Crimin, K., et al., 2007, Analyses of dynamic beat-to-beat QT-TQ interval (ECG restitution) changes in humans under normal sinus rhythm and prior to an event of torsades de pointes during QT prolongation caused by sotalol, *Annals of Noninvasive Electrocardiology*, 12:338–348.

Fossa, A.A., Wisialowski, T., Magnano, A., et al., 2005, Dynamic beat-to-beat modeling of the QT-RR interval relationship: Analysis of QT prolongation during alterations of autonomic state versus human ether a-go-go-related gene inhibition, *Journal of Pharmacology and Experimental Therapeutics*, 312:1–11.

Foster, W.R., Chen, S.J., He, A., et al., 2007, A retrospective analysis of toxicogenomics in the safety assessment of drug candidates, *Toxicologic Pathology*, 35:621–635.

Franceschi, M., Scarcelli, C., Niro, V., et al., 2008, Prevalence, clinical features and avoidability of adverse drug reactions as cause of admission to a geriatric unit: A prospective study of 1756 patients, *Drug Safety*, 31:545–556.

Freemantle, N. and Irs, A., 2008, Observational evidence for determining drug safety, *British Medical Journal*, 336:627–628.

Furberg, C.D., Levin, A.A., Gross, P.A., Shapiro, R.S., and Strom, B.L., 2006, The FDA and drug safety: A proposal for sweeping changes, *Archives of Internal Medicine*, 166:1938–1942.

Gage, B.F. and Lesko, L.J., 2008, Pharmacogenetics of warfarin: Regulatory, scientific, and clinical issues, *Journal of Thrombosis and Thrombolysis*, 25: 45–51.

Galea, S.A., Sweet, A., Beninger, P., et al., 2008, The safety profile of varicella vaccine: A 10-year review, *Journal of Infectious Diseases*, 197(Suppl. 2). S165–S169.

Ganz, P.A., Hussey, M.A., Moinpour, C.M., et al., 2008, Late cardiac effects of adjuvant chemotherapy in breast cancer survivors treated on Southwest Oncology Group protocol s8897, *Journal of Clinical Oncology*, 26:1223–1230.

Garg, D., Gandhi, T., and Gopi Mohan, C., 2008, Exploring QSTR and toxicophore of hERG K+ channel blockers using GFA and HypoGen techniques, *Journal of Molecular Graphics and Modeling*, 26:966–976.

Garnerin, P., Pellet-Meier, B., Chopard, P., Perneger, T., and Bonnabry, P., 2007, Measuring human-error probabilities in drug preparation: A pilot simulation study, *European Journal of Clinical Pharmacology*, 63:769–776.

Giacomini, K.M., Brett, C.M., Altman, R.B. et al. for the Pharmacogenetics Research Network, 2007, The pharmacogenetics research network: From SNP discovery to clinical drug response, *Clinical Pharmacology and Therapeutics*, 81:328–345.

Glantz, L.H. and Annas, G.J., 2008, The FDA, preemption, and the Supreme Court, *New England Journal of Medicine*, 358:1883–1885.

Goldfine, A.B., 2008, The rough road for rosiglitazone, *Current Opinion in Endocrinology, Diabetes, and Obesity*, 15:113–117.

Gomez-Varela, D., Zwick-Wallasch, E., Knotgen, H., et al., 2007, Monoclonal antibody blockade of the human Eag1 potassium channel function exerts antitumor activity, *Cancer Research*, 67:7343–7349.

Gonzalez, V., Salgueiro, E., Jimeno, F.J., et al., 2008, Post-marketing safety of antineoplasic monoclonal antibodies: Rituximab and trastuzumab, *Pharmacoepidemiology and Drug Safety*, March 13 [E-publication ahead of print].

Goodsaid, F. and Frueh, F., 2007, Biomarker qualification pilot process at the US Food and Drug Administration, *Journal of the AAPS*, 9:E105–E108.

Granger, C.B., Vogel, V., Cummings, S.R., et al., 2008, Do we need to adjudicate major clinical events? *Clinical Trials*, 5:56–60.

Green, J.L., Hawley, J.N., and Rask, K.J., 2007, Is the number of prescribing physicians an independent risk factor for adverse drug events in an elderly outpatient population? *American Journal of Geriatric Pharmacotherapy*, 5: 31–39.

Guergova-Kuras, M., 2007, Clinical Biomarkers Forum: Harnessing the potential of biomarkers from translational research throughout clinical trials. 13–14 September 2007, Prague, Czech Republic, *IDrugs*, 10:782–783.

Hancox, J.C. and James, A.F., 2008, Refining insights into high-affinity drug binding to the human ether-a-go-go-related gene potassium channel, *Molecular Pharmacology*, 73:1592–1595.

Hanton, G., 2007, Preclinical cardiac safety assessment of drugs, *Drugs R & D*, 8:213–218.

Hartford, C.G., Petchel, K.S., and Mickail, H., 2006, Pharmacovigilance during the pre-approval phases: An evolving pharmaceutical industry model in response to ICH E2E, CIOMS VI, FDA and EMEA/CHMP risk-management guidelines, *Drug Safety*, 29:657–673.

Hauben, M., Horn, S., and Reich, L., 2007, Potential use of data-mining algorithms for the detection of 'surprise' adverse drug reactions, *Drug Safety*, 30:143–155.

Heller, T., Kirchheiner, J., Armstrong, V.W., et al., 2006, AmpliChip CYP450 GeneChip: A new gene chip that allows rapid and accurate CYP2D6 genotyping, *Therapeutic Drug Monitoring*, 28:673–677.

Henderson, J.A., Alexander, B.C., Smith, J.J., et al., 2005, The Food and Drug Administration and molecular imaging agents: Potential challenges and opportunities, *Journal of the American College of Radiology*, 2:833–840.

Hennessy, S. and Strom, B.L., 2007, PDUFA reauthorization: Drug safety's golden moment of opportunity? *New England Journal of Medicine*, 356:1703–1704.

Herdeiro, M.T., Polonia, J., Gestal-Otero, J.J., and Figueiras, A., 2008, Improving the reporting of adverse drug reactions: A cluster-randomized trial among pharmacists in Portugal, *Drug Safety*, 31:335–344.

Hewitt, P. and Walijew, A., 2008, Toxicogenomics in drug safety assessment, *Pharmacogenomics*, 9:379–382.

Ho, P.M., Rumsfeld, J.S., Masoudi, F.A., et al., 2006, Effect of medication nonadherence on hospitalization and mortality among patients with diabetes mellitus, *Archives of Internal Medicine*, 166:1836–1841.

Hoffman, E.P., 2007, Editorial: Skipping toward personalized molecular medicine, *New England Journal of Medicine*, 357:2719–2722.

Hondeghem, L.M., 2008, QT and TdP. QT: An unreliable predictor of proarrhythmia, *Acta Cardiologica*, 63:1–7.

Hondeghem, L.M., 2006, Thorough QT/QTc not so thorough: Removes torsadogenic predictors from the T-wave, incriminates safe drugs, and misses profibrillatory drugs, *Journal of Cardiovascular Electrophysiology*, 17:337–340.

Hovor, C. and O'Donnell, L.T., 2007, Probabilistic risk analysis of medication error, *Quality Management in Health Care,* 16:349–353.

Huang, S.M., Strong, J.M., Zhang, L., et al., 2008, New era in drug interaction evaluation: US Food and Drug Administration update on CYP enzymes, transporters, and the guidance process, *Journal of Clinical Pharmacology,* March 31 [E-publication ahead of print].

Huang, S.M., Temple, R., Throckmorton, D.C., and Lesko, L.J., 2007, Drug interaction studies: Study design, data analysis, and implications for dosing and labeling, *Clinical Pharmacology and Therapeutics,* 81:298–304.

Hughes, B., 2008, 2007: Spotlight on drug safety, *Nature Reviews Drug Discovery,* 7:5–7.

Hulhoven, R., Rosillon, D., Bridson, W.E., et al., 2008, Effect of levetiracetam on cardiac repolarization in healthy subjects: A single-dose, randomized, placebo- and active-controlled, four-way crossover study, *Clinical Therapeutics,* 30: 260–270.

Hulhoven, R., Rosillon, D., Letiexhe, M., et al., 2007, Levocetirizine does not prolong the QT/QTc interval in healthy subjects: Results from a thorough QT study, *European Journal of Clinical Pharmacology,* 63:1011–1017.

Hutmacher, M.M., Chapel, S., Agin, M.A., Fleishaker, J.C., and Lalonde, R.L., 2008, Performance characteristics for some typical QT study designs under the ICH E-14 guidance, *Journal of Clinical Pharmacology,* 48:215–224.

Iwamoto, M., Kost, J.T., Mistry, G.C., et al., 2008, Raltegravir thorough QT/ QTc study: A single supratherapeutic dose of raltegravir does not prolong the QTcF interval, *Journal of Clinical Pharmacology,* April 25 [E-publication ahead of print].

James, A.F., Choisy, S.C., and Hancox, J.C., 2007, Recent advances in understanding sex differences in cardiac repolarization, *Progress in Biophysics and Molecular Biology,* 94:265–319.

Jannazzo, A., Hoffman, J., and Lutz, M., 2008, Monitoring of anthracycline-induced cardiotoxicity, *Annals of Pharmacotherapy,* 42:99–104.

Jo, S.H., Hong, H.K., Chong, S.H., and Choe, H., 2008, Protriptyline block of the human ether-a-go-go-related gene (hERG) K+ channel, *Life Sciences,* 82: 331–340.

Johansson, K., Olsson, S., Hellman, B., and Meyboom, R.H., 2007, An analysis of Vigimed, a global e-mail system for the exchange of pharmacovigilance information, *Drug Safety*, 31:883–889.

Judson, R.S., Salisbury, B.A., Reed, C.R., and Ackerman, M.J., 2006, Pharmacogenetic issues in thorough QT trials, *Molecular Diagnosis and Therapy*, 10:153–162.

Jurcut, R., Wildiers, H., Ganame, J., et al., 2008, Detection and monitoring of cardiotoxicity: What does modern cardiology offer? *Supportive Care in Cancer*, 16:437–445.

Kaitin, K.I., Obstacles and opportunities in new drug development, 2008, *Clinical Pharmacology and Therapeutics*, 83: 210–212.

Kannankeril, P.J., 2008, Understanding drug-induced torsades de pointes: A genetic stance, *Expert Opinion on Drug Safety*, 7:231–239.

Kannankeril, P.J. and Roden, D.M., 2007, Drug-induced long QT and torsades de pointes: Recent advances, *Current Opinion in Cardiology*, 22:39–43.

Keun, H.C., 2006, Metabonomic modeling of drug toxicity, *Pharmacology and Therapeutics*, 109:92–106.

Keun, H.C. and Athersuch, T.J., 2007, Application of metabonomics in drug development, *Pharmacogenomics*, 8:731–741.

Kip, K.E., Hollabaugh, K., Marroquin, O.C., and Williams, D.O., 2008, The problem with composite endpoints in cardiovascular studies: The story of major adverse events and percutaneous coronary intervention, *Journal of the American College of Cardiology*, 51:701–707.

Kola, I., 2008, The state of innovation in drug development, *Clinical Pharmacology and Therapeutics*, 83:227–230.

Kramer, C., Beck, B., Kriegl, J.M., and Clark, T., 2008, A composite model for hERG blockade, *ChemMedChem*, 3:254–265.

Kramer, J.A., Sagartz, J.E., and Morris, D.L., 2007, The application of discovery toxicology and pathology towards the design of safer pharmaceutical lead candidates, *Nature Review Drug Discovery*, 6:636–649.

Kristeller, J.L., Roslund, B.P., and Stahl, R.F., 2008, Benefits and risks of aprotinin use during cardiac surgery, *Pharmacotherapy*, 28:112–124.

Kubitza, D., Mueck, W., and Becka, M., 2008, Randomized, double-blind, crossover study to investigate the effect of rivaroxaban on QT-interval prolongation, *Drug Safety*, 31:67–77.

Kuhlmann, J., 2007, The application of biomarkers in early clinical drug development to improve decision-making processes, *Ernst Schering Research Foundation Workshop*, 59:29–45.

Kunac, D.L. and Reith, D.M., 2008, Preventable medication-related events in hospitalised children in New Zealand, *New Zealand Medical Journal*, 121:17–32.

Kurokawa, J., Tamagawa, M., Harada, N., et al., 2008, Acute effects of estrogen on the guinea pig and human I_{Kr} channels and drug-induced prolongation of cardiac repolarization, *Journal of Physiology*, April 25 [E-publication ahead of print].

Lacana, E., Amur, S., Mummanneni, P., Zhao, H., and Frueh, F.W., 2007, The emerging role of pharmacogenomics in biologics, *Clinical Pharmacology and Therapeutics*, 82:466–471.

Lacerda, A.E., Kuryshev, Y.A., Chen, Y., et al., 2008, Alfuzosin delays cardiac repolarization by a novel mechanism, *Journal of Pharmacology and Experimental Therapeutics*, 324:427–33.

Lapi, F., Cecchi, E., Pedone, C., et al., 2008, Safety aspects of iodinated contrast media related to their physiochemical properties: A pharmacoepidemiology study in two Tuscany hospitals, *European Journal of Clinical Pharmacology*, 64:723–737.

Lasser, K.E., Seger, D.L., Yu, D.T., et al., 2006, Adherence to black box warnings for prescription medications in outpatients, *Archives of Internal Medicine*, 166:338–344.

Lasseter, K.C., Shaughnessy, L., Cummings, D., et al., 2008, Ghrelin agonist (TZP-101): Safety, pharmacokinetics and pharmacodynamic evaluation in healthy volunteers: A phase I, first-in-human study, *Journal of Clinical Pharmacology*, 48:193–202.

Lerner, R.B., de Carvalho, M., Vieira, A.A., Lopes, J.M., and Moreira, M.E., 2008, Medication errors in a neonatal intensive care unit, *Jornal de Pediatria*, 84:166–170.

Letourneau, M., Wells, Walop, W., and Duclos, P., 2008, Improving global monitoring of vaccine safety: A quantitative analysis of adverse event reports in the WHO Adverse Reactions Database, *Vaccine*, 26:1185–1194.

Lonn, E., 2001, The use of surrogate endpoints in clinical trials: Focus on clinical trials in cardiovascular diseases, *Pharmacoepidemiology and Drug Safety*, 10: 497–508.

Lowes, B.D. and Buttrick, P.M., 2008, Genetic determinants of drug response in heart failure, *Current Cardiology Reports*, 10:176–181.

Lu, H.R., Vlaminckx, E., and Gallacher, D.J., 2008, Choice of cardiac tissue *in vitro* plays an important role in assessing the risk of drug-induced cardiac arrhythmias in humans: Beyond QT prolongation, *Journal of Pharmacological and Toxicological Methods*, 57:1–8.

Lu, H.R., Vlaminickx, E., Hermans, A.N., et al., 2008, Predicting drug-induced changes in QT interval and arrhythmias: QT-shortening drugs point to gaps in the ICH S7B guidelines, *British Journal of Pharmacology*, May 19 [E-publication ahead of print].

Lu, H.R., Vlaminckx, E., Van de Water, A., et al., 2007, *In-vitro* experimental models for the risk assessment of antibiotic-induced QT prolongation, *European Journal of Pharmacology*, 577:222–232.

Luo, T., Luo, A., Liu, M, and Liu, X., 2008, Inhibition of the hERG channel by droperidol depends on channel gating and involves the S6 residue F656, *Anesthesia and Analgesia*, 106:1161–1170.

Lux, R.L., Gettes, L.S., and Mason, J.W., 2006, Understanding proarrhythmic potential in therapeutic drug development: Alternate strategies for measuring and tracking repolarization, *Journal of Electrocardiology*, 39:S161–S164.

Ma, H., Smith, B., and Dmitrienko, A., 2008, Statistical analysis methods for QT/QTc prolongation, *Journal of Biopharmaceutical Statistics*, 18:553–563.

Makaryus, A.N., Bryns, K., Makaryus, M.N., et al., 2006, Effect of ciprofloxacin and levofloxacin on the QT interval: Is this a significant "clinical" event? *Southern Medical Journal,* 99:52–56.

Malhotra, B.K., Glue, P., Sweeney, K., et al., 2007, Thorough QT study with recommended and supratherapeutic doses of tolterodine, *Clinical Pharmacology and Therapeutics*, 81:377–385.

Malik, M., Hnatkova, K., Batchvarov, V., et al., 2004, Sample size, power calculations, and their implications for the cost of thorough studies of drug induced QT interval prolongation, *Pacing and Clinical Electrophysiology*, 27: 1659–1669.

Mandhane, S.N., Ayer, U.B., Midha, A.S., Rao, C.T., and Rajamannar, T., 2008, Preclinical efficacy and safety pharmacology of SUN-1334H, a potent orally active antihistamine agent, *Drugs in R & D*, 9:93–112.

Mann, R.D., 2007, Multi-criteria decision analysis—A new approach to an old problem, *Pharmacoepidemiology and Drug Safety*, 16(Suppl.1), S1.

Margulis, M. and Sorota, S., 2008, Additive effects of combined application of multiple hERG blockers, *Journal of Cardiovascular Pharmacology*, May 9 [E-publication ahead of print].

Marrer, E. and Dieterie, F., 2007, Promises of biomarkers in drug development—A reality check, *Chemical Biology and Drug Design*, 69:381–394.

Masetti, M., Cavalli, A., and Recanatini, M., 2008, Modeling the hERG potassium channel in a phospholipid bilayer: Molecular dynamics and drug docking studies, *Journal of Computational Chemistry*, 29:795–808.

Mason, J.W., Ramseth, D.J., Chanter, D.O., et al., 2007, Electrocardiographic reference ranges derived from 79,743 ambulatory subjects, *Journal of Electrocardiology*, 40:228–234.

McClellan, M., 2007, Drug safety reform at the FDA—Pendulum swing or systematic improvement? *New England Journal of Medicine*, 356:1700–1702.

Megarbane, B., Aslani, A.A., Deve, N., and Band, F.J., 2008, Pharmacokinetic/pharmacodynamic modeling of cardiac toxicity in human acute overdoses: Utility and limitations, *Expert Opinion on Drug Metabolism and Toxicology*, 4:569–579.

Meletiadis, J., Chanock, S., and Walsh, T.J., 2008, Defining targets for investigating the pharmacogenomics of adverse drug reactions to antifungal agents, *Pharmacogenomics*, 9:561–584.

Mello de Queiroz, F., Suarez-Kurtz, G., Stuhmer, W., and Pardo, L.A., 2006, Ether a go-go potassium channel expression in soft tissue sarcoma patients, *Molecular Cancer*, 5:42.

Menna, P., Salvatorelli, E., and Minotti, G., 2008, Cardiotoxicity of antitumor drugs, *Chemical Research in Toxicology*, 21:978–989.

Merlot, C., 2008, *In silico* methods for early toxicity assessment, *Current Opinion in Drug Discovery and Development*, 11:80–85.

Meyers, N.L. and Hickling, R.I., 2007, The cardiovascular safety profile of renzapride, a novel treatment for irritable bowel syndrome, *Journal of International Medical Research*, 35:848–866.

Michel, M.C., Wetterauer, U., Vogel, M., and de la Rosette, J.J., 2008, Cardiovascular safety and overall tolerability of solifenacin in routine clinical use: A 12-week, open-label, post-marketing surveillance study, *Drug Safety*, 31:505–514.

Milberg, P., Hilker, E., Ramtin, S., et al., 2007, Proarrhythmia as a class effect of quinolones: Increased dispersion of repolarization and triangulation of action potential predict torsades de pointes, *Journal of Cardiovascular Electrophysiology*, 18:647–654.

Milic, M., Bao, X., Rizos, D., Liu, F., and Ziegler, M.G., 2006, Literature review and pilot studies of the effect of QT correction formulas on reported beta2-agonist-induced QTc prolongation, *Clinical Therapeutics*, 28:582–590.

Mitcheson, J.S., 2008, hERG potassium channels and the structural basis of drug-induced arrhythmias, *Chemical Research in Toxicology*, 21:1005–1010.

Moore, T.J., Cohen, M.R., and Furberg, C.D., 2007, Serious adverse events reported to the Food and Drug Administration, 1998-2005, *Archives of Internal Medicine*, 167:1752–1759.

Morgan, J., Roper, M.H., Sperling, L., et al., 2008, Myocarditis, pericarditis, and dilated cardiomyopathy after smallpox vaccination among civilians in the United States, January-October 2003, *Clinical Infectious Diseases*, 46(Suppl. 3):S242–S250.

Morganroth, J., 2004, A definitive or thorough phase 1 QT ECG trial as a requirement for drug safety assessment, *Journal of Electrocardiology*, 37:25–29.

Morganroth, J., 2007, Cardiac repolarization and the safety of new drugs defined by electrocardiography, *Clinical Pharmacology and Therapeutics*, 81:108–113.

Morganroth, J., 2008, Response to "Design of the 'Thorough QT study,' *Clinical Pharmacology and Therapeutics*, 83:529–530.

Morganroth, J., Ilson, B.E., Shaddinger, B.C., et al., 2004, Evaluation of vardenafil and sildenafil on cardiac repolarization, *American Journal of Cardiology*, 93:1378–1383.

Mouridsen, H., Keshaviah, A., Coates, A.S., et al., 2007, Cardiovascular adverse events during adjuvant endocrine therapy for early breast cancer using letrozole or tamoxifen: Safety analysis of BIG 1-98 trial, *Journal of Clinical Oncology*, 25:5715–5722.

Mulrow, C.D., Cornell, J., and Localio, A.R., 2007, Rosiglitazone: A thunderstorm from scarce and fragile data, *Annals of Internal Medicine*, 147:585–587.

Muster, W., Breidenbach, A., Fischer, H., et al., 2008, Computational toxicology in drug development, *Drug Discovery Today*, 13:303–310.

Myokai, T., Ryu, S., Shimizu, H., and Oiki, S., 2008, Topological mapping of the asymmetric drug binding to the human ether-a-go-go-related gene product (hERG) potassium channel by use of tandem dimers, *Molecular Pharmacology*, 73:1643–1651.

Nagy, A.C., Cserep, Z., Tolnay, E., Nagykalnai, T., and Forster, T., 2008, Early diagnosis of chemotherapy-induced cardiomyopathy: A prospective tissue Doppler imaging study, *Pathology Oncology Research*, March 15 [E-publication ahead of print].

Nakagawa, M., Ooie, T., Takahashi, N., et al., 2006, Influence of menstrual cycle on QT interval dynamics, *Pacing and Clinical Electrophysiology*, 29:607–613.

Natekar, M., Mahajan, V., Satra, A., O'Kelly, M., and Karnad, D.R., 2008, Use of ANOVA to estimate inter- and intra-reader variability for a group of readers in thorough QT/QTc studies, *Clinical Pharmacology and Therapeutics*, 83: 489–91.

Need, A.C., Motulsky, A.G., and Goldstein, D.B., 2005, Priorities and standards in pharmacogenetic research, *Nature Genetics*, 27:671–681

Neilan, T.G., Jassal, D.S., Perez-Sanz, T.M., et al., 2006, Tissue Doppler imaging predicts left ventricular dysfunction and mortality in a murine model of cardiac injury, *European Heart Journal*, 27:1868–1875.

Nelson, M.R., Daniel, K.R., Carr, J.J., et al., 2008, Associations between electrocardiographic interval durations and coronary artery calcium scores: The Diabetes Heart Study, *Pacing and Clinical Electrophysiology*, 31:314–321.

Nelson, H.S., Gross, N.J., Levine, B., et al., Formoterol Study Group, 2007, Cardiac safety profile of nebulized formoterol in adults with COPD: A 12-week, multicenter, randomized, double-blind, double-dummy, placebo- and active-controlled trial, *Clinical Therapeutics*, 29:2167–2178.

Nilsson, L.J. and Regnstrom, K.J., 2008, Pharmacogenomics in the evaluation of efficacy and adverse events during clinical development of vaccines, *Methods in Molecular Biology*, 448:469–479.

Noel, G.J., Goodman, D.B., Chien, S., et al., 2004, Measuring the effects of supratherapeutic doses of levofloxacin on healthy volunteers using four methods of QT correction and periodic and continuous ECG recordings, *Journal of Clinical Pharmacology*, 44:464–473.

Noel, G.J., Natarajan, J., Chien, S., et al., 2003, Effects of three flouroquinolones on QT interval in healthy adults after single doses, *Clinical Pharmacology and Therapeutics*, 73:292–303.

Nutt, R., Vento, L.R., and Ridinger, M.H., 2007, *In vivo* molecular imaging biomarkers: Clinical pharmacology's new "PET"? *Clinical Pharmacology and Therapeutics*, 81:792–795.

O'Brien, P.J., 2008, Cardiac troponin is the most effective translational safety biomarker for myocardial injury in cardiotoxicity, *Toxicology*, 245:206–218.

Ohno, Y., Hisaka, A., and Suzuki, H., 2007, General framework for the quantitative prediction of CYP3A4-mediated oral drug interactions based on the AUC increase by coadministration of standard drugs, *Clinical Pharmacokinetics*, 46:681–696.

Oliva, A., Levin, R., Behrman, R., and Woodcock, J., 2008, Bioinformatics modernization and the critical path to improved benefit-risk assessment of drugs, *Drug Information Journal*, 42:273–279.

Olson, M.K., 2004, Are novel drugs more risky for patients than less novel drugs? *Health Economics*, 23:1135–1158.

O'Neill, R.T., 1995, Statistical concepts in planning and evaluation of drug safety from clinical trials in drug development: Issues of international harmonization, *Statistics in Medicine*, 14:117–127.

O'Neill, R.T., 1998, Biostatistical considerations in pharmacovigilance and pharmacoepidemiology: Linking quantitative risk assessment in pre-market licensure application safety data, post-market alert reports and formal epidemiological studies, *Statistics in Medicine,* 17:1851–1858.

O'Neill, R.T., 2006, FDA's critical path initiative: A perspective on contributions of biostatistics, *Biometrical Journal*, 48:559–564.

O'Neill, R.T., 2008, A perspective on characterizing benefits and risks derived from clinical trials: Can we do more? *Drug Information Journal*, 42:235–245.

Pan, N.H., Yang, H.Y., Hsieh, M.H., and Chan, Y.J., 2008, Coronary calcium score from multislice computed tomography correlates with QT dispersion and left ventricular wall thickness, *Heart Vessels*, 23:155–160.

Pardo, L.A., Contreras-Jurado, C., Zientkowska, M., Alves, F., and Stuhmer, W., 2005, Role of voltage-gated potassium channels in cancer, *Journal of Membrane Biology*, 205:115–124.

Patel, C. and Antzelevitch, C., 2008, Cellular basis for arrhythmogenesis in an experimental model of the short ST syndrome, *Heart Rhythm*, 5:585–590.

Pater, C., 2005, Methodological considerations in the design of trials for safety assessment of new drugs and chemical entities, *Current Controlled Trials in Cardiovascular Medicine*, 6:1.

Perez, A.E., Suman, V.J., Davidson, N.E., et al., 2008, Cardiac safety analysis of doxorubicin and cyclophosphamide followed by paclitaxel with or without trastuzumab in the North Central Cancer Treatment Group N9831 adjuvant breast cancer trial, *Journal of Clinical Oncology*, 26:1231–1238.

Phillips, E.J. and Mallal, S.A., 2008, Pharmacogenetics and the potential for the individualization of antiretroviral therapy, *Current Opinions in Infectious Diseases*, 21:16–24.

Pingitore, A. and Iervasi, G., 2008, Triiodothyronine (T3) effects on cardiovascular system in patients with heart failure, *Recent Patents in Cardiovascular Drug Discovery*, 3:19–27.

Pollard, C.E., Valentin, J.P., and Hammond, T.G., 2008, Strategies to reduce the risk of drug-induced QT interval prolongation: A pharmaceutical company perspective, *British Journal of Pharmacology*, May 26 [E-publication ahead of print].

Pradhan, J., Vankayala, H., Niraj, A., et al., 2008, QT dispersion at rest and during adenosine stress myocardial perfusion imaging: Correlation with myocardial jeopardy score, *Clinical Cardiology*, 31:205–210.

Prentice, R.L., 1989, Surrogate endpoints in clinical trials: Definition and operational criteria, *Statistics in Medicine*, 8:431–440.

Psaty, B.M. and Charo, R.A., 2007, FDA responds to Institute of Medicine drug safety recommendations—in part, *Journal of the American Medical Association*, 297:1917–1920.

Rajman, I., 2008, PK/PD modeling and simulations: Utility in drug development, *Drug Discovery Today*, 13:341–346.

Raschi, E., Vasina, V., Poluzzi, E., and De Ponti, F., 2008, The hERG K(+) channel: Target and antitarget strategies in drug development, *Pharmacological Research*, 57:181–195.

Ray, W.A. and Stein, C.M., 2006, Reform of drug regulation—Beyond an independent drug-safety board, *New England Journal of Medicine*, 354:194–201.

Ray, W.A. and Stein, C.M., 2008, The aprotinin story—Is BART the final chapter? *New England Journal of Medicine*, 358:2398–2400

Richter, W.S., 2006, Imaging biomarkers as surrogate endpoints for drug development, *European Journal of Nuclear Medicine and Molecular Imaging*, 33(S):S6–S10.

Robert, J., 2007, Preclinical assessment of anthracycline cardiotoxicity in laboratory animals: Predictiveness and pitfalls, *Cell Biology and Toxicology*, 23:27–37.

Robinson, S., Delongeas, J.L., Donald, E., et al., 2008, A European pharmaceutical company initiative challenging the regulatory requirement for acute toxicity studies in pharmaceutical drug development, *Regulatory Toxicology and Pharmacology*, 50:345–352.

Roden, D.M., Altman, R.B., Benowitz, N.L., et al. for the Pharmacogenetics Research Network, 2006, Pharmacogenomics: Challenges and opportunities, *Annals of Internal Medicine*, 145:749–757.

Rodriguez, I., Kilborn, M.J., Liu, X.K., Pezzullo, J.C., and Woolsey, R.L., 2001, Drug-induced QT prolongation in women during the menstrual cycle, *Journal of the American Medical Association*, 285:1322–1326.

Roncaglioni, A. and Benfenati, E., 2008, *In silico*-aided prediction of biological properties of chemicals: Oestrogen receptor-mediated effects, *Chemical Society Reviews*, 37:441–450.

Roses, A.D., 2004, Pharmacogenetics and drug development: The path to safer and more effective drugs, *Nature Reviews Genetics*, 5:645–656.

Sarapa, N., 2007, Quality assessment of digital annotated ECG data from clinical trials by the FDA ECG warehouse, *Expert Opinion on Drug Safety*, 6:595–607.

Sarapa, N. and Britto, M.R., Challenges of characterizing proarrhythmic risk due to QTc prolongation induced by nonadjuvant anticancer agents, *Expert Opinion on Drug Safety*, 7:305–318.

Sarapa, N., Mortara, J.L., Brown, B.D., Isola, L., and Badilini, F., 2008, Quantitative performance of E-Scribe warehouse in detecting quality issues with digital annotated ECG data from healthy subjects, *Journal of Clinical Pharmacology*, 48:538–546.

Sarapa, N., Nickens, D.J., Raber, S.R., Reynolds, R.R., and Amantea, M.A., 2008, Ritonavir 100 mg does not cause QTc prolongation in healthy subjects: A possible role as CYP3A inhibitor in thorough QTc studies, *Clinical Pharmacology and Therapeutics*, 83:153–159.

Sari, A.B., Sheldon, T.A., Cracknell, A., et al., 2007, Extent, nature and consequences of adverse events: Results of a retrospective casenote review in a large NHS hospital, *Quality and Safety in Health Care*, 16:434–439.

Sartipy, P., Bjorquist, P., Strehl, R., and Hyliner, J., 2007, The application of human embryonic stem cell technologies to drug discovery, *Drug Discovery Today*, 12:688–699.

Savelieva, I. and Camm, A.J., 2008, I_f inhibition with ivabradine: Electrophysiological effects and safety, *Drug Safety*, 31:95–107.

Sayers, S.L., Riegel, B., Goldberg, L.R., Coyne, J.C., and Samaha, F.F., 2008, Clinical exacerbations as a surrogate end point in heart failure research, *Heart and Lung*, 37:28–35.

Scherer, D., von Lowenstern, K., Zitron, E., et al., 2008, Inhibition of cardiac hERG potassium channels by tetracyclic antidepressant mianserin, *Naunyn-Schmiedebergs Archives of Pharmacology*, May 6 [E-publication ahead of print].

Schwarz, U.I., Ritchie, M.D., Bradford, Y., et al., 2008, Genetic determinants of response to warfarin during initial anticoagulation, *New England Journal of Medicine*, 358:999–1008.

Serra, D.B., Affrime, M.B., Bedigian, M.P., et al., 2005, QT and QTc interval with standard and supratherapeutic doses of derifenacin, a muscarinic M3 selective receptor antagonist for the treatment of overactive bladder, *Journal of Clinical Pharmacology*, 45:1038–1047.

Sethuraman, V. and Sun, Q., 2008, Impact of baseline ECG collection on the planning, analysis and interpretation of 'thorough' QT trials, *Pharmaceutical Statistics*, May 14 [E-publication ahead of print].

Shah, R.R., 2007, Cardiac repolarisation and drug regulation: Assessing cardiac safety 10 years after the CPMP guidance, *Drug Safety*, 30(12):1093–1110.

Shah, R.R., 2008, If a drug deemed 'safe' in nonclinical tests subsequently prolongs QT in phase 1 studies, how can its sponsor convince regulators to allow development to proceed? *Pharmacology and Therapeutics*, April 1 [E-publication ahead of print].

Shaikh, S.A., Jain, T., Sandhu, G., Latha, N., and Jayaram, B., 2007, From drug target to leads—Sketching a physiochemical pathway for lead molecule design *in silico*, *Current Pharmaceutical Design*, 13:3454–3470.

Shalviri, G., Mohammad, K., Majdzadeh, R., and Gholami, K., 2007, Applying quantitative methods for detecting new drug safety signals in pharmacovigilance national database, *Pharmacoepidemiology and Drug Safety*, 16:1136–1140.

Shamovsky, I., Connolly, S., David, L., et al., 2008, Overcoming undesirable hERG potency of chemokine receptor antagonists using baseline lipophilicity relationships, *Journal of Medicinal Chemistry*, 51:1162–1178.

Shen, L.Z., Coffey, T., and Deng, W., 2008, A Bayesian approach to utilizing prior data in new drug development, *Journal of Biopharmaceutical Statistics*, 18:227–243.

Shrank, W.H., Hoang, T., Ettner, S.L., et al., 2006, The implications of choice: Prescribing generic or preferred pharmaceuticals improves medication adherence for chronic conditions, *Archives of Internal Medicine*, 166:332–337.

Simpson, R.J., Jr., 2008, Assessing the safety of drugs through observational research, *Heart*, 94:129–130.

Sistare, F.D. and Degeorge, J.J., 2008, Applications of toxicogenomics to nonclinical drug development: Regulatory science considerations, *Methods in Molecular Biology*, 460:239–261.

Strnadova, C., 2005, The assessment of QT/QTc interval prolongation in clinical trials: A regulatory perspective, *Drug Information Journal*, 39:407–433.

Stafford, R.S., 2008, Regulating off-label drug use: Rethinking the role of the FDA, *New England Journal of Medicine*, 358:1427–1429.

Stockbridge, N., 2005, Points to consider in electrocardiogram waveform extraction, *Journal of Electrocardiology*, 38:319–320.

Stockbridge, N. and Brown, B.D., 2004, Annotated ECG waveform data at FDA, *Journal of Electrocardiology*, 37(S):63–64.

Stockbridge, N. and Throckmorton, D.C., 2004, Regulatory advice on evaluation of the proarrhythmic potential of drugs, *Journal of Electrocardiology*, 37(S): 40–41.

St. Clair, L. and Ballantyne, C.M., 2007, Biological surrogates for enhancing cardiovascular risk prediction in type 2 diabetes mellitus, *American Journal of Cardiology*, 99:80B–99B.

Stenver, D.I., 2008, Pharmacovigilance: What to do if you see an adverse reaction and the consequences, *European Journal of Radiology*, 66:184–186.

Strom, B.L., 2006, How the US drug safety system should be changed, *Journal of the American Medical Association*, 295:2072–2074.

Strom, B.L., Faich, G.A., Reynolds, R.F., et al., 2008, The Ziprasidone Observational Study of Cardiac Outcomes (ZODIAC): Design and baseline subject characteristics, *Journal of Clinical Psychiatry*, 69:114–121.

Stummana, T.C. and Bremer, S., 2008, The possible impact of human embryonic stem cells on safety pharmacological and toxicological assessments in drug discovery and drug development, *Current Stem Cell Research and Therapy*, 3:118–131.

Sturmer, T., Rothman, K.J., and Avorn, J., 2008, Pharmacoepidemiology and "*in silico*" drug evaluation: Is there common ground? *Journal of Clinical Epidemiology*, 61:205–206.

Synnergren, J., Adak, S., Englund, M.C., 2008, Cardiomyogenic gene expression profiling of differentiating human embryonic stem cells, *Journal of Biotechnology*, 134:162–170.

Synnergren, J., Akesson, K., Dahlenborg, K., et al., 2008, Molecular signature of cardiomyocyte clusters derived from human embryonic stem cells, *Stem Cells*, April 24 [E-publication ahead of print].

Stylianou, A., Roger, J., and Stephens, K., 2008, A statistical assessment of QT data following placebo and moxifloxacin dosing in thorough QT studies, *Journal of Biopharmaceutical Statistics*, 18(3):502–516.

Takemasa, H., Nagatomo, T., Abe, H., et al., 2008, Coexistence of hERG current block and disruption of protein trafficking in ketoconazole-induced long QT syndrome, *British Journal of Pharmacology*, 153:439–447.

Teixeira, C.E., Priviero, F.B., and Webb, R.C., 2006, Differential effects of phosphodiesterase type 5 inhibitors sildenafil, vardenafil, and tadalafil in rat aorta, *Journal of Pharmacology and Experimental Therapeutics*, 316:654–661.

Telli, M.L., Witteles, R.M., Fisher, G.A., and Srinivas, S., 2008, Cardiotoxicity associated with the cancer therapeutic agent sunitinib malate, *Annals of Oncology*, April 23 [E-publication ahead of print].

Temple, R., 2007, Quantitative decision analysis: A work in progress, *Clinical Pharmacology and Therapeutics*, 82:127–130.

Thai, K.M. and Ecker, G.F., 2007, Predictive models for hERG channel blockers: Ligand-based and structure-based approaches, *Current Medicinal Chemistry*, 14:3003–3026.

Thai, K.M. and Ecker, G.F., 2008, A binary QSAR model for classification of hERG potassium channel blockers, *Bioorganic and Medicinal Chemistry*, 16:4107–4119.

Thakrar, B.T., Grundschober, S.B., and Doessegger, L., 2007, Detecting signals of drug-drug interactions in a spontaneous reports database, *British Journal of Clinical Pharmacology*, 64:489–495.

Tian, H. and Natarajan, J., 2008, Effect of baseline measurement on the change from baseline in QTc intervals, *Journal of Biopharmaceutical Statistics*, 18:542–552.

Tsikouris, J.P., Peeters, M.J., Cox, C.D., Meyerrose, G.E., and Seifert, C.F., 2006, Effects of three flouroquinolones on QT analysis after standard treatment courses, *Annals of Noninvasive Electrocardiology*, 11:52–56.

Tsong, Y., Shen, M., Zhong, J., and Zhang, J., 2008, Statistical issues of QT prolongation assessment based on linear concentration modeling, *Journal of Biopharmaceutical Statistics*, 18(3):564–84.

Tsong, Y., Zhong, J., and Chen, W.J., 2008, Validation testing in thorough QT/QTc clinical trials, *Journal of Biopharmaceutical Statistics*, 18:529–541.

Tsong, Y. and Zhang, J., 2008, Guest editors' notes on statistical issues in design and analysis of thorough QTc studies, *Journal of Biopharmaceutical Statistics*, 18:405–407.

van der Hooft, C.S., Dieleman, J.P., Siemes, C., et al., 2008, Adverse drug reaction-related hospitalisations: A population-based cohort study, *Pharmacoepidemiology and Drug Safety*, 17:365–371.

van Staa, T.P., Smeeth, L., Persson, I., Parkinson, J., and Leufkens, H.G., 2008, Evaluating drug toxicity signals: Is a hierarchical classification of evidence useful or a hindrance? *Pharmacoepidemiology and Drug Safety*, 17:475–484.

Vargas, H.M., Bass, A.S., Breidenbach, A, et al., 2008, Appraisal—State of the Art: Scientific review and recommendations on preclinical cardiovascular safety evaluation of biologics, *Journal of Pharmacological and Toxicological Methods*, April 18 [E-publication ahead of print].

Vedani, A., Dobler, M., and Lill, M.A., 2006, The challenge of predicting drug toxicity *in silico*, *Basic and Clinical Pharmacology and Toxicology*, 99:195–208.

Viskin, S. and Rosovski, U., 2005, The degree of potassium channel blockade and the risk of torsades de pointes: The truth, nothing but the truth, but not the whole truth, *European Heart Journal*, 26:536–537.

Vladutiu, G.D., 2008, The FDA announces new drug labeling for pharmacogenetic testing: Is personalized medicine becoming a reality? *Molecular Genetics and Metabolism,* 93:1–4.

Volpi, S., Heaton, C., Mack, K., et al., 2008, Whole genome association study identifies polymorphisms associated with QT prolongation during iloperidone treatment of schizophrenia, *Molecular Psychiatry*, June 3 [E-publication ahead of print].

Wang, Y., Pan, G., and Balch, A., 2008, Bias and variance evaluation of QT interval correction methods, *Journal of Biopharmaceutical Statistics*, 18:427–450.

Wang, D., Patel, C., Cui, C., and Yan, G.X., 2008, Preclinical assessment of drug-induced proarrhythmias: Role of the arterially perfused rabbit left ventricular wedge preparation, *Pharmacology and Therapeutics*, March 15 [E-publication ahead of print].

Weaver, J., Willy, M., and Avigan, M., 2008, Informatic tools and approaches in postmarketing pharmacovigilance used by FDA, *AAPS Journal*, 10:35–41.

Weintraub, W.S. and Diamond, G.A., 2008, Predicting cardiovascular events with coronary calcium scoring, *New England Journal of Medicine*, 358:1394–1396.

Weir, A.B., 2008, Hazard identification and risk assessment for biologics targeting the immune system, *Journal of Immunotoxicology*, 5:3–10.

Wilke, R.A., Lin, D.W., Roden, D.M., et al., 2007, Identifying genetic risk factors for serious adverse drug reactions: Current progress and challenges, *Nature Reviews Drug Discovery*, 6:904–916.

Winterstein, A.G., Gerhard, T., Shuster, J., et al., 2007, Cardiac safety of central nervous system stimulants in children and adolescents with attention-deficit/ hyperactivity disorder, *Pediatrics*, 120:1494–1501.

Wittes, J., Lakatos, E., and Probstfield, J., 1989, Surrogate endpoints in clinical trials: Cardiovascular diseases, *Statistics in Medicine*, 8:415–425.

Wolfstadt, J.I., Gurwitz, J.H., Field, T.S., et al., 2008, The effect of computerized physician order entry with clinical decision support on the rates of adverse drug events: A systematic review, *Journal of General Internal Medicine*, 23:451–458.

Wood, A.J.J., 2006, Sounding board: A proposal for radical changes in the drug-approval process, *New England Journal of Medicine*, 355:618–623.

Woodcock, J. and Woosley, R., 2008, The FDA critical path initiative and its influence on new drug development, *Annual Reviews of Medicine*, 59:1–12.

Woosley, R. and Cossman, J., 2007, Drug development and the FDA's Critical Path Initiative, *Clinical Pharmacology and Therapeutics*, 81:129–133.

Wu, S., Chen, J.J., Kudelka, A., Lu, J., and Zhu, X., 2008, Incidence and risk of hypertension with sorafenib in patients with cancer: A systematic review and meta analysis, *Lancet Oncology*, 9:117–123.

Yin, T. and Miyata, T., 2007, Warfarin dose and the pharmacogenomics of CYP2C9 and VKORC1: Rationale and perspectives, *Thrombosis Research*, 120:1–10.

Young, H.M., Gray, S.L., McCormick, W.C., et al., 2008, Types, prevalence, and potential clinical significance of medication administration errors in assisted living, *Journal of the American Geriatrics Society*, May 14 [E-publication ahead of print].

Yusuf, S., Bosch, J., Devereaus, P.J., et al., 2008, Sensible guidelines for the conduct of large randomized trials, *Clinical Trials*, 5:38–39.

Zemrak, W.R. and Kenna, G.A., 2008, Association of antipsychotic and antidepressant drugs with QT interval prolongation, *American Journal of Health-system Pharmacy*, 65:1029–1038.

Zeng, H., Penniman, J.R., Kinose, F., et al., 2008, Improved throughput of PatchXpress hERG assay using intracellular potassium fluoride, *Assay and Drug Development Technologies*, 6:235–241.

Zhang, J., 2008, Testing for positive control activity in a thorough QTc study, *Journal of Biopharmaceutical Statistics*, 18(3):517–528.

Zhang, J. and Machado, S.G., 2008, Statistical issues including design and sample size calculation in thorough QT/QTc studies, *Journal of Biopharmaceutical Statistics*, 18(3):451–467.

Zhang, L., Chappell, J., Gonzales, C.R., et al., 2007, QT effects of duloxetine at supratherapeutic doses: A placebo and positive controlled study, *Journal of Cardiovascular Pharmacology*, 49:146–153.

Zhang, L., Dmitrienko, A., and Luta, G., 2008, Sample size calculations in thorough QT studies, *Journal of Biopharmaceutical Statistics* 2008, 18(3):468-482.

Zhang, X., Crespo, A., and Fernandez, A., 2008, Turning promiscuous kinase inhibitors into safer drugs, *Trends in Biotechnology*, April 8 [E-publication ahead of print].

Zhao, X.L., Qi, Z.P., Fang, C., et al., 2008, hERG K+ channel blockade by the novel antiviral drug sophocarpine, *Biological and Pharmaceutical Bulletin*, 31: 627–663.

REFERENCES

American Heart Association/American Stroke Association, 2007, *Heart disease and stroke statistics: 2007 update at-a-glance.* http://www.americanheart.org/downloadable/heart/1166711577754HS_StatsInsideText.pdf, accessed November 19, 2007.

Anantharam, A. and Abbott, G.W., 2005, Does hERG coassemble with a β subunit? Evidence for roles of MinK and MiRP1. In Chadwick, D.J. and Goode, J. (Eds.), *The hERG cardiac potassium channel: Structure, function, and long QT syndrome,* Chichester, UK: John Wiley & Sons, 100–112.

Anderson, R.H. and Ho, S.Y., 2003, The morphology of the cardiac conduction system. In Chadwick, D.J. and Goode, J. (Eds.), *Development of the cardiac conduction system,* Chichester, UK: John Wiley & Sons, 6–24.

Anson, B.D., Weaver, J.G., Ackerman, M.J., et al., 2005, Blockade of HERG channels by HIV protease inhibitors, *Lancet,* 365:682–686.

Arlett, P., Moseley, J., and Seligman, P.J., 2005, A view from regulatory agencies. In Strom, B.L. (Ed.), *Pharmacoepidemiology,* 4th edition, Chichester, UK: John Wiley & Sons, 103–130.

Arnold, B.D.C., 2004, Regulatory aspects of pharmacovigilance. In Talbot, J. and Waller, P. (Eds.), *Stephens' detection of new adverse drug reactions,* 5th edition, Chichester, UK: John Wiley & Sons, 375–451.

Asano, K., Bohlmeyer, T.J., Westcott, J.Y., et al., 2002, Altered expression of endothelin receptors in failing human left ventricles, *Journal of Molecular and Cellular Cardiology,* 34:833–846.

Ascher-Svanum, H., Zhu, B., Faries, D., Lacro, J.P., and Dolder, C.R., 2006, A prospective study of risk factors for nonadherence with antipsychotic medication in the treatment of schizophrenia, *Journal of Clinical Psychiatry,* 67:1114–1123.

Ascione, F.J., 2001, *Principles of scientific literature evaluation: Critiquing clinical drug trials,* Washington, DC: American Pharmaceutical Association.

Integrated Cardiac Safety: Assessment Methodologies for Noncardiac Drugs in Discovery, Development, and Postmarketing Surveillance. By J. Rick Turner and Todd A. Durham
Copyright © 2009 John Wiley & Sons, Inc.

Augen, J., 2004, *Bioinformatics in the post-genomic era: Genome, transcriptome, proteome, and information-based medicine*, Boston: Addison-Wesley.

Avorn, J., 2006, Dangerous deception—Hiding the evidence of adverse drug effects, *New England Journal of Medicine*, 355:2169–2171.

Avorn, J., 2007, In defense of pharmacoepidemiology—Embracing the yin and yang of drug research, *New England Journal of Medicine*, 357:2219–2221.

Bader, G.D. and Enright, A.J., 2005, Intermolecular interactions and biological pathways. In Baxevanis, A.D. and Ouellette, B.F.F. (Eds.), *Bioinformatics: A practical guide to the analysis of genes and proteins,* 3rd edition, Hoboken, NJ: Wiley-Interscience, 253–291.

Balkrishnan, R., Arondekar, B.V., Camacho, F.T., et al., 2007, Comparisons of rosiglitazone versus pioglitazone monotherapy introduction and associated health care utilization in Medicaid-enrolled patients with type 2 diabetes mellitus, *Clinical Therapeutics*, 29:1306–1315.

Ball, P., 2000, Moxifloxacin (Avelox): An 8-methoxyquinolone antibacterial with enhanced potency, *International Journal of Clinical Practice*, 54:329–332.

Barbey, J.T., Pezzullo, J.C., and Soignet, S.L., 2003, Effect of arsenic trioxide on QT interval in patients with advanced malignancies, *Journal of Clinical Oncology*, 21:3609–3615.

Bates, D.W., Cullen, D.J., Laird, N., et al., 1995, Incidence of adverse drug events and potential adverse drug events, *Journal of the American Medical Association*, 274:29–34.

Bates, D.W., Spell, N., Cullen, D.J., et al., 1997, The costs of adverse drug events in hospitalized patients, *Journal of the American Medical Association*, 277:307–311.

Berneis, K., Rizzo, M., Stettler, C., et al., 2008, Comparative effects of rosiglitazone and pioglitazone on fasting and postprandial low-density lipoprotein size and subclasses in patients with type 2 diabetes, *Expert Opinion on Pharmacotherapy*, 9:343–349.

Bernot, A., 2004, *Genome, transcriptome and proteome analysis*, Chichester, UK: John Wiley & Sons. [First published in French in 2001: Translated into English by J. McClellan and S. Cure.]

Biomarkers Definitions Working Group, 2001, Biomarkers and surrogate endpoints: Preferred definitions and conceptual framework, *Clinical Pharmacology and Therapeutics*, 69:89–95.

Bjerregaard, P. and Gussak, I., 2008, Short QT syndrome. In Gussak, I. and Antzelevitch, C., (Eds.), *Electrical diseases of the heart: Genetics, mechanisms, treatment, prevention*, London: Springer-Verlag, 554–563.

Blackshear, K.L. and Kantor, B., 2007, Pathogenesis of atherosclerosis. In Murphy, J.G. and Lloyd, M.A. (Eds.), *Mayo Clinic cardiology: Concise textbook,* 3rd edition, Rochester, MN: Mayo Clinic Scientific Press, 699–714.

Bloomfield, D. and Krishna, R., 2008, Commentary on the clinical relevance of concentration/QTc relationships for new drug candidates, *Journal of Clinical Pharmacology*, 48:6–8.

Bock, G. and Goode, J. (Eds.), 2006, *Heart failure: Molecules, mechanisms and therapeutic targets,* Chichester, UK: John Wiley & Sons.

Bogardus, S.T., Holmboe, E., and Jekel, J.F., 1999, Perils, pitfalls, and possibilities in talking about medical risk, *Journal of the American Medical Association*, 28:1037–1041.

Bombardier, C., Laine, L., Reicin, A., et al. for the VIGOR Study Group, 2000, Comparison of upper gastrointestinal toxicity of rofecoxib and naproxen in patients with rheumatoid arthritis, *New England Journal of Medicine*, 343:1520–1528.

Bond, C. (Ed.), 2004, *Concordance*, London: Pharmaceutical Press.

Borer, J.S., Pouleur, H., Abadie, E., et al., 2007, Cardiovascular safety of drugs not intended for cardiovascular use: Need for a new conceptual basis for assessment and approval, *European Heart Journal*, 28:1904–1909.

Bosworth, H.B., Oddone, E.Z., and Weinberger, M. (Eds.), 2005, *Patient treatment adherence: Concepts, interventions, and measurement,* Mahwah, N.J.: Lawrence Erlbaum Associates.

Bosworth, H.B., Weinberger, M, and Oddone, E.Z., 2006, Introduction. In Bosworth, H.B., Oddone, E.Z., and Weinberger, M. (Eds.), *Patient treatment adherence: Concepts, interventions, and measurement,* Mahwah, N.J.: Lawrence Erlbaum Associates.

Bowers, D., House, A., and Owens, D, 2006, *Understanding clinical papers,* 2nd edition, Chichester, UK: John Wiley & Sons.

Bradford Hill, A., (1965), The environment and disease: Association or causation? *Proceedings of the Royal Society of Medicine*, 58:285–300.

Brass, E.P., Lewis, R.J., Lipicky, R., Murphy, J., and Hiatt, W.R., 2006, Risk assessment in drug development for symptomatic indications: A framework for the prospective exclusion of unacceptable cardiovascular risk, *Clinical Pharmacology and Therapeutics*, 79:165–172.

Breckenridge, A., 2004, Foreword. In Talbot, J. and Waller, P. (Eds.), 2004, *Stephens' detection of new adverse drug reactions,* 5th edition, Chichester, UK: John Wiley & Sons, xi–xii.

Brenner, G.M. and Stevens, C.W., 2006, *Pharmacology,* 2nd edition, Philadelphia: Saunders/Elsevier.

Britten, N. and Weiss, M., 2004, What is concordance? In Bond, C. (Ed.), *Concordance*, London: Pharmaceutical Press, 9–28.

Bryson, B., 2004, *A short history of nearly everything*, New York: Black Swan.

Bunch, T.J. and Ackerman, M.J., 2007, Cardiac channelopathies. In Murphy, J.G. and Lloyd, M.A. (Eds.), *Mayo clinic cardiology: Concise Textbook,* 3rd edition, Rochester, MN: Mayo Clinic Scientific Press, 335–344.

Byerly, M.J., Nakonezny, P.A., and Lescouflair, E., 2007, Antipsychotic medication adherence in schizophrenia, *Psychiatry Clinical North America*, 30:437–452.

Cabell, C.H., Noto, T.C., and Krucoff, M.W., 2005, Clinical utility of the Food and Drug Administration Electrocardiogram Warehouse: A paradigm for the critical pathway initiative, *Journal of Electrocardiography*, 38(4 Suppl):175–179.

Camm, A.J., Malik, M., and Yap, Y.G., 2004, *Acquired long QT syndrome,* Malden, MA: Futura/Blackwell Publishing.

Campbell, M.J., Machin, D., and Walters, S.J., 1999, *Medical statistics,* 3rd edition, Chichester, UK: John Wiley & Sons.

Campbell, M.J. and Machin, D., 2005, *Design of studies for medical research*, Chichester, UK: John Wiley & Sons.

Catterall, W.A., 2006, The voltage-gated ion channel superfamily. In Triggle, D.J., Gopalakrishnan, M., Rampe, D., and Zheng, W. (Eds.), *Voltage-gated ion channels as drug targets*, Manheim, Germany: Wiley-VCH, 7–18.

Cavalli, A., Poluzzi, E., De Ponti, F., and Recanatini, M., 2002, Toward a pharmacophore for drugs inducing the long QT syndrome: Insights from a CoMFA study of hERG K(+) channel blockers, *Journal of Medicinal Chemistry*, 45:3844–3853.

Chadwick, D.J. and Goode, J. (Eds.), 2003, *Development of the cardiac conduction system,* Chichester, UK: John Wiley & Sons. (Novartis Foundation Symposium 266.)

Chadwick, D.J. and Goode, J. (Eds.), 2005, *The hERG cardiac potassium channel: Structure, function, and long QT syndrome,* Chichester, UK: John Wiley & Sons.

Chan, K.A. and Jones, S.C., 2007, NSAIDS—COX-2 Inhibitors—Risks and benefits. In Mann, R. and Andrews, E. (Eds.), *Pharmacovigilance,* 2nd edition, Chichester, UK: John Wiley & Sons, 583–602.

Chen, F.C. and Brozovich, F.W., 2007, Chronic stable angina. In Murphy, J.G. and Lloyd, M.A. (Eds.), *Mayo clinic cardiology: Concise textbook,* 3rd edition, Rochester, MN: Mayo Clinic Scientific Press.

Chernew, M.E., Shah, M.R., Wegh, A., et al., 2008, Impact of decreasing copayments on medication adherence within a disease management environment, *Health Affairs*, 27:103–112.

Chow, S-C. and Liu, J-P., 2004, *Design and analysis of clinical trials: Concepts and methodologies,* 2nd edition, Hoboken, NJ: John Wiley & Sons.

Chuang-Stein, C., 1992, Summarizing laboratory data with different reference ranges in multi-center trials, *Drug Information Journal*, 26:77–84.

Clatworthy, J., Bowskill, R., Rank, T., Parham, R., and Horne, R., 2007, Adherence to medication in bipolar disorder: A qualitative study exploring the role of patients' beliefs about the condition and its treatment, *Bipolar Disorders*, 9:656–664.

Clemen, R.T., 1996, *Making hard decisions: An introduction to decision analysis,* 2nd edition, Belmont, CA:Duxbury Press.

Cobert, B., 2007, *Manual of drug safety and pharmacovigilance,* Sudbury, MA: Jones and Bartlett Publishers.

Cohen, M.R. (Ed.), 2007a, *Medication errors,* 2nd edition, Washington, DC: American Pharmacists Association.

Cohen, M.R., 2007b, Causes of medication errors. In Cohen, M.R. (Ed.), *Medication Errors,* 2nd edition, Washington, DC: American Pharmacists Association, 55–66.

Couderc, J-P. and Zareba, W., 2005, Assessment of ventricular repolarization from body-surface ECGs in humans. In Morganroth, J.M. and Gussak, I. (Eds.), *Cardiac safety of noncardiac drugs: Practical guidelines for clinical research and drug development,* Totowa, NJ: Humana Press Inc., 107–129.

Culley, C.M., Lacy, M.K., Klutman, N., and Edwards, B., 2001, Moxifloxacin: Clinical efficacy and safety, *American Journal of Health Systems Pharmacists,* 58:379–388.

Curran, M.E., Splawski, I., Timothy, K.W., Vincent, G.M., Green, E.D., and Keating, M.T., 1995, A molecular basis for cardiac arrhythmia: HERG mutations cause long QT syndrome, *Cell,* 80:795.

Dale, J.W. and von Schantz, M., 2002, *From genes to genomes: Concepts and applications of DNA technology,* Chichester, UK: John Wiley & Sons.

Davis, N.M. and Cohen, M.R., 1981, *Medication errors: Causes and prevention,* Philadelphia: George F. Stickley.

Dawkins, R., 1999, *The blind watchmaker: Why the evidence of evolution reveals a universe without design,* New York: W.W. Norton & Company.

Dayan, C.M. and Wraith, D.C., 2008, Preparing for first-in-man studies: The challenges for translational immunology post-TGN1412, *Clinical Experimental Immunology,* 151:231–234.

De Ponti, F., 2008, Pharmacological and regulatory aspects of QT prolongation. In Vaz, R.J. and Klabunde, T. (Eds.), *Antitargets: Prediction and Prevention of drug side effects,* Weinheim, Germany: Wiley-VCH.

De Smet, P.A., Denneboom, W., Kramers, C., and Grol, R., 2007, A composite screening tool for mediation reviews of outpatients: General issues with specific examples, *Drugs & Aging,* 24:733–760.

Dessertenne, F., 1966, La tachycardia ventriculaire a deux foyers opposees variable, *Arch Mal Coeur Vaiss,* 59:263–272.

Devlin, T.M., 2006, Eukaryotic cell structure. In Devlin, T.M. (Ed.), *Textbook of biochemistry with clinical correlations,* 6th edition, Hoboken, NJ: John Wiley & Sons, 1–22.

Dhillon, S. and Gill, K., 2006, Basic pharmacokinetics. In Dhillon, S. and Kostrzewski, A. (Eds.), *Clinical pharmacokinetics*, London: Pharmaceutical Press.

Diamond, G.A., Bax, L., and Kaul, S., 2007, Perspective: Uncertain effects of rosiglitazone on the risk for myocardial infarction and cardiovascular death, *Annals of Internal Medicine,* 147:578–581.

Doering, C. and Zamponi, G., 2006, Overview of voltage-gated calcium channels. In Triggle, D.J., Gopalakrishnan, M., Rampe, D., and Zheng, W. (Eds.), 2006, *Voltage-gated ion channels as drug targets*, Weinheim, Germany: Wiley-VCH, 65–99.

Doggrell, S.A., 2008, Clinical trials with thiazolidinediones in subjects with type 2 diabetes—Is pioglitazone any different from rosiglitazone? *Expert Opinion on Pharmacotherapy*, 9:405–420.

Dormandy, J.A., Charbonnel, B., Eckland, D.J., et al., 2005, Secondary prevention of macrovascular events in patients with type 2 diabetes in the PROactive Study (PROspective pioglitAzone Clinical Trial in macroVascular Events): A randomised controlled trial, *Lancet*, 366:1279–1289.

Dowell, J., 2004, The prescriber's perspective. In Bond, C. (Ed.), *Concordance*, London: Pharmaceutical Press, 49–70.

Durham, T.A. and Turner, J.R., 2008, *Introduction to statistics in pharmaceutical clinical trials*, London: Pharmaceutical Press.

Edelson, E., 1999, *Gregor Mendel and the roots of genetics*, New York: Oxford University Press.

Elkins, S., Crumb, W.J., Sarazan, R.D., Wikel, J.H., and Wrighton, S.A., 2002, Three-dimensional quantitative structure-activity relationship for inhibition of human ether-a-go-go-related gene potassium channel, *Journal of Pharmacology and Experimental Therapeutics*, 301:427–434.

[EMEA CPMP] European Medicines Agency, Committee for Proprietary Medicinal Products, 2001, *Points to Consider on Application with 1. Meta-Analyses and 2. One Pivotal Study,* http://www.emea.europa.eu/pdfs/human/ewp/233099fen.pdf.

Epstein, R.J., 2003, *Human molecular biology: An introduction to the molecular basis of health and disease,* Cambridge, UK: Cambridge University Press.

Extramiana, F., Haggui, A., Maison-Blanche, P., et al., 2007, T-wave morphology parameters based on principal component analysis reproducibility and dependence on T-offset position, *Annals of Noninvasive Electrocardiology,* 12: 354–363.

Faich, G.A. and Stemhagen, A., 2005, Cardiac arrhythmia assessments in Phase IV clinical studies. In Morganroth, J.M. and Gussak, I., (Eds.), *Cardiac safety of noncardiac drugs: Practical guidelines for clinical research and drug development,* Totowa, NJ: Humana Press Inc., 229–237.

FDA, 2005a, White Paper: Prescription Drug User Fee Act (PDUFA): Adding Resources and Improving Performance in FDA Review of New Drug Applications [see www.fda.gov].

FDA, 2005b, *Guidance for Industry: Premarketing risk assessment* [see www.fda.gov].

FDA, 2005c, *Guidance for Industry: Good pharmacovigilance practices and pharmacoepidemiologic assessment* [see www.fda.gov].

FDA, 2005d, *Guidance for Industry: Development and use of risk minimization action plans* [see www.fda.gov].

FDA, 2006, *Guidance for Industry: Reports on the status of postmarketing study commitments—Implementation of Section 130 of the Food and Drug Administration Modernization Act of 1997* [see www.fda.gov].

FDA, 2007, *Guidance for clinical investigators, sponsors, and IRBs (Draft): Adverse event reporting—Improving human subject protection* [see www.fda.gov].

FDA, 2008, *The Sentinel Initiative: National Strategy for Monitoring Medical Product Safety,* http://www.fda.gov/oc/initiatives/advance/reports/report0508.pdf, accessed August 1, 2008.

Ficker, E., Dennis, A., Kuryshev, Y., Wible, B.A., and Brown, A.M., 2005, hERG channel trafficking. In Chadwick, D.J. and Goode, J. (Eds.), *Symposium on the hERG cardiac potassium channel: Structure, function, and long QT syndrome,* Chichester, UK: John Wiley & Sons, 57–69.

Finkle, J., 2008, QT assessment for oncology drugs. Presentation given during a Webinar entitled *Cardiac safety in large molecules: New regulatory expectations, new strategies*, February 26 [see Section 7.20 for more details.]

FitzGerald, G.A., 2003, COX-2 and beyond: Approaches to prostaglandin inhibition in human disease, *Nature Review Drug Discovery*, 2:879–890.

Fletcher, R.H. and Fletcher, S.W., 2005, *Clinical epidemiology: The essentials,* 4th edition, Baltimore, MD: Lippincott Williams & Wilkins.

Fogoros, R.N., 2006, *Electrophysiologic testing,* 4th edition, Malden, MA: Blackwell Publishing.

Folb, P.I., 2006, Animal tests as predictors of human response. In Lee, C-J., Lee, L.H., Wu, C.L., Lee, B.R., and Chen, M-L. (Eds.), *Clinical trials of drugs and biopharmaceuticals*, Boca Raton, FL: Taylor & Francis, 31–55.

Friedman, L.M., Furberg, C.D., and DeMets, D.L., 1998, *Fundamentals of clinical trials*, 3rd edition, New York: Springer.

Gad, S.C., 2002, *Drug safety evaluation*, Hoboken, NJ: John Wiley & Sons.

Gad, S.C., 2006, *Statistics and experimental design for toxicologists and pharmacologists*, 4th edition, Boca Raton, FL: CRC Press.

Gaita, F., Giustetto, C., Bianchi, F., et al., 2003, Short QT syndrome: A familial cause of sudden death, *Circulation*, 108:965–970.

Gallin, J.I. (Ed.), 2002, *Principles and practice of clinical research*, Burlington, MA: Academic Press.

Gallion, S.L., Beresford, A., and Bey, P., 2005, Parallel lead optimization. In Handen, J.S. (Ed.), *Industrialization of drug discovery: From target selection through lead optimization*, Boca Raton, FL: Taylor & Francis, 137–163.

Garattini, S. and Liberati, A., 2000, The risk of bias from omitted research, *British Medical Journal*, 321:845–846.

Gardner, S.N. and Schultz, D., 2007, The postmarket surveillance of medical devices: Meeting the challenge. In Brown, S.L., Bright, R.A., and Tavris, D.R. (Eds.), *Medical device epidemiology and surveillance,* Chichester: John Wiley & Sons, 482–486.

Garnett, C.E., Beasley, N., Bhattaram, V.A., et al., 2008, Concentration-QT relationships play a key role in the evaluation of proarrhythmic risk during regulatory review, *Journal of Clinical Pharmacology*, 48:13–8.

Gauvin, D.V., Tilley, L.P., Smith, F.W., Jr., and Baird, T.J., 2006, Electrocardiogram, hemodynamics, and core body temperatures of the normal freely moving laboratory beagle dog by remote radiotelemetry, *Journal of Pharmacological and Toxicological Methods*, 53:128–139.

Gerstein, H.C., Yusuf, S., Bosch, J. et al. for the DREAM Trial Investigators, 2006, Effect of rosiglitazone on the frequency of diabetes in patients with impaired glucose tolerance or impaired fasting glucose: A randomised controlled trial, *Lancet*, 368:1096–1105. [Erratum, *Lancet*, 368:1170]

Ghose, A.K., Viswanadhan, V.N., and Wendoloski, J.J., 1999, A knowledge-based approach in designing combinatorial or medicinal chemistry libraries for drug discovery. 1. A qualitative and quantitative characterization of known drug databases, *Journal of Combinatorial Chemistry*, 1:55–68.

Glantz, L.H. and Annas, G.J., 2008, The FDA, preemption, and the Supreme Court, New England Journal of Medicine, 358:1883–1885.

Glasser, S.P., Salas, M., and Delzell, E., 2007, Importance and challenges of studying marketed drugs: What is a Phase IV study? Common clinical research designs, registries, and self-reporting systems, *Journal of Clinical Pharmacology*, 47:1074–1086.

Glitz, D., 2006, Protein synthesis: Translation and posttranslational modifications. In Devlin, T.M. (Ed.), *Textbook of biochemistry with clinical correlations,* 6th edition, Hoboken, NJ: John Wiley & Sons, 201–244.

Goldstein, D.B., Tate, S.K., and Sisodiya, S.M., 2003, Pharmacogenetics goes genomic, *Nature Reviews Genetics*, 4:937–947. [Erratum in *Nature Reviews Genetics*, 5:76]

Gopalakrishnan, M., Shieh, C-C., and Chen, J., 2006, Potassium channels: Overview of molecular, biophysical, and pharmacological properties. In Triggle, D.J., Gopalakrishnan, M., Rampe, D., and Zheng, W. (Eds.), *Voltage-gated ion channels as drug targets*, Manheim, Germany: Wiley-VCH, 193–213.

Gordon-Lubitz, R.J., 2003, Risk communication: Problems of presentation and understanding, *Journal of the American Medical Association*, 289:95.

Greaves, P., 2007, *Histopathology of preclinical toxicity studies,* 3rd edition, New York: Academic Press/Elsevier.

Guess, H.A., 2005, Premarketing applications of pharmacoepidemiology. In Strom, B.L. (Ed.), *Pharmacoepidemiology,* 4th edition, Chichester, UK: John Wiley & Sons, 391–400.

Gussak, I., Brugada, P., Brugada, J., et al., 2000, Idiopathic short QT interval: A new clinical syndrome? *Cardiology,* 94:99–102.

Gussak, I. and Antzelevitch, C. (Eds.), 2003, *Cardiac repolarization: Bridging basic and clinical science,* New York: Springer-Verlag.

Halpern, S.D. and Berlin, J.A., 2005, Beyond conventional publication bias: Other determinants of data suppression. In Rothstein, H.R., Sutton, A.J., and Borenstein, M., (Eds.), *Publication bias in meta-analysis: Prevention, assessment and adjustments,* Chichester, UK: John Wiley & Sons, 303–317.

Hancox, J.C. and Mitcheson, J.S., 2006, Combined hERG channel inhibition and disruption of trafficking in drug-induced long QT syndrome by fluoxetine: A case-study in cardiac safety pharmacology, *British Journal of Pharmacology,* 149:457–459.

Harman, R.J., 2004, *Development and control of medicines and medical devices,* London: Pharmaceutical Press.

Harrison-Woolrych, M. and Coulter, D.M., 2007, PEM in New Zealand. In Mann, R. and Andrews, E. (Eds.), *Pharmacovigilance,* 2nd edition, Chichester, UK: John Wiley & Sons, 317–332.

Haverkamp, W., Breithardt, G., Camm, A.J., et al., 2000, The potential for QT prolongation and proarrhythmia by non-antiarrhythmic drugs: Clinical and regulatory implications. Report on a policy conference of the European Society of Cardiology, *European Heart Journal,* 21:1216–1231. [This paper was also published in *Cardiovascular Research,* 2000, 47:219–233.]

Haynes, R.B., Sackett, D.L., Guyatt, G.H., and Tugwell, P., 2006, *Clinical epidemiology: How to do clinical practice research,* 3rd edition, Philadelphia: Lippincott Williams & Wilkins.

Hellman, B., 2006, General toxicology. In Mulder, G.J. and Denker, L. (Eds.), *Pharmaceutical Toxicology,* London: Pharmaceutical Press, 1–39.

Herxheimer, A., 1986, Consumer organizations. In Inman, W.H.W. (Ed.), *Monitoring for drug safety,* 2nd edition, Hingham, MA: MTP Press, 699–704.

Hiatt, W.R., 2006, Observational studies of drug safety—Aprotinin and the absence of transparency, *New England Journal of Medicine,* 355:2171–2173.

Ho, R.J.Y. and Gibaldi, G., 2003, *Biotechnology and biopharmaceuticals: Transforming proteins and genes into drugs,* Weinheim: Wiley-LISS.

Hollister, A.S. and Montague, T.H., 2005, Statistical analysis plans for ECG data: Controlling the intrinsic and extrinsic variability in QT data. In Morganroth, J.M. and Gussak, I. (Eds.), *Cardiac safety of noncardiac drugs: Practical guidelines for clinical research and drug development,* Totowa, NJ: Humana Press Inc., 239–257.

Holmes, M.R., Ramkissoon, K.R., and Giddings, M.C., 2005, Proteomics and protein identification. In Baxevanis, A.D. and Ouellette, B.F.F. (Eds.), *Bioinformatics: A practical guide to the analysis of genes and proteins,* 3rd edition, Hoboken, NJ: Wiley-Interscience, 445–472.

Home, P.D., Pocock, S.J., Beck-Nielsen, H., et al. for the RECORD Study Group, 2005, Rosiglitazone Evaluated for Cardiac Outcomes and Regulation of Glycaemia in Diabetes (RECORD): Study design and protocol, *Diabetologia,* 48:1726–1735.

Home, P.D., Pocock, S.J., Beck-Nielsen, H., et al. for the RECORD Study Group, 2007, Rosiglitazone evaluated for cardiovascular outcomes: An interim analysis, *New England Journal of Medicine,* 357:28–38.

Homon, C.A. and Nelson, R.M., 2006, High-throughput screening: Enabling and influencing the process of drug discovery. In Smith, C.G. and O'Donnell, J.T. (Eds.), *The process of new drug discovery and development,* 2nd edition, New York: Informa Healthcare, 79–102.

Hondeghem, L.M., 2005, TRIad: Foundation for proarrhythmia (triangulation, reverse use dependence and instability). In Chadwick, D.J. and Goode, J. (Eds.), *The hERG cardiac potassium channel: Structure, function, and long QT syndrome,* Chichester, UK: John Wiley & Sons, 235–244.

Hondeghem, L.M., 2007, Relative contributions of TRIad and QT to proarrhythmia, *Journal of Cardiovascular Electrophysiology,* 18:655–657.

Hondeghem, L.M., 2008, Use and abuse of QT and TRIaD in cardiac safety research: Importance of study design and conduct, *European Journal of Pharmacology*, 584:1–9.

Hondeghem, L.M., De Clerk, F., and Camm, J., 2007, Short patent lives jeopardize drug and patient safety, *Journal of Cardiovascular Pharmacology*, 50:353–357.

Horne, R. and Weinman, J., 2004, The theoretical basis of concordance and issues for research. In Bond, C., (Ed.), *Concordance*, London: Pharmaceutical Press, 119–145.

Huttmacher, M.M., Chapel, S., Agin, M.A., Fleishaker, J.C., and Lalonde, R.L., 2008, Performance characteristics for some typical QT study designs under the ICH-E14 guidance, *Journal of Clinical Pharmacology,* 48:215–224.

ICH Guidance E14, 2005, The clinical evaluation of QT/QTc interval prolongation and proarrhythmic potential for non-antiarrhythmic drugs (see http://www.ich.org/LOB/media/MEDIA1476.pdf)

ICH Guidance S7A, 2001, Safety pharmacology studies for human pharmaceuticals (see http://www.ich.org/LOB/media/MEDIA504.pdf).

ICH Guidance S7B, 2005, The non-clinical evaluation of the potential for delayed ventricular repolarization (QT interval prolongation) by human pharmaceuticals (see http://www.ich.org/LOB/media/MEDIA2192.pdf).

[IHGS] International Human Genome Sequencing Consortium, 2001, Initial sequencing and analysis of the human genome, *Nature*, 409:860–921.

[IHGS] International Human Genome Sequencing Consortium, 2004, Finishing the euchromatic sequence of the human genome, *Nature*, 431:931–945.

Ingelman-Sundberg, M., 2008, Editorial: Pharmacogenomic biomarkers for prediction of severe adverse drug reactions, *New England Journal of Medicine*, 358:637–639.

Inman, W.H.W., 1981a, Postmarketing surveillance of adverse drug reactions in general practice. I: Search for new methods, *British Medical Journal*, 282:1131–1132.

Inman, W.H.W., 1981b, Postmarketing surveillance of adverse drug reactions in general practice. II: Prescription-event monitoring at the University of Southampton, *British Medical Journal*, 282:1126–1127.

Inman, W.H.W., Rawson, N.S.B., and Wilton, L.V., 1986, Prescription-event monitoring. In Inman, W.H.W. (Ed.), *Monitoring for drug safety,* 2nd edition, Hingham, MA: MTP Press, 213–235.

Inman, W.H.W. and Weber, J.C.P., 1986, The United Kingdom. In Inman, W.H.W. (Ed.), *Monitoring for drug safety,* 2nd edition, Hingham, MA: MTP Press, 13–47.

Institute of Medicine of the National Academies, 2000, *To err is human: Building a safer health system*, Washington, DC: National Academies Press.

Institute of Medicine of the National Academies, 2001, *Crossing the quality chasm: A new health care system for the 21st century,* Washington, DC: National Academies Press.

Institute of Medicine of the National Academies, 2004, *Patient safety: Achieving a new standard for care,* Washington, DC: National Academies Press.

Institute of Medicine of the National Academies, 2007a, *Preventing medication errors,* Washington, DC: National Academies Press.

Institute of Medicine of the National Academies, 2007b, *The future of drug safety: Promoting and protecting the health of the public,* Washington, DC: National Academies Press.

Ioannidis, J.P.A., 2005, Why most published research findings are false, *PLoS Medicine*, 2(8):e124.

Jamshidi, N., Vo, T.D., and Palsson, B.O., 2007, *In silico* analysis of SNPs and other high-throughput data. In Zhang, J. and Rokosh, G. (Eds.), *Cardiac gene expression: Methods and protocols*, Totowa, NJ: Humana Press, 267–285.

JNC 7 Express, 2003, *Seventh report of the Joint National Committee on prevention, detection, evaluation, and treatment of high blood pressure (Express version).* http://www.nhlbi.nih.gov/guidelines/hypertension/express.pdf, accessed April 29, 2008.

JNC 7, 2004, *Seventh Report of the Joint National Committee on prevention, detection, evaluation, and treatment of high blood pressure.* http://www.nhlbi.nih.gov/guidelines/hypertension/jnc7full.pdf, accessed April 29, 2008.

Jongeneel, C.V., Iseli, C., Stevenson, B.J., et al., 2003, Comprehensive sampling of gene expression in human cell lines with massively parallel signature sequencing, *Proceedings of the National Academy of Sciences,* 100:4702–4705.

Jost, N., Papp, J.G., and Varro, A., 2007, Slow delayed rectifier potassium current (I_{Ks}) and the repolarization reserve, *Annals of Noninvasive Electrocardiology*, 12:64–78.

Kahn, S.E., Haffner, S.M., Heise, M.A., et al., 2006, Gycemic durability of rosiglitazone, metformin, or glyburide monotherapy, *New England Journal of Medicine*, 355:2427–2443. [Erratum, *New England Journal of Medicine*, 2007, 356:1387–1388.]

Kaitin, K.I., 2008, *Tufts CSDD annual report on trends in drug development: Are efforts to books R&D efficiency working?* Presentation given at the 6th Annual Partnering with Central Labs, ECG, and Imaging Labs Conference, Orlando, Florida, January 24th.

Kanagala, R., 2007, Sudden cardiac death. In Murphy, J.G. and Lloyd, M.A. (Eds.), *Mayo clinic cardiology: Concise textbook,* 3rd edition, Rochester, MN: Mayo Clinic Scientific Press, 493–505.

Kang, J., Chen, X.L., Wang, H., et al., 2005, Discovery of a small molecule activator of the human ether-a-go-go-related gene (hERG) cardiac K+ channel, *Molecular Pharmacology*, 67:827–836.

Kannel, W.B. and Sorlie, P., 1975, Hypertension in Framingham. In Paul, O. (Ed.), *Epidemiology and control of hypertension*, New York: Grune & Stratton/ Intercontinental Medical Book Corporation.

Kaplan, E.L. and Meier, P., 1958, Nonparametric estimation from incomplete observations, *Journal of the American Statistical Association*, 53:457–481.

Karkouti, K., Beattie, W.S., Dattilo, K.M., et al., 2006, A propensity score case-control comparison of aprotinin and tranexamic acid in high-transfusion-risk cardiac surgery, *Transfusion*, 46:327–338.

Katz, D.L., 2001, *Clinical epidemiology & evidence-based medicine: Fundamental principles of clinical reasoning & research,* Thousand Oaks, CA: Sage Publications.

Kay, R., 2007, *Statistical thinking for non-statisticians in drug regulation*, Chichester, UK: John Wiley & Sons.

Kennelly, P.J. and Rodwell, V.W., 2006a, Proteins: higher orders of structure. In Murray, R.K., Granner, D.K., and Rodwell, V.W. (Eds.), *Harper's illustrated biochemistry,* 27th edition, New York: Lange Medical Books/McGraw-Hill, 30–40.

Kennelly, P.J. and Rodwell, V.W., 2006b, Enzymes: Mechanisms of action. In Murray, R.K., Granner, D.K., and Rodwell, V.W. (Eds.), *Harper's illustrated biochemistry,* 27th edition, New York: Lange Medical Books/McGraw-Hill, 49–60.

Kim, E.Y., Han, H.R., Jeong, S., et al., 2007, Does knowledge matter? Intentional medication nonadherence among middle-aged Korean Americans with high blood pressure, *Journal of Cardiovascular Nursing,* 22:397–404.

Korobkin, R., 2007, Perspective: Who should protect the public? The Supreme Court and medical device regulation, *New England Journal of Medicine,* 357: 1680–1681.

Korolkova, Y.V., Tseng, G.N., and Grishin, E.V., 2004, Unique interaction of scorpion toxins with the hERG channel, *Journal of Molecular Recognition,* 17: 209–217.

Kovacs, R.J., 2008, Clinical reality. Presentation given at a workshop conducted by Biomedical Sciences entitled *Current issues in drug development from a cardiac safety perspective,* Durham, NC, March 6, 2008.

Krall, M.D., 2007, Letter to the Editor, *New England Journal of Medicine,* 357: 1776–1777.

Krynetskiy, E. and McDonnell, P., 2007, Building individualized medicine: Prevention of adverse reactions to warfarin therapy. *Journal of Pharmacology and Experimental Therapeutics,* 322:427–434.

Lagrutta, A.A. and Salata, J.J., 2006, Ion channel safety issues in drug development. In Triggle, D.J., Gopalakrishnan, M., Rampe, D., and Zheng, W. (Eds.), 2006, *Voltage-gated ion channels as drug targets,* Manheim: Wiley-VCH, 444–465.

Lasser, K.E., Seger, D.L., Yu, D.T., et al., 2006, Adherence to black box warnings for prescription medications in outpatients, *Archives of Internal Medicine,* 166: 338–344.

Layton, D., Key, C., and Shakir, S.A., 2003, Prolongation of the QT interval and cardiac arrhythmias associated with cisapride: Limitations of the pharmacoepidemiological studies conducted and proposals for the future, *Pharmacoepidemiology and Drug Safety,* 12:31–40.

Leader, B., Baca, Q.J., and Golan, D.E., 2008, Protein therapeutics: A summary and pharmacological classification, *Nature Reviews Drug Discovery,* 7:21–39.

Leape, L.L., 2007, Systems analysis and redesign: The foundation of metical error prevention. In Cohen, M.R. (Ed.), *Medication Errors,* 2nd edition, Washington, DC: American Pharmacists Association

Leishman, D. and Waldron, G., 2006, Assay technologies: Techniques available for quantifying drug-channel interactions. In Triggle, D.J., Gopalakrishnan, M., Rampe, D., and Zheng, W. (Eds.), *Voltage-gated ion channels as drug targets,* Manheim, Germany: Wiley-VCH, 37–63.

Li, J. and Hidalgo, I.J., 2006, The evolving role of the Caco-2 cell model to estimate intestinal absorption potential and elucidate transport mechanisms. In Smith, C.G. and O'Donnell, J.T. (Eds.), *The process of new drug discovery and development,* 2nd edition, New York: Informa Healthcare USA, 161–186.

Li, Y., Cianchetta, G., and Vaz, R.J., 2006, Structural and ligand-based models for hERG and their application in medicinal chemistry. In Triggle, D.J., Gopalakrishnan, M., Rampe, D., and Zheng, W. (Eds.), *Voltage-gated ion channels as drug targets,* Manheim, Germany: Wiley-VCH, 428–443.

Lin, Y-L. and Chan, K., 2008, Pharmacokinetic and pharmacodynamic characterization of non-antiarrhythmic QT-prolonging drugs associated with torsades de pointes, *Drug Information Journal,* 42:211–219.

Lipinski, C.A., Lombardo, F., Dominy, B.W., and Feeney, P.J., 2001, Experimental and computational approaches to estimate solubility and permeability in drug discovery and development settings, *Advanced Drug Delivery Reviews,* 46: 3–26.

Litwin, J.S., Kleiman, R.B., and Gussak, I., 2008, Acquired (drug-induced) long QT syndrome. In Gussak, I. and Antzelevitch, C. (Eds.), *Electrical diseases of the heart: Genetics, mechanisms, treatment, prevention,* London: Springer-Verlag, 705–718.

Lo Re, V., III and Strom, B.L., 2007, The role of academia and the research community in assisting the Food and Drug Administration to ensure US drug safety, *Pharmacoepidemiology and Drug Safety,* 16:818–825.

Lohr, K.N., 2007, Emerging methods in comparative effectiveness and safety: Symposium overview and summary, *Medical Care,* 45(S):S5–S8.

Lowes, B.D., Gilbert, E.M., Abraham, W.T., et al, 2002, Myocardial gene expression in dilated cardiomyopathy treated with beta-blocking agents, *New England Journal of Medicine,* 346:1357–1365.

442 REFERENCES

Machin, D. and Campbell, M.J., 2005, *Design of studies for medical research*, Chichester, UK: John Wiley & Sons.

Malik, M. and Camm, A.J., 2001, Evaluation of drug-induced QT interval prolongation: Implications for drug approval and labelling, *Drug Safety*, 24: 323–351.

Mallal, S., Phillips, E., Carosi, G., et al. for the PRECICT-1 Study Team, 2008, HLA-B*5701 screening for hypersensitivity to abacavir, *New England Journal of Medicine*, 358:568–579.

Mangano, D.T., Tudor, I.C., and Dietzel, C., for the Multicenter Study of Perioperative Ischemia Research Group and the Ischemia Research and Education Foundation, 2006, The risk associated with aprotinin in cardiac surgery, *New England Journal of Medicine*, 354:353-365.

Mann, R., and Andrews, E. (Eds.), 2002, Preface. *Pharmacovigilance*, Chichester, UK: John Wiley & Sons, xvii.

Mann, R. and Andrews, E. (Eds.), 2007a, *Pharmacovigilance,* 2nd edition, Chichester, UK: John Wiley & Sons.

Mann, R. and Andrews, E., 2007b, Introduction. In Mann, R. and Andrew, E. (Eds.), *Pharmacovigilance*, 2nd edition, Chichester, UK: John Wiley & Sons.

Marinker, M., 2004, From compliance to concordance: A personal view. In Bond, C. (Ed.), *Concordance*, London: Pharmaceutical Press, 1–7.

Marino, P., Simoni, J.M., and Silverstein, L.B., 2007, Peer support to promote medication adherence among people living with HIV/AIDS: The benefits to peers, *Social Work in Health Care*, 45:67–80.

Martin, E.W., 1978, *Hazards of medications*, Philadelphia, PA: J.B. Lippincott Company.

Martinez, M.N., 2005, Interspecies differences in physiology and pharmacology: Extrapolating preclinical data to human populations. In Rogge, M.C. and Taft, D.R. (Eds.), *Preclinical drug development*, Boca Raton, FL: Taylor & Francis, 11–66.

Mason, J.W., 2008, *Reduce the number of ECGs: Definitive QT study design*, Presentation given at the CBI Second Annual Cardiac Safety Summit, Alexandria, VA, January 15, 2008.

Matthews, J.N.S., 1999, *Introduction to randomized controlled clinical trials*, London: Edward Arnold.

Matthews, J.N.S., 2006, *Introduction to randomized controlled clinical trials*, 2nd edition, Boca Raton, FL: Chapman & Hall/CRC.

Mead, N. and Bower, P., 2000, Patient-centredness: A conceptual framework and review of the empirical literature, *Social Science and Medicine*, 51:1087–1110

Meyer, U.A., 2002, Introduction to pharmacogenomics: Promises, opportunities, and limitations. In Licinio, J. and Wong, M-L. (Eds.), *Pharmacogenomics: The search for individualized therapies*, Manheim: Wiley-VCH, 1–8.

Meyer, T., Sartipy, P., Blind, F., Leisgen, C., and Guenther, E., 2007, New cell models and assays in cardiac safety profiling, *Expert Opinion on Drug Metabolism and Toxicology*, 3:507–517.

Mitcheson, J., Perry, M., Stansfeld, P., et al., 2005, Structural determinants for high-affinity block of hERG potassium channels. In Chadwick, D.J. and Goode, J. (Eds.), *Symposium on the hERG cardiac potassium channel: Structure, function, and long QT syndrome,* Chichester, UK: John Wiley & Sons, 136–150.

Monkhouse, D.C., 2006, Manufacturing and clinical medicine trends for the clinical trial material professional. In Monkhouse, D.C., Carney, C.F., and Clark, J.L. (Eds.), *Drug products for clinical trials,* 2nd edition, Boca Raton: Taylor & Francis, 21–68.

Moore, T.J., Cohen, M.R., and Furberg, C.D., 2007, Serious adverse drug events reported to the Food and Drug Administration 1998–2005, *Archives of Internal Medicine*, 167:1752–1759.

Moorman, A.F.M. and Christoffels, V.M., 2003, Development of the cardiac conduction system: A matter of chamber development. In Chadwick, D.J. and Goode, J. (Eds.), *Development of the cardiac conduction system,* Chichester, UK: John Wiley & Sons, 25–43.

Morganroth, J., Brozovich, F.V., McDonald, J.T., and Jacobs, R.A., 1991, Variability of the QT measurement in healthy men: With implications for selection of an abnormal QT value to predict drug toxicity and proarrhythmia, *American Journal of Cardiology*, 67:774–776.

Morganroth, J., 1993, Relations of QTc prolongation on the electrocardiogram to torsades de pointes: Definitions and mechanisms, *American Journal of Cardiology*, 72: 10B–13B.

Morganroth, J., 2005, Design and conduct of the Thorough Phase I ECG trial for new bioactive drugs. In Morganroth, J.M. and Gussak, I. (Eds.), *Cardiac safety of noncardiac drugs: Practical guidelines for clinical research and drug development,* Totowa, NJ: Humana Press Inc., 205–222.

Morganroth, J.M. and Gussak, I. (Eds.), 2005, *Cardiac safety of noncardiac drugs: Practical guidelines for clinical research and drug development,* Totowa, NJ: Humana Press Inc.

Mortara, J.L., 2005, ECG acquisition and signal processing: 12-lead ECG acquisition. In Morganroth, J.M. and Gussak, I. (Eds.), *Cardiac safety of noncardiac drugs: Practical guidelines for clinical research and drug development,* Totowa, NJ: Humana Press Inc., 131–145.

Mukherjee, D., Nissen, S.E., and Topol, E.J., 2001, Risk of cardiovascular events associated with selective COX-2 inhibitors, *Journal of the American Medical Association,* 286:954–959.

Mulder, G.J., 2006, Drug metabolism: Inactivation and bioactivation of xenobiotics. In Mulder, G.J. and Dencker, L. (Eds.), *Pharmaceutical toxicology,* London: Pharmaceutical Press, 41–66.

Murray, R.K., 2006, Glycoproteins. In Murray, R.K., Granner, D.K., and Rodwell, V.W. (Eds.), *Harper's illustrated biochemistry,* 27th edition, New York: Lange Medical Books/McGraw-Hill, 523–544.

Murray, R.K. and Granner, D.K., 2006, Membranes: Structure and function. In Murray, R.K., Granner, D.K., and Rodwell, V.W. (Eds.), *Harper's illustrated biochemistry,* 27th edition, New York: Lange Medical Books/McGraw-Hill, 422–441.

Nada, A. and Somberg, J., 2007, First-in-man (FIM) clinical trials post-TeGenero: A review of the impact of the TeGenero trial on the design, conduct, and ethics of FIM trials, *American Journal of Therapeutics,* 14:594–604.

Nerbonne, J.M. and Kass, R.S., 2005, Molecular physiology of ion channels that control cardiac repolarization. In Morganroth, J.M. and Gussak, I. (Eds.), *Cardiac safety of noncardiac drugs: Practical guidelines for clinical research and drug development,* Totowa, NJ: Humana Press Inc., 13–36.

Nesto, R.W., Bell, D., Bonow, R.O., et al., 2003, Thiazolidinedione use, fluid retention, and congestive heart failure: A consensus statement from the American Heart Association and the American Diabetes Association, October 7, 2003, *Circulation,* 108:2941–2948.

Nissen, S.E. and Wolski, K., 2007, Effect of rosiglitazone on the risk of myocardial infarction and death from cardiovascular causes, *New England Journal of Medicine*, 356:2457–2471.

Norgrady, T. and Weaver, D.F., 2005, *Medicinal chemistry: A molecular and biochemical approach,* 3rd edition, Oxford: Oxford University Press.

Norris, S.L., Carson, S., and Roberts, C., 2007, Comparative effectiveness of pioglitazone and rosiglitazone in type 2 diabetes, prediabetes, and the metabolic syndrome: A meta-analysis, *Current Diabetes Reviews*, 3:127–140.

Obrist, P.A., 1981, *Cardiovascular psychophysiology: A perspective*, New York: Plenum Press.

O'Donohue, W.T. and Levensky, E.R. (Eds.), 2006, *Promoting treatment adherence: A practical handbook for health care providers*, Thousand Oaks, CA: Sage Publications.

Ofran, Y. and Rost, B., 2005, Predictive methods using protein sequences. In Baxevanis, A.D. and Ouellette, B.F.F. (Eds.), *Bioinformatics: A practical guide to the analysis of genes and proteins,* 3rd edition, Hoboken, NJ: Wiley-Interscience, 197–221.

Ohnishi, K., Yoshida, H., Shigeno, K., et al., 2000, Prolongation of the QT interval and ventricular tachycardia in patients treated with arsenic trioxide for acute promyelocytic leukemia, *Annals of Internal Medicine*, 133:881–885.

Oliver, J.J. and Webb, D.J., 2003, Surrogate endpoints. In Wilkins, M.R. (Ed.), *Experimental therapeutics*, London: Martin Dunitz/Taylor & Francis Group, 145–165.

Olsson, S. and Meyboom, R., 2006, Pharmacovigilance. In Mulder, G.J. and Dencker, L. (Eds.), *Pharmaceutical toxicology*, London: Pharmaceutical Press, 229–241.

O'Neill, R.T., 1987, Statistical analyses of adverse event data from clinical trials: Special emphasis on serious events, *Drug Information Journal*, 21:9–20.

O'Neill, R.T., 1995, Statistical concepts in the planning and evaluation of drug safety from clinical trials in drug development: Issues of international harmonization, *Statistics in Medicine*, 14:1117–1127.

O'Neill, R.T., 1998, Biostatistical considerations in pharmacovigilance and pharmacoepidemiology: Linking quantitative risk assessment in pre-market licensure application safety data, post-market alert reports, and formal epidemiological studies, *Statistics in Medicine*, 17:1851–1858.

O'Neill, R.T., 2008, A perspective on characterizing benefits and risks derived from clinical trials: Can we do more? *Drug Information Journal*, 42:235–245.

Osterberg, L. and Blaschke, T., 2005, Adherence to medication, *New England Journal of Medicine*, 353:487–497.

Palladino, M.A., 2006, *Understanding the human genome project*, 2nd edition, San Francisco: Pearson/Benjamin Cummings.

Park, D.C. and Liu, L.L. (Eds.), 2007, *Medical adherence and aging: Social and cognitive perspectives*, Washington, DC: American Psychological Association.

Pasternak, J.J., 1999, *Introduction to human molecular genetics: Mechanisms of inherited diseases*, Hoboken, NJ: John Wiley & Sons.

Perrio, M., Voss, S., and Shakir, S.A., 2007, Application of the Bradford Hill criteria to assess the causality of cisapride-induced arrhythmia: A model for assessing causal association in pharmacovigilance, *Drug Safety*, 30:333–346.

[PhRMA] Pharmaceutical Research and Manufacturers of America QT Statistics Expert Working Team, 2005, Investigating drug-induced QT and QTc prolongation in the clinic: Review of statistical design and analysis considerations. Report from the Pharmaceutical Research and Manufacturers of America QT Statistics Expert Team, *Drug Information Journal*, 39:243–266.

Piantadosi, S., 2005, *Clinical trials: A methodologic perspective,* 2nd edition, Hoboken, NJ: Wiley-Interscience.

Pignone, M., 2007, Rosiglitazone appears to be associated with an increased risk of cardiovascular events, *Clinical Diabetes*, 25:123–124.

Piper, D.R., Sanguinetti, M.C., and Tristani-Firouzi, M., 2005, Voltage sensor movement in the hERG K^+ channel. In Chadwick, D.J. and Goode, J. (Eds.), *Symposium on the hERG cardiac potassium channel: Structure, function, and long QT syndrome*, Chichester, UK: John Wiley & Sons, 46–52.

Primrose, S.B. and Twyman, R.M., 2006, *Principles of gene manipulation and genomics,* 7th edition. Malden, MA: Blackwell Publishing.

Rabinowitz, M. and Shankley, N., 2006, The impact of combinatorial chemistry on drug discovery. In Smith, C.G. and O'Donnell, J.T. (Eds.), *The process of new drug discovery and development,* 2nd edition, New York: Informa Healthcare, 55–77.

Raffa, R.B., Rawls, S.M., and Beyzarov, E.P., 2005, *Netter's illustrated pharmacology*, Philadelphia: Saunders/Elsevier.

Ray, W.A., 2008, Learning from aprotinin—Mandatory trials of comparative efficacy and safety are needed, *New England Journal of Medicine*, 358:840–842.

Recanatini, M., Cavalli, A., and Masetti, M., 2005, *In silico* modeling— Pharmacophores and hERG channel models. In Chadwick, D.J. and Goode, J. (Eds.), *Symposium on the hERG cardiac potassium channel: Structure, function, and long QT syndrome,* Chichester, UK: John Wiley & Sons, 171–180.

Regulatory Affairs Professionals Society, 2005, *Fundamentals of US regulatory affairs*, Rockville, MD: Regulatory Affairs Professionals Society.

Regulatory Affairs Professionals Society, 2007, *Fundamentals of US regulatory affairs,* 5th edition, Rockville, MD: Regulatory Affairs Professionals Society.

Rentschler, S., Morley, G.E., and Fishman, G.I., 2003, Patterning of the mouse conduction system. In Chadwick, D.J. and Goode, J. (Eds.), *Development of the cardiac conduction system,* Chichester, UK: John Wiley & Sons, 194–209.

Roberts, R.J., 1993, An amazing distortion in DNA induced by a methyltransferase. Nobel Lecture (Nobel Prize for Medicine), December 8. (http://nobelprize.org/ nobel_prizes/medicine/laureates/1993/roberts-lecture.pdf, accessed March 17, 2008.)

Robertson, G.A., Jones, E.M.C., and Wang, J., 2005, Gating and assembly of heteromeric hERG1a/1b channels underlying I_{Kr} in the heart. In Chadwick, D.J. and Goode, J. (Eds.), *Symposium on the hERG cardiac potassium channel: Structure, function, and long QT syndrome,* Chichester, UK: John Wiley & Sons, 4–13.

Rodeheffer, R.J. and Redfield, M.M., 2007, Heart failure: Diagnosis and evaluation. In Murphy, J.G. and Lloyd, M.A. (Eds.), *Mayo clinic cardiology: Concise textbook,* 3rd edition, Rochester, MN: Mayo Clinic Scientific Press, 1101–1112.

Roden, D.M., 2004, Drug-induced prolongation of the QT interval, *New England Journal of Medicine,* 350:1013–1022.

Rogge, M.C. and Taft, D.R. (Eds.), 2005, *Preclinical drug development,* Boca Raton, FL: Taylor & Francis

Rolan, P.E. and Molnar, V., 2006, The assessment of pharmacokinetics in early-phase drug evaluation. In Lee, C-J., Lee, L.H., Wu, C.L., Lee, B.R., and Chen, M-L. (Eds.), *Clinical trials of drugs and biopharmaceuticals,* Boca Raton, FL: Taylor & Francis, 123–132.

Rosen, C.J., 2007, Perspective: The rosiglitazone story—Lessons from and FDA advisory committee meeting, *New England Journal of Medicine,* 357:844–846.

Routledge, P., 2004, Adverse drug reactions and interactions: Mechanisms, risk factors, detection, management and prevention. In Talbot, J. and Waller, P. (Eds.), *Stephens' detection of new adverse drug reactions,* 5th edition, Chichester, UK: John Wiley & Sons, 91–125.

Sager, P.T., Nebout, T., and Darpo, B., 2005, ICH E14: A new regulatory guidance on the clinical evaluation of QT/QTc interval prolongation and proarrhythmic potential for non-antiarrhythmic drugs, *Drug Information Journal,* 39:387–394.

Sarapa, N., 2005, Digital 12-lead holter vs standard resting supine electrocardiogram for the assessment of drug-induced QTc prolongation: Assessment by different recording and measurement methods. In Morganroth, J.M. and Gussak, I. (Eds.), *Cardiac safety of noncardiac drugs: Practical guidelines for clinical research and drug development,* Totowa, NJ: Humana Press Inc., 147–166.

Satin, L., 2008, *Issues in the Thorough QT Trial.* Presentation given at the CBI 3rd Annual Conference on Cardiac Safety, Washington, DC, January 2008.

Schneeweiss, S., Seeger, J.D., Landon, J., and Walker, A.M., 2008, Aprotinin during coronary-artery bypass drafting and risk of death, *New England Journal of Medicine,* 358:771–783.

Schultz, R.M., 2006, Proteins II: Structure-function relationships in protein families. In Devlin, T.M. (Ed.), *Textbook of biochemistry with clinical correlations,* 6th edition, Hoboken, NJ: John Wiley & Sons, 319–363.

Schultz, W.B., 2007, Perspective: Bolstering the FDA's drug-safety authority, *New England Journal of Medicine,* 357:2217–2219.

Schuster, D.P., 2005, Introduction: The value of translational and experimental clinical research. In Schuster, D.P. and Powers, W.J., Eds, *Translational and experimental clinical research*, Philadelphia: Lippincott Williams & Wilkins, xv–xxi.

Schwartz, P.J., 2005, The long QT syndrome: A clinical counterpart of *hERG* mutations. In Chadwick, D.J. and Goode, J. (Eds.), *Symposium on the hERG cardiac potassium channel: Structure, function, and long QT syndrome,* Chichester, UK: John Wiley & Sons, 186–198.

Senn, S., 2007, *Statistical issues in drug development,* 2nd edition, Chichester, UK: John Wiley & Sons.

Shah, R.R, 2005a, Interpretation of clinical ECG data: Understanding the risk from non-antiarrhythmic drugs. In Morganroth, J.M. and Gussak, I. (Eds.), *Cardiac safety of noncardiac drugs: Practical guidelines for clinical research and drug development,* Totowa, NJ: Humana Press Inc., 259–298.

Shah, R.R., 2005b, Drug-induced QT interval prolongation: Regulatory guidance and perspectives on hERG channel studies. In Chadwick, D.J. and Goode, J. (Eds.), *Symposium on the hERG cardiac potassium channel: Structure, function, and long QT syndrome,* Chichester, UK: John Wiley & Sons, 251–280.

Shah, R.R., 2007a, Cardiac repolarisation and drug regulation: Assessing cardiac safety 10 years after the CPMP guidance, *Drug Safety*, 30:1093–1110.

Shah, R.R., 2007b, Withdrawal of terodiline: A tale of two toxicities. In Mann, R. and Andrews, E. (Eds.), *Pharmacovigilance,* 2nd edition, Chichester, UK: John Wiley & Sons, 109–136.

Shakir, S.A.W., 2007, PEM in the UK. In Mann, R. and Andrews, E. (Eds.), *Pharmacovigilance,* 2nd edition, Chichester, UK: John Wiley & Sons, 307–316.

Shakir, S.A. and Layton, D., 2002, Causal association in pharmacovigilance and pharmacoepidemiology: Thoughts on the application of the Austin Bradford-Hill criteria, *Drug Safety*, 25:467–471.

Silverstein, F.E., Faich, G., Goldstein, J.L., et al., 2000, Gastrointestinal toxicity with celecoxib vs. nonsteroidal anti-inflammatory drugs of osteoarthritis and rheumatoid arthritis. The CLASS study: A randomized controlled trial, *Journal of the American Medical Association*, 284:1247:1255.

Simko, J., Csilek, A., Karaszi, and Lorincz, I., 2008, Proarrhythmic potential of antimicrobial agents, *Infection*, May 3 [E-publication ahead of print].

Simoni, J.M., Pantalone, D.W., Plummer, M.D., and Huang, B., 2007, A randomized controlled trial of a peer support intervention targeting antiretroviral medication adherence and depressive symptomatology in HIV-positive men and women, *Health Psychology*, 26:488–495.

Simons, L.E. and Blount, R.L., 2007, Identifying barriers to medication adherence in adolescent transplant recipients, *Pediatric Psychology*, 32:831–844.

Singh, S., Loke, Y.K., and Furberg, C.D., 2007, Long-term risk of cardiovascular events with rosiglitazone: A meta-analysis, *Journal of the American Medical Association*, 298:1189–1195.

Smetzer, J.L., 2007, Managing medication risks through a culture of safety. In Cohen, M.R. (Ed.), *Medication Errors,* 2nd edition, Washington, DC: American Pharmacists Association, 605–654.

Smith, C.G. and O'Donnell, J.T. (Eds.), 2006, *The process of new drug discovery and development,* 2nd edition, New York: Informa Healthcare USA.

Soloviev, M.V., Barry, R., and Terrett, J., 2004, Chip based proteomics technology. In Rapley, R. and Harbron, S. (Eds.), *Molecular analysis and genome discovery*, Chichester, UK: John Wiley & Sons, 217–249.

Soloviev, M.V., Hamlin, R.L., Shellhammer, L.J., et al., 2006, Variations in hemodynamic and ECG in healthy, conscious, freely moving telemetrized beagle dogs, *Cardiovascular Toxicology*, 6:51–62.

Stephens, M.D.B., 2004, Introduction. In Talbot, J. and Waller, P. (Eds.), *Stephens' detection of new adverse drug reactions,* 5th edition, Chichester, UK: John Wiley & Sons, 1–90.

Stevens, M. and Roberts, C., 2007, The impact of future trends in new sciences on the practising pharmacist, *The Pharmaceutical Journal*, 279:273–274.

Stevenson, F., 2004, The patient's perspective. In Bond, C. (Ed.), *Concordance*, London: Pharmaceutical Press, 29–47.

Stewart, L.A. and Clarke, M.J., 1995, Practical methodology of meta-analyses (overviews) using updated individual patient data, *Statistics in Medicine*, 14: 2057–2079.

Stewart, L., Tierney, J., and Burdett, S., 2005, Do systematic reviews based on individual patient data offer a means of circumventing biases associated with trial publications? In Rothstein, H.R., Sutton, A.J., and Borenstein, M., (Eds.), *Publication bias in meta-analysis: Prevention, assessment and adjustments,* Chichester, UK: John Wiley & Sons, p. 262–286.

Stewart, L.A. and Clarke, M.J., 1995, Practical methodology of meta-analyses (overviews) using updated individual patient data, *Statistics in Medicine,* 14: 2057–2079.

Strom, B.L. (Ed.), 2005a, *Pharmacoepidemiology,* 4th edition, Chichester, UK: John Wiley & Sons, 29–36.

Strom, B.L., 2005b, Sample size considerations for pharmacoepidemiology studies. In Strom, B.L. (Ed.), *Pharmacoepidemiology,* 4th edition, Chichester, UK: John Wiley & Sons, 29–36.

Strom, B.L., 2007, Methodologic challenges to studying patient safety and comparative effectiveness, *Medical Care,* 45(10 Suppl. 2):S13–S15.

Sullivan, S.D., Kreling, D.H., Hazlet, T.K., et al., 1990, Noncompliance with medication regimes and subsequent hospitalizations: A literature analysis and cost of hospitalization estimate, *Journal of Research in Pharmaceutical Economics,* 2:19–33.

Takemasa, H., Nagatomo, T., Abe, H., et al., 2008, Coexistence of hERG current block and disruption of protein trafficking in ketoconazole-induced long QT syndrome, *British Journal of Pharmacology,* 153:439–447.

Talbot, J. and Stephens, M.D.B., 2004, Clinical trials: Collection of safety data and establishing the adverse drug reaction profile. In Talbot, J. and Waller, P. (Eds.), *Stephens' detection of new adverse drug reactions,* 5th edition, Chichester, UK: John Wiley & Sons, 167–242.

Talbot, J. and Waller, P. (Eds.), 2004, *Stephens' detection of new adverse drug reactions,* 5th edition, Chichester, UK: John Wiley & Sons.

Taylor, M.R. and Bristow, M.R., 2006, Alterations in myocardial gene expression as a basis for cardiomyopathies and heart failure. In Bock, G. and Goode, J. (Eds.), *Heart failure: Molecules, mechanisms and therapeutic targets,* Chichester, UK: John Wiley & Sons, 73–89.

Thomas, G., 2003, *Fundamentals of medicinal chemistry*, Chichester, UK: John Wiley & Sons.

Tisdale, J.E., Kovacs, R., Mi, D., et al., 2007, Accuracy of uncorrected versus corrected QT interval for prediction of torsade de pointes associated with intravenous haloperidol, *Pharmacotherapy*, 27:175–182.

Tozer, T.N. and Rowland, M., 2006, *Introduction to pharmacokinetics and pharmacodynamics: The quantitative basis of drug therapy*, Lippincott Williams & Wilkins.

Triggle, D.J., Gopalakrishnan, M., Rampe, D., and Zheng, W. (Eds.), 2006, *Voltage-gated ion channels as drug targets*, Weinheim, Germany: Wiley-VCH.

Tseng, G.N. and Guy, H.R., 2005, Structure-function studies of the outer mouth and voltage sensor domain of hERG. In Chadwick, D.J. and Goode, J. (Eds.), *Symposium on the hERG cardiac potassium channel: Structure, function, and long QT syndrome,* Chichester, UK: John Wiley & Sons, 19–35.

Tsong, Y., Shen, M., Zhong, J., and Zhang, J., 2008, Statistical issues of QT prolongation assessment based on linear concentration modeling, *Journal of Biopharmaceutical Statistics*, 18(3):564–84.

Turner, J. R., 1994, *Cardiovascular reactivity and stress: Patterns of physiological response,* New York: Plenum Press.

Turner, J.R., 2007, *New drug development: Design, methodology, and analysis,* Hoboken, NJ: John Wiley & Sons.

van der Heyden, M.A., Smits, M.E., and Vos, M.A., 2008, Drugs and trafficking of ion channels: A new proarrhythmic threat on the horizon, *British Journal of Pharmacology*, 153:406–409.

van der Laan, J.W., 2006, Safety assessment of pharmaceuticals: Regulatory aspects. In Mulder, G.J. and Dencker, L. (Eds.), *Pharmaceutical toxicology*, London: Pharmaceutical Press, 209–227.

Vargas, H., 2008, Proarrhythmic liability of large-molecule drugs. Presentation given during a Webinar entitled *Cardiac safety in large molecules: New regulatory expectations, new strategies*, February 26 [see Section 7.20 for more details].

Vargas, H.M., Bass, A.S., Breidenbach, A., et al., 2008, Scientific review and recommendations on preclinical cardiovascular safety evaluation of biologics, *Journal of Pharmacological and Toxicological Methods*, April 18 [E-publication ahead of print].

Venter, J.C., Adams, M.D., Myers, E.W., et al., 2001, The sequence of the human genome, *Science*, 291:1304–1351.

Vlahakes, G.J., 2006, Editorial: The value of Phase 4 clinical testing, *New England Journal of Medicine*, 354:413–415.

Wadman, M., 2007, Experts call for active surveillance of drug safety, *Nature*, 446: 358–359.

Walsh, G., 2003, *Biopharmaceuticals: Biochemistry and biotechnology*, 2nd edition, Chichester, UK: John Wiley & Sons.

Walsh, G., 2007, *Pharmaceutical biotechnology: Concepts and applications*, Chichester, UK: John Wiley & Sons.

Wang, Q., Shen, J., Splawski I., et al., 1995, SCN5A mutations associated with an inherited cardiac arrhythmia, long QT syndrome, *Cell*, 80:805–811.

Watson, J.D., 2004, *DNA: The secret of life,* New York: Alfred A. Knopf.

Weaver, K.E., Llabre, M.M., Duran, R.E, et al., 2005, A stress and coping model of medication adherence and viral load in HIV-positive men and women on highly active antiretroviral therapy (HAART), *Health Psychology*, 24:385–392.

Webb, P., Bain, C., and Pirozzo, S., 2005, *Essential epidemiology: An introduction for students and health professionals,* Cambridge, UK: Cambridge University Press.

Weiner, H, 2006, Enzymes: Classification, kinetics, and control. In Devlin, T.M. (Ed.), *Textbook of biochemistry with clinical correlations,* 6th edition, Hoboken, NJ: Wiley-LISS, 365–412.

Weir, M.R., Sperling, R.S., Reicin, A., and Gertz, B.J., 2003, Selective COX-2 inhibition and cardiovascular effects: A review of the rofecoxib development program, *American Heart Journal*, 146:591–604.

West, L.J., 1991, Medicines Control Agency (MCA) and other regulatory authorities. In International Drug Surveillance Department (IDSD), Glaxo Group Research, *Drug safety: A shared responsibility,* New York: Churchill Livingstone, 89–97.

Westfall, P.H., Tobias, R.D., Rom, D., Wolfinger, R.D., and Hochberg, Y., 1999, *Multiple comparisons and multiple tests using SAS®,* Cary, NC: SAS Institute.

Whitehead, A., 2002, *Meta-analysis of controlled clinical trials,* Hoboken, NJ: John Wiley & Sons.

WHO, 2002, *The importance of pharmacovigilance: Safety monitoring of medicinal products,* Geneva: World Health Organization (see http://www.who.int/en/).

WHO, 2003, *Adherence to long-term therapies: Evidence for action,* Geneva: World Health Organization (see http://www.who.int/en/).

WHO, 2004, *Pharmacovigilance: Ensuring the safe use of medicines,* Geneva: World Health Organization (see http://www.who.int/en/).

Wijnen, P.A., Op den Buijsch, R.A., Drent, M., et al., 2007, Review article: The prevalence and clinical relevance of cytochrome P450 polymorphisms, *Aliment Pharmacology and Therapeutics,* 26(S2):211–219.

Wild, R.N., 2007, Micturin and torsades de pointes. In Mann, R. and Andrews, E. (Eds.), *Pharmacovigilance,* 2nd edition, Chichester, UK: John Wiley & Sons, 105–108.

Wishart, D., 2005, protein structure and analysis. In Baxevanis, A.D. and Ouellette, B.F.F. (Eds.), *Bioinformatics: A practical guide to the analysis of genes and proteins,* 3rd edition, Hoboken, NJ: Wiley-Interscience, 223–251.

Wolfe, M.M., Ding, E.L., and Song, Y., 1999, Gastrointestinal toxicity of nonsteroidal anti-inflammatory drugs, *New England Journal of Medicine,* 340: 1888–1899.

Wood, A.J.J., 2006, Sounding board: A proposal for radical changes in the drug-approval process, *New England Journal of Medicine,* 355:618–623.

Woodward, M., 2005, *Epidemiology: Study design and data analysis,* 2nd edition, Boca Raton, FL: Chapman & Hall/CRC.

Wozniacka, A., Cygankiewicz, I., Chudzik, M., Sysa-Jedrzejowska, A., and Wranicz, J.K., 2006, The cardiac safety of chloroquine phosphate treatment in patients with systemic lupus erythematosus: The influence on arrhythmia, heart rate variability and repolarization parameters, *Lupus*, 15:521–525.

Yap, Y.G. and Camm, A.J., 2002, *Drug-induced long QT syndrome,* Armonk, NY: Futura Publishing Company.

Yasumura, Y., Takemura, K., Sakamoto, A., Kitakaze, M., and Miyatake, K., 2003, Changes in myocardial gene expression associated with beta-blocker therapy in patients with chronic heart failure, *Journal of Cardiac Failure*, 9:469–474.

Yi, H., Cao, Z., Dai, C., Wu, Y., and Li, W., 2007, Interaction simulation of hERG K+ channel with its specific BeKm-1 peptide: Insights into the selectivity of molecular recognition, *Journal of Proteome Research*, 6:611–620.

Yilmaz, U., Oztop, I., Ciloglu, A., et al., 2007, 5-flourouracil increases the number and complexity of premature complexes in the heart: A prospective study using ambulatory ECG monitoring, *International Journal of Clinical Practice*, 61: 795–801.

Zhang, J., 2008, *Study design, sample size and assay sensitivity in TQT studies*, Presentation given at the 2nd Annual Summit on Cardiac Safety, Alexandria, VA, January 14–15.

Zhang, M., Korolkova, Y.V., Liu, J., et al., 2003, BeKm-1 is a hERG-specific toxin that shares the structure with ChTx but the mechanism of action with ErgTx1, *Biophysical Journal*, 84:3022–3036.

Zhou, J., Augelli-Szafran, C.E., Bradley, J.A., et al., 2005, Novel potent human ether-a-go-go-related gene (hERG) potassium channel enhancers and their *in vitro* anti-arrhythmogenic activity, *Molecular Pharmacology*, 68:876–884.

INDEX

*Integrated Cardiac Safety: Assessment Methodologies for Noncardiac Drugs in Discovery,
Development, and Postmarketing Surveillance.* By J. Rick Turner and Todd A. Durham
Copyright © 2009 John Wiley & Sons, Inc.

null hypothesis 170
numerator, use in ratios 12
nurses 329

O

observational studies. *See*
nonexperimental
studies
odds ratio 218, 247, 306
Office of Drug Safety 271, 299
Office of New Drugs 272
Office of Surveillance and
Epidemiology 271
oncology, pharmacotherapy for
316-318
optimal responders, to drug 383
optimization, of drug molecule.
See lead optimization
oral, drug administration route
98
osteoarthritis 294
overuse, of health care
services 334

P

palpitations 293
pancreas 301
parallel design, use in TQT
study 151, 181
participant-level (patient-level)
data. *See* individual
patient/participant data
patch clamp technique 120
patent life, drug 319
patient-centered care 341
patient interviews 276
Patient Safety, report by the
Institute of Medicine
342-344
patient-years
events per 309
of follow-up 321
PDUFA. *See* Prescription Drug

User Fee Act
perfect storm scenario, occurrence of
torsades de pointes 358
pericardial/pleural effusion 317, 318
period effects, parallel study
design 151
peristaltic contractions, in tubular
hearts 56
peroxisome proliferator-activated
receptor-gamma
(PPAR-γ) 302
Per-protocol analysis population 314
Peto fixed-effects model, in
meta-analysis 313
pharmaceutical biotechnology,
terminology 126
Pharmaceutical Research and
Manufacturers of America
(PhRMA) 7
pharmacists 329
pharmacodynamics 136
genetic influence 383
pharmacoepidemiology 263, 273, 378
pharmacogenetics 383f
pharmacogenomics 383f
pharmacokinetics 99, 113-114
pharmacokinetic/pharmacodynamic
modeling 178, 362
pharmacology studies 114
pharmacophore 95
pharmacoproteomics 384
pharmacotherapeutic continuum 385
pharmacovigilance 262, 270
pharmacovigilance plan, in ICH
Guidance E2E 278-279
phase 0 to 4, action potential 65
phases I-III nomenclature, clinical
trials 4-5
phase IV nomenclature, clinical trial
232-233
phenylpropanolamine 294
phosphorylation 50
PhRMA's QT Statistics Expert